Using Literature to Help
Troubled Teenagers
Cope with Health Issues

Recent Titles in
The Greenwood Press "Using Literature to Help Troubled Teenagers"
Series

Using Literature to Help Troubled Teenagers Cope with Family Issues
Joan F. Kaywell, editor

Using Literature to Help Troubled Teenagers Cope with Societal Issues
Pamela S. Carroll, editor

Using Literature to Help Troubled Teenagers Cope with Identity Issues
Jeffrey S. Kaplan, editor

Using Literature to Help Troubled Teenagers Cope with Health Issues

Edited by
Cynthia Ann Bowman

Foreword by Jan Cheripko

The Greenwood Press "Using Literature to
Help Troubled Teenagers" Series
Joan F. Kaywell, Series Adviser

Greenwood Press
Westport, Connecticut • London

Library of Congress Cataloging-in-Publication Data

Using literature to help troubled teenagers cope with health issues /
    edited by Cynthia Ann Bowman ; foreword by Jan Cheripko.
        p.   cm.—(The Greenwood Press "Using literature to help troubled
    teenagers" series)
    Includes bibliographical references and index.
    ISBN 0–313–30531–5 (alk. paper)
    1. Bibliotherapy for teenagers.   2. Teenagers—Diseases.   3. Young
adult literature—Study and teaching (Secondary)   I. Bowman,
Cynthia Ann, 1958– .   II. Series.
RJ505.B5U843   2000
615.8'516'0835—dc21   99–36669

British Library Cataloguing in Publication Data is available.

Library of Congress Catalog Card Number: 99–36669
ISBN: 0–313–30531–5

First published in 2000

Greenwood Press, 88 Post Road West, Westport, CT 06881
An imprint of Greenwood Publishing Group, Inc.
www.greenwood.com

Printed in the United States of America

The paper used in this book complies with the
Permanent Paper Standard issued by the National
Information Standards Organization (Z39.48–1984).

10 9 8 7 6 5 4 3 2 1

Dedicated with love and gratitude to
Dr. Robert Waddell
and all physicians who truly care for their patients and families

Contents

Series Foreword   *Joan F. Kaywell*   ix

Foreword   *Jan Cheripko*   xvii

Introduction   xix

CHAPTER 1   *Freak the Mighty*: Birth Defects and Disability in a Literary Friendship
Kathleen Carico and Paula Stanley   1

CHAPTER 2   *Izzy, Willy-Nilly*: Issues of Disability for Adolescents and Their Families
Cynthia Ann Bowman and Phyllis A. Gordon   27

CHAPTER 3   Bridging the Alone Space: Fiction for Young People with Sensory Impairments
Kim McCollum-Clark and Kelsey Backels   51

CHAPTER 4   Tracking Adolescent Responses to Cancer
Jim Powell and Nancy Lafferty   77

CHAPTER 5   Normalcy Was All She Wanted: Learning to Live with Diabetes
Sue F. Johnson and Claire J. Dandeneau   97

CHAPTER 6   Focusing Our Attention: Reading about
ADHD
A. Lee Williams and Albert Scott   111

CHAPTER 7   *The Friends*: Promoting Adolescent Mental
Health Through Awareness and Literature
Karen L. Ford and Charlene Alexander   135

CHAPTER 8   The Craziness Within and the Craziness
Without: Depression and Anger in *Ironman*
*John Noell Moore and David William
Hartman*   151

CHAPTER 9   Dying to Be Thin: Eating Disorders in Young
Adult Literature
Patricia P. Kelly and Marshall D. Tessnear   175

CHAPTER 10   Reading Anorexia in *Nell's Quilt*
Nancy Mellin McCracken and Jan Carli   197

CHAPTER 11   HIV/AIDS: *What You Don't Know Can
Kill You*
*Nancy Prosenjak, and Laura Sullivan and
Diane Hartman*   217

CHAPTER 12   Conquering Alcoholism in *Imitate the Tiger*
Margaret Ford and Danna Bozick   243

CHAPTER 13   *Going Backwards*: A Family Systems View
of Alzheimer's
Joyce Graham and Scott Johnson   265

Index   291

About the Editor and Contributors   309

Series Foreword

The idea for this six-volume series—addressing family issues, identity issues, social issues, abuse issues, health issues, and death and dying issues—came while I, myself, was going to a therapist to help me deal with the loss of a loved one. My therapy revealed that I was a "severe trauma survivor" and I had to process the emotions of a bad period of time during my childhood. I was amazed that a trauma of my youth could be triggered by an emotional upset in my adult life. After an amazing breakthrough that occurred after extensive reading, writing, and talking, I looked at my therapist and said, "My God! I'm like the gifted child with the best teacher. What about all of those children who survive situations worse than mine and do not choose education as their escape of choice?" I began to wonder about the huge number of troubled teenagers who were not getting the professional treatment they needed. I pondered about those adolescents who were fortunate enough to get psychological treatment but were illiterate. Finally, I began to question if there were ways to help them while also improving their literacy development.

My thinking generated two theories on which this series is based: (1) Being literate increases a person's chances of emotional health, and (2) Twenty-five percent of today's students are "unteachable." The first theory was generated by my pondering these two statistics: 80% of our prisoners are illiterate (Hodgkinson, 1991), and 80% of our prisoners have been sexually abused (Child Abuse Council, 1993). If a correlation actually exists between these two statistics, then it suggests a strong need for literacy skills in order for a person to be able to address emotional turmoil in healthy or constructive ways. The second theory came out of work I did for my book, *Adolescents at Risk: A Guide to Fiction and Nonfiction for Young Adults, Parents and Professionals* (Greenwood Press, 1993), and my involvement in working with teachers and students in middle and secondary schools. Some of the emotional baggage our youth bring to school is way too heavy for them to handle without help. These students simply cannot handle additional academic responsibilities when they are "not right" emotionally.

THEORY ONE: BEING LITERATE INCREASES A PERSON'S CHANCES OF EMOTIONAL HEALTH

Well-educated adults who experience intense emotional pain, whether it is from the loss of a loved one or from a traumatic event, have several options available for dealing with their feelings. Most will find comfort in talking with friends or family members, and some will resort to reading books to find the help they need. For example, reading Dr. Elizabeth Kübler-Ross's five stages for coping with death—denial, anger, bargaining, depression, and acceptance or growth—might help a person understand the various stages he or she is going through after the death of a friend or relative. Sometimes, however, additional help is needed when an individual is experiencing extreme emotions and is unable to handle them.

Consider a mother whose improper left-hand turn causes the death of her seven-year-old daughter and the injury of her four-year-old daughter. It is quite probable that the mother will need to seek additional help from a therapist who will help her deal with such a trauma. A psychologist or psychiatrist will, more than likely, get her to talk openly about her feelings, read some books written by others who have survived such a tragedy, and do regular journal writing. A psychiatrist may also prescribe some medication during this emotionally challenging time. This parent's literacy skills of talking, reading, and writing are essential to her getting through this difficult period of her life.

Now, consider her four-year-old daughter who is also experiencing extreme grief over the loss of her beloved older sister. If this child is taken to counseling, the therapist will probably get her to talk, role-play, and draw out her feelings. These are the literacy skills appropriate to the developmental level of a four-year-old child. Such a child, if not taken to a counselor when needed, will manifest her emotions in one of two ways—either by acting out or by withdrawing.

Lev Vygotsky, a well-respected learning theorist, suggests that without words there could be no thoughts and the more words a person has at his or her disposal, the bigger that person's world. If what Vygotsky suggests is true, then a person with a limited or no vocabulary is only capable of operating at an emotional level. *The Story of My Life* by Helen Keller adds credibility to that view. In the introduction to the biography, written by Robert Russell, he describes Helen Keller's frustration at not being able to communicate:

> Perhaps the main cause for her early tantrums was plain frustration at not being able to communicate. . . . Not being able to hear, Helen had nothing to imitate, so she had no language. This meant more than simply not being able to talk. It meant having nothing clear to talk about because for her things had no names. Without names, things have no distinctness or individuality. Without language, we could not describe the difference between an elephant and an egg. Without the words we would have no clear conception of either elephant or egg. The name of a thing confers identity upon it and makes it possible for us to think about it. Without names for love or sorrow, we do not know we are experiencing them. Without words, we could not say, "I love you," and human beings need to say this and much more. Helen had the need, too, but she had not the means. As she grew older and the need increased, no wonder her fits of anger and misery grew. (pp. 7–9)

Helen, herself, writes,

> [T]he desire to express myself grew. The few signs I used became less and less adequate, and my failures to make myself understood were invariably followed by outbursts of passion. I felt as if invisible hands were holding me, and I made frantic efforts to free myself. I struggled—not that struggling helped matters, but the spirit of resistance was strong within me; I generally broke down in tears and physical exhaustion. If my mother happened to be near I crept into her arms, too miserable even to remember the cause of the tempest. After awhile the need of some means of communication became so urgent that these outbursts occurred daily, sometimes hourly. (p. 28)

If Vygotsky's theory reflected by the illuminating words of a deaf, blind, and mute child is true, then it is no wonder that 80% of our prisoners are illiterate victims of abuse.

THEORY TWO: 25% OF TODAY'S TEENAGERS ARE "UNTEACHABLE" BY TODAY'S STANDARDS

Teachers are finding it increasingly difficult to teach their students, and I believe that 25% of teenagers are "unteachable" by today's standards. A small percentage of these troubled youth do choose academics as their escape of choice, and they are the overachievers to the "nth" degree. That is not to say that all overachievers are emotionally disturbed teenagers, but some of them are learning, not because of their teachers, but because their very survival depends upon it. I know. I was one of them. The other adolescents going through inordinately difficult times (beyond the difficulty inherent in adolescence itself) might not find the curriculum very relevant to their lives. Their escapes of choice include rampant sex, drug use, gang membership, and other self-destructive behaviors. Perhaps the violence permeating our schools is a direct result of the utter frustration of some of our youth.

Consider these data describing the modern teenage family. At any given time, 25% of American children live with one parent, usually a divorced or never-married mother (Edwards & Young, 1992). Fifty percent of America's youth will spend some school years being raised by a single parent, and almost four million school-age children are being reared by neither parent (Hodgkinson, 1991). In 1990, 20% of American children grew up in poverty, and it is probable that 25% will be raised in poverty by the year 2000 (Howe, 1991). Children in homeless families often experience developmental delays, severe depression, anxiety, and learning disorders (Bassuk & Rubin, 1987).

Between one-fourth and one-third of school-aged children are living in a family with one or more alcoholics (Gress, 1988). Fourteen percent of children between the ages of 3 and 17 experience some form of family violence (Craig, 1992). Approximately 27% of girls and 16% of boys are sexually abused before the age of 18 (Krueger, 1993), and experts believe that it is reasonable to say that 25% of children will be sexually abused before adulthood (Child Abuse Council, 1993). Remember to note that eight out of ten criminals in prison were abused when they were children (Child Abuse Council, 1993).

Consider these data describing the modern teenager. Approximately two out of ten school-aged youth are affected by anorexia nervosa and bulimia (Phelps & Bajorek, 1991) and between 14% to 23% have vomited to lose weight (National Centers for Disease Control, 1991). By the time students become high school seniors, 90% have experimented with alcohol use and nearly two-thirds have used drugs (National Institute on Drug Abuse, 1992). In 1987, 40% of seniors admitted they had used dangerous drugs and 60% had used marijuana (National Adolescent Student Health Survey). In 1974, the average age American high school students tried marijuana was 16; in 1984, the average age was twelve (Nowinski, 1990).

By the age of 15, a fourth of the girls and a third of the boys are sexually active (Gibbs, 1993), and three out of four teenagers have had sexual intercourse by their senior year (Males, 1993). Seventy-five percent of the mothers who gave birth between the ages of 15 and 17 are on welfare (Simkins, 1984). In 1989, AIDS was the sixth leading cause of death for 15- to 24-year-olds (Tonks, 1992–1993), and many AIDS experts see adolescents as the third wave of individuals affected by HIV (Kaywell, 1993). Thirty-nine percent of sexually active teenagers said they preferred not to use any method of contraception (Harris Planned Parenthood Poll, 1986).

Ten percent of our students are gay (Williams, 1993), and the suicide rate for gay and lesbian teenagers is two to six times higher than that of heterosexual teens (Krueger, 1993). Suicide is the second leading cause of teenage deaths; "accidents" rated first (National Centers for Disease Control, 1987). An adolescent commits suicide every one hour and 47 minutes (National Center for Health Statistics, 1987), and nine children die from gunshot wounds every day in America (Edelman, 1989). For those children growing up in poor, high crime neighborhoods, one in three has seen a homicide by the time they reach adolescence (Beck, 1992).

Consider these data describing the dropout problem. In 1988, the dropout rate among high school students was 28.9% (Monroe, Borzi, & Burrell, 1992). More than 80% of America's one million prisoners are high school dropouts (Hodgkinson, 1991). We spend more than $20,000 per year per prisoner (Hodgkinson, 1991) but spend less than $4,000 per year per student. Forty-five percent of special education students drop out of high school (Wagner, 1989).

Numbers and statistics such as these are often incomprehensible, but consider the data in light of a 12th grade classroom of 30 students. Eight to 15 are being raised by a single parent, six are in poverty, eight to ten are being raised in families with alcoholics, four have experienced some form of family violence, and eight of the female and five of the male students have been sexually violated. Six are anorectic or bulimic, 27 have used alcohol, 18 have used marijuana, and 12 have used dangerous drugs. Twenty-two have had sexual intercourse and 12 of them used no protection. Three students are gay. Eight will drop out of school, and six of those eight will become criminals. Everyday in our country, two adolescents commit suicide by lunchtime.

These are the students that our teachers must teach every day, and these are the students who need help beyond what schools are currently able to provide. Think about the young adults who are both illiterate and in pain! Is there anything that can be done to help these young people with their problems while increasing their literacy skills? Since most of our nation's prisoners are illiterate—the acting out side—and most homeless people are not exactly Rhodes scholars—the withdrawal side— it seems logical to try to help these adolescents while they are still within the educational system.

Perhaps this series, which actually pairs literacy experts with therapists, can help the caretakers of our nation's distraught youth—teachers, counselors, parents, clergy, and librarians—acquire understanding and knowledge on how to better help these troubled teenagers. The series provides a unique approach to guide these caretakers working with troubled teenagers. Experts discuss young adult literature, while therapists provide analysis and advice for protagonists in these novels. Annotated bibliographies provide the reader with similar sources that can be used to help teenagers discuss these issues while increasing their literacy skills.

Joan F. Kaywell

REFERENCES

Bassuk, E. L. & Rubin, L. (1987). Homeless children: A neglected population. *American Journal of Orthopsychiatry, 57* (2), p. 279 ff.

Beck, J. (1992, May 19). Inner-city kids beat the odds to survive. *The Tampa Tribune.*

Craig, S. E. (1992, September). The educational needs of children living with violence. *Phi Delta Kappan, 74* (1), p. 67 ff.

Edelman, M. W. (1989, May). Defending America's children. *Educational Leadership, 46* (8), p. 77 ff.

Edwards, P. A. & Young, L. S. J. (1992, September). Beyond parents: Family, community, and school involvement. *Phi Delta Kappan, 74* (1), p. 72 ff.

Gibbs, N. (1993, May 24). How should we teach our children about sex? *Time, 140* (21), p. 60 ff.

Gress, J. R. (1988, March). Alcoholism's hidden curriculum. *Educational Leadership, 45* (6), p. 18 ff.

Hodgkinson, H. (1991, September). Reform versus reality. *Phi Delta Kappan, 73* (1), p. 9 ff.

Howe II, H. (1991, November). America 2000: A bumpy ride on four trains. *Phi Delta Kappan, 73* (3), p. 192 ff.

Kaywell, J. F. (1993). *Adolescents at risk: A guide to fiction and nonfiction for young adults, parents and professionals.* Westport, CT: Greenwood Press.

Keller, H. (1967). *The story of my life.* New York: Scholastic.

Krueger, M. M. (1993, March). Everyone is an exception: Assumptions to avoid in the sex education classroom. *Phi Delta Kappan, 74* (7), p. 569 ff.

Males, M. (1993, March). Schools, society, and "teen" pregnancy. *Phi Delta Kappan, 74* (7), p. 566 ff.

Monroe, C., Borzi, M. G., & Burrell, R. D. (1992, January). Communication apprehension among high school dropouts. *The School Counselor, 39* (4), p. 273 ff.

Nowinski, J. (1990). *Substance abuse in adolescents and young adults.* New York: Norton.

Phelps, L. & Bajorek, E. (1991). Eating disorders of the adolescent: Current issues in etiology, assessment, and treatment. *School Psychology Review, 20* (1), p. 9 ff.

Simkins, L. (1984, spring). Consequences of teenage pregnancy and motherhood. *Adolescence, 19* (73), p. 39 ff.

Tonks, D. (1992–1993, December–January). Can you save your students' lives? Educating to prevent AIDS. *Educational Leadership, 50* (4), p. 48 ff.

Wagner, M. (1989). *Youth with disabilities during transition: An overview of descriptive findings from the national longitudinal transition study.* Stanford, CA: SRI International.

Williams, R. F. (1993, spring). Gay and lesbian teenagers: A reading ladder for students, media specialists, and parents. *The ALAN Review, 20* (3), p. 12 ff.

Foreword

Jan Cheripko

When I first started writing *Imitate the Tiger* I had no sense that this would be a book to be used by educators to help teens in trouble. It was simply a story—my story. I see my job as an educator as doing exactly what the Latin root of education states: to lead from darkness into light. And my job as a writer I see as following the dictum a wise mentor once told me: "Writing is an experiment in telling the truth." To lead from darkness into light demands truth-telling. Adolescents trying to make sense out of this world need light, and they can only find light if others hold up the light for them to see. The light the educator and writer holds must be the truth. If what is offered is false, then young people remain in darkness—although sometimes convinced they are indeed enlightened—and the educator and writer who has offered the false light of lies, self-aggrandizement, self-indulgence, and victimization has made the darkness even deeper. The truth, I will add, always offers hope—not sentimentality, but real hope born from facing the suffering in life. It's up to the educator to offer a way out—a valid, tangible, realistic, achievable, high-principled way out. Similarly, writers for a young adult audience have a moral responsibility to tell the whole truth—that people do suffer, but that suffering is the price to pay to gain great wisdom and compassion for others. Too many YA writers are stuck at "We're all victims of suffering." It is a monogram worn well, too, by addicts, addicts who never get past that lie, who never gain the promises of sanity and serenity.

There are many, many drugs by which this generation is anesthetizing itself: alcohol, sex, food, gambling, narcotics, money, and power. And now there is a rising interest in an old drug—violence. More and more young people, at younger and younger ages, have discovered that doing violence to others can get you high, that acting out one's hate can make one feel good. What lies at the heart of the intrigue with all of these drugs is fear—fear of not getting what one wants when one wants it. In *Macbeth*, Hecate, goddess of the witches, says it this way:

> He shall spurn fate, scorn death, and bear
> His hopes 'bove wisdom, grace and fear;
> And you all know security
> Is mortals' chiefest enemy.

There is no thought of consequences, no thought of getting caught, no thought of what the future holds, no thought that one will eventually die. Instead we trust our own hopes, our thoughts, our beliefs, our ego to the exclusion of the wisdom of others and the grace of a power greater than ourselves; and we never face our fears, including the fear of not being comfortable; not being taken care of, not being happy, excited, healthy, mesmerized. We fear that life will short-change us; so instead we seek security in what we know—our own ideas, self-assuredness, self-deceived belief that somehow we'll get out of this jam and cheat death. We are out of control, and our self-deceptions eventually destroy us.

If, right now, you can think of some who fit Hecate's description—who spurn fate and trust only their own lies—what will you say to them? How will you reach out to bring them from darkness into light? What truth from your own life will you offer them? What lamp of hope will you use to show them the way? Will you tell them the truth about themselves and run the risk of losing your security and comfort when they spurn you as well?

Education really is a life-or-death art.

Introduction

I am continually one of adolescents' most interested students. From them I have learned, in addition to what's popular or trendy, how adolescents respond to literature and how to make assignments relevant. Most important, they have taught me lessons about life, hope, and courage—lessons I will never forget.

Dave, a high school senior, swaggered into my third-period class with an impish grin and a mischievous attitude. The girls adored him and he reveled in his popularity. On that first day, I didn't know Dave had any health issues until, after lunch, my fifth-period class laughingly began recounting the lunchroom scenario. When most of the seniors were trying to sell passes for a nonexistent elevator or maps to the secret Olympic pool to the naïve freshmen, Dave strolled up to a table of freshmen eating lunch, sat down with them, and removed his prosthetic leg, placing it on the table. Dave lost his leg when he was hit by a drunk driver. He had learned to adjust, although he openly discussed his feelings of depression when he went to the beach or was stared at by strangers. Dave lived life in the present and enjoyed playing on the basketball team even though he knew he would never have the professional career he dreamed of. During one game when our team was behind, Dave detached his leg, causing the opposing team to lose concentration and give us the ball. In a class picture, Dave waved his leg triumphantly in the air.

Jan learned as a middle schooler that she had cancer and began chemotherapy treatments in the eighth grade. She came into class wearing a bandana around her head and a smile that touched my heart. Due to extensive treatments and hospital stays, she was absent often, yet always returned eager to make up any work she missed. As her absences became longer, we had to prepare her classmates for her inevitable death.

Terri was a fun-loving and vivacious freshman who wanted to write books for children. With the onset of juvenile diabetes in sixth grade, she knew she had to watch her diet regularly. Terri never wanted anyone to treat her differently from her peers; however, we knew when she left the classroom that she needed her medication. Her extracurricular activities illustrated her tenacity and spirit, and as the diabetes worsened, her eyesight rapidly began failing. Although she eventually lost her sight, her interest in helping others with diabetes led her to become a counselor at a camp for adolescents with the disease.

Bill spent his entire middle school and high school years fighting leukemia—enduring chemotherapy, radiation, blood transfusions, and bone marrow transplants. Although the prognosis wasn't good, he continued in school. Touched by his courage and strength, his classmates celebrated his first girlfriend, his first school dance, and his academic accomplishments. I still have his reader-response journal in which his perspectives on coming of age were insightful and tearful.

All of these students found strength, wisdom, or comfort in the pages of a book, escaping from pain, fear, and anger through literature. Good literature that gives adolescents the truth has incredible power to heal and renew. As their teacher, I witnessed their struggles; through my own experiences, I understood the impact of their health conflicts.

When Joan Kaywell asked me to do this volume, I began to juxtapose scenes of doctors' offices and pain with those of the normal educational and social aspects of school. Poor health interferes with learning, and good health facilitates it. With the advancements in medicine, the focus has shifted from traditional health problems, like those described above, to behavior-related problems such as motor vehicle accidents, substance abuse, eating disorders, sexually transmitted diseases, depression, and gun-related violence. Adolescents are in a state of crisis. The traditional illnesses and high-risk behaviors have become interrelated through the multitude of physical, social, and emotional changes adolescents are experiencing, and I have attempted to capture this broad spectrum. As I read through the chapters in this volume, I observed that serious problem behaviors tend to cluster and reinforce one another, and that they often have roots in family/childhood experiences. No chapter stands alone—each has connections to other chapters, suggested treatment plans, and young adult literature. Each seeks to illuminate knowledge, skills, and values that foster physical and mental health. This series is a step to reach outside formal system boundaries to strengthen and heal our American youth today.

CHAPTER 1

Freak the Mighty: Birth Defects and Disability in a Literary Friendship

Kathleen Carico and Paula Stanley

Freak the Mighty by Rodman Philbrick (1993) is a powerful novel about love, loss, imagination, and courage. It is the story of two boys with great needs, one of the spirit and one of the body, whose gifts of friendship to each other transform their lives. We chose to discuss this book because of its powerful messages: how to recognize human potential, especially in those who seem to possess few of what we might ordinarily think of as the seeds of success; how to recognize true friendship even when it appears in the form of "freakish" pairings; how love and support can make people valiant; and how resilience in the face of adversity makes life rich and, against impossible odds, happy.

Before we examine the book in depth, however, a word about the purpose of the chapter is in order. As we sat down together to discuss the task before us, we recognized the following:

- Every person in the entire school, including the teacher, provides guidance. The classroom teacher has many opportunities to support, advise, and listen, and teachers can use many strategies, including the ones we share in this chapter, to create a positive learning environment for all students. Teachers provide important interpersonal support.

- Teachers and counselors are trained to work with students in different ways and have specialized roles. These roles should be complementary, especially because teachers and counselors are working for the same goal—a healthy pattern of cognitive, personal, and social growth.

And so it is in this spirit that we offer our thoughts, our strategies, and our resources—that each of us can see in our own situations how we can be more helpful to the people in our lives, especially the children. First, Kathleen will look at the book and the characters through a summary and a discussion of its literary merits. Paula will then describe the characters from a psychosocial perspective; present possibilities for schoolwide interventions, including strategies for teachers dealing with disabled students; and offer specific counseling strategies. Kathleen will follow up with strategies for using *Freak the Mighty* in the classroom.

FREAK THE MIGHTY

Freak the Mighty is a story about two young adolescent boys who, each dealing with a disability, enrich and change each other's lives through their friendship. The main character and narrator is Max, whose life in school is difficult because of a learning disability and because of his perception of himself as a "butthead" and a "goon." He lives with his maternal grandparents, Grim and Gram, as they all struggle with his emergence into adolescence, a process complicated by memories of a horrible crime that took place when Max was four—his father's murder of his mother.

Max lives an inward, solitary life, spending most of his time reading comic books or hanging out in what he calls "down under," the basement room at his grandparents' house. His life changes when Kevin moves in next door. Suffering from mourquis disease, a congenital defect that allows his organs to grow, but not his skeleton, Kevin has spent his life equipping his bright mind by reading, studying books and reference materials, and experimenting with chemistry sets and mechanical toys. Kevin's enthusiasm for learning presents Max with opportunities to learn—about King Arthur, quests, bionics, reading, and, most of all, about the joy of finding acceptance. Kevin seems not to see what others see in Max as problematic: his inability to read and comprehend beyond a rudimentary level; his traumatic past; his cloudy future; and, not least important, his awkward but "mighty" body that seems to grow daily out of Max's control. Kevin seems to change neither his language nor his manner to accommodate Max's problems, but simply sweeps Max along with him in his quest to live life as an adventure.

In turn, Max gives Kevin the gift of mobility and a sense of normalcy as he carries the disabled boy on his shoulders and as he quietly and simply both accepts and admires his new friend. As they realize that the power of two is greater than their individual powers, "Freak the Mighty," Kevin's nickname for the two of them together, is born. Thereafter, as Freak the Mighty, Kevin and Max will face life's difficulties together, "slaying dragons and fools and walking high above the world" (1), as Max will later say. For each of them, there will be various dragons and fools to encounter and overcome in the world, and their friendship, both psychologically and physically, keeps them from being overwhelmed by their foes.

LITERARY MERITS

Freak the Mighty tells a powerful story through the words of a fourteen-year-old boy. Max, as narrator, speaks in the vernacular of a kid of the late twentieth century, but the vernacular is not overpowering, nor does it potentially outdate the story. Even though most of the action takes place between Kevin and Max, many of the other characters have fairly rounded personalities, which contributes to the sense of Max's authenticity as a character. In addition, because Max's narration advances the plot so skillfully in short chapters (none longer than ten pages), this book would make a great read-aloud.

Because Max is the narrator, the reader experiences the events of his life through his eyes and through his language:

> Grim out in the kitchen one night, after supper whispering to Gram had she noticed how much Maxwell was getting to look like *Him*? Which is the way he always talked about my father, who had married his dear departed daughter and produced, eek, eek, Maxwell. Grim never says my father's name, just *Him*, like his name is too scary to say. (3)

Max's humor as a narrator is sometimes sarcastic and often directed at himself in an attempt to handle new emotions. After he is credited with saving Kevin from Tony D. ("Blade") and his gang, he has difficulty dealing with the response of his grandparents:

> Next thing [Grim is] clearing his throat and coughing into his fist and Gram is looking at at the two of us and she gets this Gram-like glow, like this is how it's *supposed* to be, the way things always happen on *The Wonder Years*, with the family getting all gooey and sentimental about some dumb thing the bratty kid did while he's having all his wonderful years or whatever. (43)

One of the most striking literary merits of *Freak the Mighty* is that throughout the book language itself is significant. First, language is primary in both boys' experiences, although with opposite results. Kevin, obviously verbally gifted, enjoys learning new words, experimenting with them, playing with them. Whenever he looks up a word in the dictionary he carries in his backpack, he underlines it in red. Max is impressed with the amount of red underlining he sees in it when Kevin loans it to him to look up *archetype*, a word Kevin must also spell for him. Max, diagnosed with a language learning disability and in special classes at school, has not been able to use language well, let alone manipulate it as Kevin does—that is, until Kevin shows him how. Kevin shares his love of language and his abilities with Max, teaching him to view reading and writing in new and fresh ways from his own perspective as a reader and writer, and not, as Max seems to think, as processes that cannot be understood or controlled.

Second, the importance of identity, particularly of naming, is very important throughout the story. Rodman Philbrick uses names—"sobriquets," as Kevin calls them—to define his characters and shape the story. Grim and Gram, Kicker, Killer Kane, Fair Gwen of Air, Freak the Mighty—Max sees himself, those around him, and even the events of his life through those names. He sees his life as the "grim" past and future of his hapless grandparents, whose daughter's murder leaves them not only in deep grief but in deep distress over the future of their grandson. As for himself, Max sees his own future as a "Killer," like "Killer Kane," his father, whom he clearly resembles and whose life he fears he will also imitate, a fear he may have picked up from his grandparents. He sees himself as "Kicker," the nickname he earned as an angry daycare child whose horror at his mother's death was expressed through violent behavior. And he worries that he might live up to the other label the children gave him in school—"Mad Max"—and live life as a criminal.

When Kevin enters his life, however, a more optimistic future is personified by Kevin's supportive, lovely mother, Gwen; and even her nickname, the "Fair Gwen of Air," a play on Queen Guenevere, suggests adventure, love, and hope. When Max and Kevin become known as Freak the Mighty, Max begins to see himself differently: "I like how it feels to have a really smart brain on my shoulders, helping me think" (64).

Kevin, unlike Max, has a control of language that includes the ability to name—he is the one who christens the two of them Freak the Mighty—and to read into his own life the interpretations for the names he and Max are called. He takes no offense at the name "Freak," seeming to see with a mature eye that yes, his friendship with Max makes them freakish by some standards, but mighty by any standard. He defines words and people the way he wants and needs to. In the face of what he doesn't understand as real danger, he calls Tony D., a cruel older boy who is a dangerous bully, a "cretin," a term he must define (and spell) for Tony. His last gift to Max is a dictionary of words he has defined personally. All of the words reflect his understanding of their "true" meaning, but his interpretations reveal his ability to use literacy for his own purposes, a very sophisticated act.

Third, the flexibility of language is important; it is evident throughout Kevin's discourse, and, finally, in Max's as we see him express his life's story through his writing. It is clear that Max has had a major breakthrough in his language skills and understanding, and that in itself is a worthy topic to highlight. The book is replete with Max's newfound ability to work *with* language in ways that he had never dreamed possible.

UNDERSTANDING KEVIN AND MAX: A NEEDS ASSESSMENT FROM A PSYCHOSOCIAL PERSPECTIVE

Over 2 million children in the United States under the age of seventeen have a condition that, like Kevin's, limits their participation in school (Gerber & Okinow 1991). Many adolescents like Max have poor self-concepts that operate as barriers to their success. Adolescents like Kevin often have social and emotional adjustment difficulties due to their chronic health problems (Gerber & Okinow 1991); individuals like Max have social and emotional adjustment difficulties due to traumatic experiences and other psychosocial stressors. Individuals with chronic disabilities like Kevin and those with poor self-concepts like Max could potentially experience even more difficulty as they enter adolescence, a period of rapid growth and change. It is difficult enough for adolescents to deal with the physical, emotional, social, and psychological changes of their age. A child with a disability, whether it be physical or psychological, may find it even more difficult to resolve the developmental tasks of adolescence. Children with physical disabilities, especially ones as severe as Kevin's, may have fewer chances to participate in the social interactions that help people develop a sense of identity and relationships with peers. In addition, an adolescent with disabilities may develop negative self-perceptions and low feelings of self-worth which can result in the expectation of being rejected by others. The fear of rejection by others may lead to limited social interactions. Because of advances in cognitive development, as adolescents Kevin and Max are more likely than younger children to be aware of the implications of their disabilities, but must also be able to develop more strategies for dealing with them. However, adolescents often need encouragement and assistance in learning ways to deal with their disabilities.

The psychosocial tasks of adolescence involve changing relationships with family, peers, school, and self (Wallander & Varni 1995). Emerging cognitive abilities and physical changes in early adolescence result in a reexamination of oneself in these relationships. The major psychosocial task of adolescence, identity formation, begins with identification with the peer group (Erikson 1980). Identification with the peer group acts as a bridge to an independent identity, which develops later in adolescence. Kevin and Max, who are entering adolescence, are beginning to deal with these tasks.

PEER GROUP

Kevin and Max are about thirteen years old in the book and through their friendship demonstrate an important aspect of adolescence: peer relationships. Kevin, fortunately, seems to have a mother who is not overprotective, encouraging her son to engage in friendships and other activities important for adolescents. Both Kevin and Max seem lonely as the book begins, chiefly occupied with solitary activities. As the story unfolds, Kevin and Max develop a friendship that helps each of them gain a strength that, alone, they did not possess.

Individuals who study adolescents place great emphasis on peer relationships, and individuals who work in schools recognize the centrality of friendships in adolescent life. There is some evidence that disabled adolescents with non-disabled friends are less self-conscious than adolescents without non-disabled friends (Gerber & Okinow 1991). Kevin seems to benefit from his relationship with Max. His self-worth may be enhanced by what he can offer Max and by the acceptance and admiration he receives from him. Max expresses an appreciation for Kevin's abilities and treats him like a friend and equal rather than focusing on his disability. This allows Kevin to express aspects of his personality not related to his disability and to experience greater exploration of his identity.

Kevin and Max also are dealing with two characteristics of this psychosocial stage that are examples of adolescent egocentrism: personal fable and imaginary audience. Personal fable is a belief that one is invulnerable. Kevin seems to display a sense of invulnerability by being involved in as many activities as possible, some of which could be dangerous. For example, Kevin and Max confront gangs and encounter individuals who could do them harm. Kevin, the usual instigator of these events, focuses on the adventure rather than the dangers. The imaginary audience is especially evident in Max, who is critical of his appearance, a projection of Max's own preoccupations. He believes others are judging him as he judges himself. Kevin may deal with his concern over appearance by denying its importance and fantasizing about getting a new body, which is in reality a coping mechanism for facing not just his physical disability but the inevitability of an early death. Kevin, either consciously or unconsciously, compensates for his physical disability by highly developing his cognitive and verbal abilities. Kevin seems to experience a sense of accomplishment and high self-worth because of his talents in this area.

It is important for adolescents at Kevin's age to feel that they fit into their peer group. Both Kevin and Max have difficulty fitting in because of their uniqueness. Max withdraws from his peer group, rejecting others before they reject him; Kevin makes himself stand out by demonstrating his special gifts and demonstrating an invulnerability to the opinions of others. Studies indicate that adolescents who have physical disabilities often have adjustment problems, in large measure due to societal attitudes that value beauty and lack of physical disabilities (Wallander & Varni 1995). Adolescents have more adjustment difficulties than younger children because of the emphasis on physical appearance. Max feels uncomfortable with his large size and continual growth, as he keeps tripping over his own feet; Kevin, although he never mentions his physical appearance, does whatever it takes to accomplish what he wants. Sometimes he crawls to reach someplace faster, and at other times he uses his crutches to obtain things beyond his reach. He seems to focus less on his disability than on his interest in a project or an activity. As Gerber & Okinow (1991) note, some adolescents may have a greater appreciation for life if they have a disability. Kevin would seem to be one of those adolescents.

Individuals with physical disabilities often have difficulty with social skills (Griffin, Gerber, & Rotatori, 1986). They often need to learn to be more cooperative and how to share and make initial attempts at meeting others and improving interactions with peers. When Max first attempts to speak to Kevin, Max describes him as having the look of wanting to kill him. It is hard to know if this is Max's perception or Kevin's defense to keep others at a distance for fear of rejection. Kevin and Max help each other develop better social skills through their friendship.

IDENTITY AND SELF-CONCEPT

It is helpful for teachers and counselors to consider a disabled child's frame of reference, which can provide important information about origins of behavior. Without an understanding of a disabled child's frame of reference, it is easy to apply stereotypes and miss out on the uniqueness of each disabled person. Kevin, for example, copes with his health difficulties by distracting himself with interesting activities and imbuing his physical disability with a special status, a bionic potential. Other disabled children may underachieve due to their perceptions of the meaning of their disability. The perceptual tradition supports the view that individuals create a unique reality for themselves in understanding the world (Purkey & Novak 1996; Purkey & Schmidt 1996). An event or situation is not as significant as the meaning of that event or situation to the person. We can create our own attitudes toward a situation or event, as Kevin did in living life to the fullest even though he knew his life was going to be short. Intentionally or unintentionally, he chose a specific attitude toward his disability and how he would deal with it. We know others and ourselves based on our specific reality construction.

Self-concept theory proposes that we behave in ways that are consistent with the beliefs we have about ourselves. Self-concept refers to who we believe ourselves to be or how we would describe ourselves. Self-esteem is the value we place on who we believe ourselves to be. Max believed himself to be "brainless," which affected his performance in school and his relationships with others. He devalued himself because of his physical size and the fact that he was the son of a killer. Kevin valued his intellect, which was an important aspect of his self-concept. Many adolescents who have disabilities may develop poor self-concepts and low self-esteem because they perceive themselves to be defective or physically unattractive and unacceptable. These adolescents need help in identifying their strengths and defining personal values that transcend physical appearance and societal messages about being disabled. It is helpful for counselors and teachers to help disabled students focus on their strengths and help them think of what they *can* do rather than what they cannot do.

People tend to behave in ways that are consistent with their self-concepts. To have one's self-concept challenged can create cognitive dissonance, which can lead to further growth and integration of new conceptions of self. Kevin helped Max learn to read and therefore to perceive himself as a reader rather than a nonreader. The self-concept may have components that have no basis in reality. Like Max, one may think one cannot read, but there may be no real evidence to support this self-perception. Purkey & Schmidt (1996) suggest three ways that self-concept can be changed: (1) through a dramatic or traumatic experience, (2) through a professional relationship such as counseling, and (3) through everyday experiences. Through everyday experiences, Kevin and Max helped each other to feel more competent and self-accepting. They learned what it meant to be loyal to another person and to feel valued for who they were separately and together.

SCHOOL-WIDE INTERVENTIONS: INVITATIONAL EDUCATION

Many factors are involved in planning interventions that will be helpful for students like Kevin and Max. Counseling interventions with Kevin and Max might include individual and group counseling but also consultation with individuals who interact with them frequently. Parents, teachers, school staff, and peers are all involved in meeting an adolescent's needs. The school environment itself could be examined to determine its health in terms of meeting the needs of individuals with disabilities.

Invitational education is one approach that can be helpful in examining the health of a school environment or climate. Proponents of invitational education propose that everything and everyone in a school has an influence on how well the school functions (Purkey & Novak 1996). Schools are systems in which everyone plays a part. Invitational education proposes four basic assumptions:

- People are able, valuable, and capable of self-direction, and they should be treated accordingly.

- Education is a cooperative, collaborative activity in which the learning process is as important as the product.

- People possess relatively untapped potential in all areas of human development.
- This potential can best be realized by places, policies, and programs that are intentionally designed to invite development, and by people who consistently seek to realize this potential in themselves and others, personally and professionally.

Kevin and Max will both benefit if others treat them as if they were able, valuable, and capable of self-direction and if they experience themselves in the same manner. Kevin and Max can be assisted in realizing their potential, which may involve many people and aspects of the school and home environment. To achieve this, students, teachers, and staff need to examine their own attitudes about disabilities and disabled persons.

It can be helpful for individuals who work with disabled children to develop a greater awareness of how the physically disabled person experiences the school and the world. To achieve this goal, staff and students might try getting around the school in a wheelchair or on crutches as part of an in-service program or school project. Impediments to movement and access to school services will quickly become apparent. To explore attitudes one might have toward physically disabled persons and disabilities, one could ask questions such as these:

- Do I treat disabled persons differently from non-disabled persons? If so, how?
- Do I believe that physical disabilities would keep me from being friends with a person? Why or why not?
- How do I think physically disabled persons are different from other individuals beyond their physical disability?
- Can I see the abilities and strengths of a child with a physical disability rather than just his or her disability?
- When I see a disabled child, do I feel and respond to the child as if he or she were helpless and encourage dependent behavior, or do I see the potential and possibilities that exist for the child?

THE FIVE P's

The school environment can be seen as composed of the five "P's" or five areas: People, Places, Programs, Policies, and Processes. Each of these five areas can be a source of health or frustration for students like Kevin and Max.

People

This area refers to the quality of interactions among people. How do other people in the school interact with students like Kevin and Max? Are they valued for the persons they are and the abilities they demonstrate? Or are they treated with fear or distance by peers or school staff because of their disabilities? Can people see beyond the disability to the person and the abilities demonstrated? Individuals within the school can benefit from examining their own beliefs concerning the life of a disabled person. One view of Kevin would be to concentrate on what he can't do. This approach focuses on his disability to the exclusion of his other attributes. Another view of Kevin would be to focus on the qualities and abilities he has beyond the handicap: that he is able, valuable, and capable.

Disabled students like Kevin often wish they were like non-disabled so that they could do the things others do (Griffin, Sexton, et al., 1986). Kevin's friendship with Max helped him to experience some of what it might be like to get around quickly and see the world from a "higher view." To help a student like Kevin deal with his feelings of wanting to be like other students, one could talk with him about what he perceives to be his limitations and help him realize his strengths and abilities (Griffin, Sexton, et al. 1986). Luckily, Kevin has developed strengths that don't depend on physical agility. He is very bright and creative and has much support for development of his strengths from his mother.

Because Kevin is also terminally ill, he has additional concerns. It appears that children who are nine and older understand the finality and universality of death. Griffin, Sexton, et al. (1986) suggest that one can meet the needs of terminally ill students like Kevin by using the following ideas:

- Provide honest answers to students' questions such as "Am I going to die?"
- Provide information about the illness.
- Encourage the student to continue as "normal" a life as possible. This involves a careful balance between a "hopeful" approach to quality of life and the evidence of foolish optimism that the student will recover.

- Establish and hold "normalized" expectations for behavior and discipline for the terminally ill student. (204)

Places

The places in a school building need to be considered both in terms of their functional nature and their attractiveness. What physical barriers exist for students like Kevin within the school? Are buildings handicapped accessible? Do handicapped students have access to the equipment they need in school, such as an appropriate classroom chair or appropriate bathroom facilities? Are water fountains too high? What is the lunchroom like? Concerns for students like Kevin in this area would be transportation and access within the school. Are they restricted when it comes to going outside during school hours? What restrictions are there on participation in extracurricular activities?

Programs

Programs include opportunities for students to be involved in activities that help meet their needs. Is the counseling program trained to assist students such as Kevin with their disabilities? Are disabled students intentionally or unintentionally separated from other students? Research indicates that disabled teenagers benefit from socializing with non-disabled students as well as disabled students (Gerber & Okinow 1991). Are there physical education classes or experiences for disabled students that help them develop physically? Are social events available to disabled students? Kevin is in a class for the gifted and is mainstreamed in terms of his disability. More programs that teach school personnel how to work with disabled children would be helpful.

Policies

School policies are the rules and regulations that govern behavior. One would hope that school policies would take into consideration the needs of disabled children. For example, Max was allowed to take classes with Kevin. Are there considerations given to absences that students like Kevin might need from school? Are there policies that create barriers for disabled students and keep them separate from other children or activities?

Processes

The last area is that of processes, which describes how people work together to make decisions. Are the processes in a school democratic or autocratic? Do children and adolescents have a chance to provide input into how the school functions? Are parents and the community involved as volunteers and invited to participate in discussions about school matters?

STRATEGIES FOR THE SCHOOL COUNSELOR

Working with students like Kevin and Max from a counseling point of view would concern such areas as self-concept, coping styles, self-talk, social skill development, physical health, and psychosocial development. Both Kevin and Max have concerns which could be helped through a counseling relationship.

Kevin might benefit from discussing concerns about his health and anxieties about his future. It might be helpful for Kevin to discuss his feelings and thoughts about being disabled and what that means to him. It would be important for him to talk about negative interactions with others, such as name-calling, and he could learn other ways of dealing with the hurtful behaviors of others. Kevin has already developed some good coping skills. He appears to stay focused in the present and perceives the future as a fantasy in order to cope with the finality of his death. He has developed self-confidence through developing his cognitive and verbal strengths. Kevin could benefit from identifying his current coping skills and possibly learn new ones. He might also benefit from teaching or tutoring others in school or work on special projects to express his strengths.

It might be helpful if Kevin could discuss his father's rejection and to try to understand what that means. It would be helpful to ensure that Kevin does not take responsibility for his father's rejection of him. Kevin's relationship with his mother could also be emphasized to help Kevin realize the social supports he has. Kevin comes across as tough and invulnerable. A counseling relationship would provide additional support for Kevin as he deals with his disabilities and the short nature of his life.

Max would benefit from discussing his concern with being his father's child. He could be helped to see that just because he looks like his father doesn't mean he will be like him. He has many self-doubts that create anxiety for him. A counselor could explore his feelings and beliefs about himself. When did he first begin feeling "brainless"?

A major concern for Max is his experience in viewing the death of his mother. This could have an effect on his school performance and relationship with others. It would help for him to talk about his father killing his mother. The trauma associated with viewing such an event can produce symptoms such as anxiety, guilt, and flashbacks (Steiner & Matthews 1996). If positive emotional support is received by a person after observing a traumatic event, he or she may not experience as many negative aftereffects.

Much of what one could get from a counseling relationship Max and Kevin experienced in friendship with each other, including acceptance, consistency, and a challenge to growth. Teachers, counselors, and other staff can provide additional support and opportunities for growth that help students like Max and Kevin reach their potential.

STRATEGIES FOR TEACHING *FREAK THE MIGHTY*

In their book *Using Young Adult Literature in the Classroom* (1997), John Bushman and Kay Parks Bushman offer what Kathleen considers to be an excellent strategy for teaching various aspects of a work—the responding report. (See the description on pages 62–63 of their book and a sample on page 64.) In this strategy, an alternative to the book report, the student always works in a response mode, but moves further and further into various aspects of structure, theme, or other literary elements and devices that have the potential to enhance the reading experience. The responding report is one framework for teaching *Freak the Mighty*, because it allows teachers and students to delve into personal issues on a one-on-one basis. In the following sample, students will be able to examine their beliefs and attitudes about friendships and differences (and the teacher will be able to meet several language arts objectives). During the planning stages of the unit containing this report, teachers may wish to consult with the school counselor or invite the counselor's participation if there are any concerns about the task.

Responding Report for *Freak the Mighty*

1. Respond briefly to the following:

   - What are your reactions after reading *Freak the Mighty*?
   - What feelings or emotions does the book evoke in you?
   - Do Kevin and Max remind you of anyone you know? If so, who?

2. Kevin and Maxwell are different in almost every way, and yet they become close friends. Why do you suppose they've become so close? Think about friendships you know about, either you and a friend of yours or other friendship pairings you see. Why do you think those people are friends? Do you admire those friendships?

3. Kevin loves to play with language. Here are some examples of his puns, quotes, and misquotes:

   - After escaping from the dangerous punk Tony (the Blade), Kevin says, "Whew! That was a close encounter of the turd kind" (31).
   - When Max tells Kevin he saw something about robotics on TV, Kevin sighs, "Ah, yes . . . television, the opiate of the massives" (19).
   - In the cafeteria, when Kevin wants a second helping, as he often does, he asks Max, "Please, sir, more gruel" (86).
   - He calls his mother "Fair Gwen of Air."

   Many of these are allusions (references) to other stories and books that Max is unfamiliar with. Kevin explains most, but not all of them, to Max. Max, though not completely understanding his friend's language, enjoys it. Do you? Which lines did you particularly like, and why? Find others in the book (at least two more), write them down, including the page numbers, and tell why you liked them. Through research (in the library or through conversations with people who might know), find out the references for at least three allusions (either the ones given above or ones you find) Kevin makes to other works.

4. Themes usually deal with ideas that are universal, understandable by most readers. However, people might disagree about the major theme of a book. In *Freak the Mighty*, the theme might involve ideas about friendship, appearances, acceptance, or coping with problems. What do you believe to be the theme of this novel? Why?

5. In this novel Rodman Philbrick uses Max as the first-person narrator, the one who tells the story and whose thoughts we as readers are able to know. Although we know what happens only from Max's perspective, we can make some inferences about how the other characters view their lives and each other. Choose one of the prompts below to use in considering how the other characters think and feel.

- Imagine that Kevin is the narrator and is describing Max to the reader. In one or two paragraphs, write down how he would describe Max. You may include physical characteristics, but you must also let the reader know what Kevin thinks of Max as a person or friend.

- Imagine a scene in which the Fair Gwen and Gram are talking about Max in Gram's kitchen. Gram is confiding to Gwen that she is worried about Max's future. Gwen responds to Gram by telling her what she thinks of Max. What does she say to encourage Gram?

- Imagine a scene at lunch in the middle school Kevin and Max attend, soon after the beginning of the year when "Freak the Mighty" is born. A few of their classmates are talking about the two boys. Write out a conversation to show the reader what the students are saying about them.

6. Choose one of the following two activities to complete.

- In the end we discover that Max has written the story down in the year following Kevin's death. However, we do not know what will happen to him. What are your predictions about his future? What will happen to Max now that Kevin is dead? Is "Freak the Mighty" also dead? Will Max recover from the loss? Will he revert to his former solitary way of living in the "down under," not communicating with anyone other than for basic necessities, or will he continue to progress to maturity, as he seemed to through his friendship with Kevin?

- After Kevin dies, Max is understandably devastated and spends a year trying to recover. What advice would you give Max now that Kevin is gone? What kinds of things will help him recover even more and live a happy life? To answer this question you might want to consider this: What did Max learn from the friendship with Kevin that he could use now to establish other relationships?

Follow-up Activities

After all of the reports are in and read by the teacher, she can use the information to structure further whole-class, small-group, and individual activities as indicated and as appropriate. The following samples allow the teacher, students, and, when appropriate, the counselor to discuss personal and social concerns of the disabled and those who relate to them in the context of a book rather than through direct probing of individual opinions.

- After reading and responding to *Freak the Mighty*, a study of multiple intelligences and their uses in schools might be useful. The teacher could begin by discussing Kevin's obvious knack for language, or highly developed verbal-linguistic intelligence. She could then move to a discussion of Gardner's (1983) conception of the other various intelligences that students possess, focusing on the fact that certain ones are rewarded more than others in schools, but that that doesn't make the others less important.

- Construct class charts to illustrate the numbers of themes individuals identified in the reports; small groups could decide on what they consider the top three or work on combining and refining the list. Charts or graphs could also be used to illustrate the motivations for friendships.

- Using the responses to #5 in the responding report students can create reader's theater presentations to dramatize the perspectives of the characters, particularly perspectives of Gwen and Kevin. It would be informative to hear the many perspectives on Max and Kevin that the students will share and to discuss why the characters hold the views they do (and why the students made the inferences they did about the characters' perspectives).

- The conversations between the students about Max and Kevin (the third option in #5) could be expanded and dramatized as brief role plays. Following the dramatizations, the teacher and a school counselor could ask students to analyze the various interpretations. To facilitate discussion the teacher could ask these questions about the scenario: What is the problem or concern in this scene? How do each of the characters probably feel? Why is this problem occurring? What are some solutions to the problem?

- In small groups students can discuss Max's options for the future (from #6 in the responding report) and come to a consensus about the best course of action and/or response for him to take.

- An activity similar to the one suggested as a schoolwide intervention would be to put self-selected students in the position of being physically challenged in some way: blindfolded, in a wheelchair, given earplugs or crutches, or other aids that would simulate a physical handicap. Reflecting on the experience of maneuvering as a physically challenged person through school for one day might allow the students to identify more with the concerns, feelings, and needs of their disabled peers.

- Appropriate follow-up activities would include reflection on literary elements and devices. For example, after discussing points #5 and #6 from the responding report, students could reflect on the way the author uses the narrator to direct (and restrict) information given to the reader. After discussing Kevin's language abilities in relation to point #4, students can discuss their individual perceptions of language learning and literacy itself.

CLOSING THOUGHTS

Freak the Mighty is a powerful book and can be used as a tool not just for studying language, but for studying ourselves and our relationships with others, particularly those who have physical differences. Many of the activities in the responding report will allow students to examine the issues in the relatively safe context of a classroom book study. However, those and other activities suggested in this chapter may trigger in students feelings associated with their personal lives. That is where the school counselor may be most helpful, either in giving advice to the teacher or in an actual counseling relationship with the student. We think the important thing to remember is that the student benefits most when all the stakeholders work together in informed and compassionate ways. This collaboration is not a simple one; it takes time, resources, and support. The alternative, it seems, is to keep the disabled student in the position of "other," on the fringes of participation and involvement; and to keep the non-disabled student uninformed or misinformed and bereft of the benefits of interacting with and understanding classmates with disabilities.

RECOMMENDED READINGS

Birth Defects: Fiction

Blume, J. (1991). *Deenie*. New York: Dell. ISBN: 0–440–93259–9. 159 pp. MS, HS.

Deenie is diagnosed with scoliosis. She wants to be treated the same as other kids, and she acknowledges all of her fears about people who once appeared to be different.

Brown, C. (1991). *My left foot*. Portsmouth, NH: Heinemann. ISBN: 0–749–39177–4. 137 pp. HS.

Christy Brown is born with cerebral palsy in Dublin, Ireland, to a working-class family. His mother, cautioned against hope for his future, teaches him to write with his left foot. He continues to learn, and one of his greatest triumphs is the writing of this book, which was eventually adapted for the screen, becoming an Oscar-winning movie.

Cleaver, V., and B. Cleaver. (1973). *Me too*. Philadelphia: Lippincott. ISBN: 0–397–31485–X. 158 pp. MS, HS.

Lydia becomes the tutor of her twin Lorna, who is intellectually impaired. Lydia tries to make Lorna acceptable so that their father will return and friends will accept Lorna as well.

Corcoran, B. (1969). *A row of tigers*. New York: Atheneum. ISBN: 0–689–20070–6. 165 pp. MS.

After Jackie runs away from home she meets up with Gene, whose body is misshapen by his curved spine. They form a friendship that changes Gene's perception of himself to a more positive, hopeful image.

Cormier, R. (1991). *The bumblebee flies anyway*. New York: Dell. ISBN: 0–440–90871–X. 241 pp. HS.

The Complex is full of patients facing and dealing with their terminal illnesses. Barney falls for patient Mazzo's twin sister, Cassie, and develops a plan to help Mazzo end his suffering. With the help of other patients, Barney builds "The Bumblebee," a car he puts together and intends to use to commit suicide.

Doherty, B. (1988). *Granny was a buffer girl*. New York: Orchard. ISBN: 0–531–08354–3. 160 pp. MS. Audiocassette. ed. (1988). G. K. Hall Audio Books. ISBN: 0–816–17771–6.

Jess is getting ready to leave her family for school in France. The love of her disabled brother and the stories of her family (including the title story) teach her lessons that enable her to part with her family.

Eliot, G. (1987/1860). Reprint ed. *The mill on the floss*. New York: Penguin USA. ISBN: 0–140–43120–9. HS. Audiocassette (1997). New York: Penguin. ISBN: 0–140–86181–5. VHS tape (1997). Los Angeles: Anchor Bay. ISBN: 0–764–00112–4.

Maggie, caught in the customs of her time and place (nineteenth century England), is forbidden by her brother Tom to associate with Philip, a hunchback who loves her and appreciates her intelligence.

Ethridge, K. (1985). *Toothpick*. New York: Holiday. ISBN: 0–823–40585–0. 118 pp. MS.

Janice has cystic fibrosis, a condition that keeps her very thin. She finds a friend in Jamie, who is naturally thin. Both encounter teasing from their classmates. As Janice's disease progresses, Jamie learns how to give the gift of his friendship, and, as a result, learns to accept himself for who he is.

Gould, M. (1982). *Golden daffodils*. New York: Harper. ISBN: LB 0–201–1157–9. 172 pp. MS.

Janis has cerebral palsy and decides in fifth grade to go to a mainstreamed school instead of her special school. She finds some people to be too helpful and others too cruel. Janis has to find a balance between what she can and cannot do to feel happy and normal.

Harnishfeger, L. (1973). *Prisoner of the Mound Builders*. Minneapolis: Lerner. ISBN: 0–822–50754–4. 141 pp. MS.

O-Tah-Wah has a leg deformity that the Indian tribe sees as unique. The tribe wants to bury O-Tah-Wah with the medicine man to assist him in the afterlife, but O-Tah-Wah and a fellow captive escape to found a new nation.

Holman, F. (1968). *A year to grow*. New York: Norton. 100 pp. MS.

Julia befriends a young retarded boy while trying to find her place in the world. She and Jimmy develop a way to communicate between themselves and spend every afternoon together until Jimmy dies. Julia finds connection and purpose through her relationship with Jimmy.

Howard, E. (1984). *Circle of giving*. New York: Atheneum. ISBN: 0–689–31027–7. 112 pp. MS.

Jeannie and Marguerite move to a new neighborhood in California during the 1920s. They discover that physical differences can unite rather than divide. Marguerite helps Francie, a severely disabled neighbor, learn to write, and Marguerite learns to play the piano.

Howe, N. (1984). *God, the universe, and hot fudge sundaes*. New York: Houghton Mifflin. ISBN: 0–395–35483–8. 182 pp. MS, HS.

Seventeen-year-old Alfie confronts issues of abortion, religious faith and conflict, divorce, and death in this story about her little sister's illness.

Hugo, V. (1995). *The hunchback of Notre Dame*. Reprint ed. New York: Bantam Books. ISBN: 0–553–21370–9. HS.

This is the classic tale of the hunchbacked bellringer Quasimodo and his love for the beautiful gypsy girl Esmeralda.

Hunt, I. (1993). *Up a road slowly*. New York: Silver Burdett. ISBN: 0–382–24366–8. 192 pp. MS.

Julia goes to live with her schoolteacher aunt Cordelia. Julia's relationship with Agnes, a retarded pupil of Aunt Cordelia's, gives Cordelia the opportunity to instill compassion into her niece for other people despite their situations.

Jewett, E. (1946). *The hidden treasure of Glaston*. New York: Viking. ISBN: 0–670–37081–9. 307 pp. HS.

Hugh is left in a monastery by his father, a knight, because he cannot bear Hugh's lameness. Hugh discovers the underground treasures at the monastery and gains healing and happiness with his discovery.

Knowles, A. (1983). *Under the shadow*. New York: Harper and Row. ISBN: LB 0–060–23222–6. 128 pp. MS.

Cathy moves to a new house in the countryside and finds a friend who has muscular dystrophy. Cathy learns a lot from Mark, who, even though physically limited, has a great imagination.

Laird, E. (1989). *Loving Ben*. New York: Delacorte. ISBN: 0–385–29810–2. 183 pp. MS.

Anna and her family must deal with the birth of her younger brother Ben, born with hydrocephalus. Anna loves Ben deeply and tries to deal honestly with what seems to be her preference for him, a preference that makes her little sister jealous. Ben dies after contracting the flu. After his death, Anna uses what she has learned from Ben to help a Down syndrome child and the child's family.

Leonard, A. (1988). *Tina's chance*. New York: Viking. ISBN: 0–670–82430–5. 187 pp. MS.

Tina learns of a hereditary illness she has after searching for information about her mother and her mother's premature death.

Newth, M. (1989). *The abduction*. New York: Farrar, Strauss and Giroux. ISBN: 0–374–30008–9. 248 pp. HS.

In this historically based novel, a young betrothed Inuit couple is kidnapped and forced to board a ship on a mission for the English queen. The woman is raped and the man is beaten. Eventually, the couple comes in contact with Christine, a young crippled woman, and Henrik, a scholar who studies their language. The story features the tragedy of a society's misunderstanding and mistreatment of those who are different, such as the Inuit couple, Christine, and Henrik, who stutters.

Philbrick, R. (1993). *Freak the mighty*. New York: Scholastic. ISBN: 0–590–47412–X. 169 pp. MS.

Rabe, B. (1987). *Margaret's moves*. New York: Dutton. ISBN: 0–525–44271–5. 105 pp. MS.

Margaret has spina bifida and wants a faster, more maneuverable wheelchair to be able to participate in life. There are financial strains on the family due to her situation, and her parents would rather buy her a waterbed to prevent bedsores. Margaret takes the initiative to earn money herself and save up for the new wheelchair.

Radley, G. (1984). *CF in his corner*. LaGrange, GA: Four Winds. ISBN: 0–02–777390–6. 128 pp. MS.

When Jeff discovers that his younger brother Scotty's health problems are caused by fibrosis and not asthma, as their mother has told them, he feels that Scotty should know. Their mother feels betrayed by Jeff after she finds out that he tells Scotty the truth. Scotty's doctor helps her come to terms with the idea that Scotty should know about his terminal illness.

Snyder, Z. (1990). *Libby on Wednesday*. New York: Delacorte. ISBN: 0–385–29979–6. 196 pp. MS.

At a new school Libby is placed in a writing group with four other seventh graders, including Alex, a boy with cerebral palsy. The group clashes at first, but as they get to know each other better, they begin to respect and learn from each other.

Stallings, G., and S. Cook (1997). *Another season: A coach's story of raising an exceptional son*. Boston: Little, Brown. ISBN: 0–316–81196–3. 256 pp. HS.

Coach Gene Stallings of the University of Alabama tells the story of his and his wife's struggles and victories in raising a child with Down syndrome after being counseled to put him in an institution.

Stein, S. (1974). *About handicaps: An open family book for parents and children together.* New York: Walker. ISBN: 0–802–77225–0. 47 pp. ES, MS.

Matthew is frightened by Joe's cerebral palsy and fears that his own slight physical ailment might turn into a dreadful disease. Through patience, talking, and an encounter with an older man who has a disability, Matthew's father eventually helps him understand disabilities better and paves the way for a positive relationship with Joe.

Birth Defects: Nonfiction

Baskin, B., and K. Harris. (1977). *Notes from a different drummer: A guide to juvenile fiction portraying the handicapped.* New Providence, NJ: R. R. Bowker. ISBN: 0–835–20978–4. 375 pp. HS.

This is a valuable guide to fiction written between 1940 and 1975 portraying the handicapped. The lengthy annotations, accompanied by analyses of the books, provide extensive information about their content and usefulness.

Kingley, J., and M. Levitz (1994). *Count us in: Growing up with Down syndrome.* New York: Harvest Books. ISBN: 0–1562–2660–X. 182 pp. MS, HS. (Equality, Dignity, and Independence of People with Disabilities Award from the National Easter Seal Society; Media Award from the National Down Syndrome Congress; Washington Irving Best Books of 1993–94; Best Books of 1994 for Teenagers by the New York Public Library; and inclusion on the Recommended Reading List for High School Students by the New York State Department of Education). See the "Count us in" web page at http://brugold.com/count.html

This is the true story of Jason and Mitchell, two young men born with Down syndrome, and their families. Friends since childhood, the two men share their perspectives on their friendship as well as on growing up, girls, sex, marriage, and many other issues confronting most children growing into young adulthood, with the additional perspective of people with obvious physical and mental differences.

Robertson, D. (1992). 3rd ed. *Portraying persons with disabilities: An annotated bibliography of fiction for children and teenagers.* New Providence, NJ: R. R. Bowker. ISBN: 0–835–23023–6.

Like *Notes from a Different Drummer* and *More Notes from a Different Drummer*, this volume provides annotations for numerous categories of fiction portraying persons with disabilities. In addition to the annotations, Robertson gives a historical account of the portrayal of the disabled in the media.

REFERENCES

Bushman, J., and K. Bushman (1997). *Using young adult literature in the English classroom.* Englewood Cliffs, NJ: Prentice-Hall.

Erikson, E. H. (1980). *Identity and the life cycle.* New York: W. W. Norton.

Gardner, H. (1983). *Frames of mind.* New York: Basic Books.

Gerber, G., and N. Okinow (1991). "Chronic illness and disability." In William Hendee, ed., *The health of adolescents: Understanding and facilitating biological, behavioral, and social development.* San Francisco: Jossey-Bass, 282–301.

Griffin, H., P. Gerber, and A. Rotatori (1986). "Counseling the health-impaired child." In A. Rotatori, P. Gerber, F. Litton, and R. Fox, eds., *Counseling exceptional students.* New York: Human Sciences Press, 213–231.

Griffin, H., D. Sexton, P. Gerber, and A. Rotatori (1986). "Counseling the physically handicapped child." In A. Rotatori, P. Gerber, F. Litton, and R. Fox, eds., *Counseling exceptional students.* New York: Human Sciences Press, 197–212.

Purkey, W. W., and J. M. Novak (1996). *Inviting school success: A self-concept approach to teaching, learning, and demographic practice.* Belmont, CA: Wadsworth.

Purkey, W. W., and J. J. Schmidt (1990). *Invitational learning for counseling and development.* Ann Arbor, MI: ERIC/CASS.

Purkey, W. W., and J. J. Schmidt (1996). *Invitational counseling: A self-concept approach to professional practice.* Pacific Grove, CA: Brooks/Cole.

Purkey, W. W., and P. H. Stanley (1994). *The inviting school treasury: 1001 ways to invite student success.* New York: Scholastic.

Steiner, H., and S. Feldman (1996). "General principles and special problems." In H. Steiner, ed., *Treating adolescents.* San Francisco: Jossey-Bass, 1–41.

Steiner, H., and Z. Matthews (1996). "Psychiatric trauma and related psychopathologies." In H. Steiner, ed., *Treating adolescents.* San Francisco: Jossey-Bass, 345–393.

Wallander, J., and J. Varni (1995). "Appraisal, coping, and adjustment in adolescents with a physical disability." In J. Wallander and L. Siegel, eds., *Adolescent health problems: Behavioral perspectives.* New York: Guilford Press, 209–231.

CHAPTER 2

Izzy, Willy-Nilly: Issues of Disability for Adolescents and Their Families

Cynthia Ann Bowman and Phyllis A. Gordon

When I was very young, people called me crippled. During my high school years, I was labeled handicapped. Today I am considered disabled, except by those people who stop me on the street to tell me that God must love me very much to give me such a special gift—A gift I received when I was five years old, a gift that would forever change the person I would become and the experiences I would have. Disability shapes identity, both perceived and real.

One morning I was running and playing with my friends; the next morning I was completely paralyzed with swollen, inflamed, and painful joints. I was scared and confused, and the worry and anxiety were reflected on the faces of my parents. When the doctors at the Cleveland Clinic gave us the diagnosis of juvenile rheumatoid arthritis (JRA) after a weeklong barrage of tests, X-rays, and joint scans, the dynamics of my entire family were changed. I was an interesting case, a thick medical chart useful for training new doctors, as rheumatoid arthritis is not commonly associated with children. The doctors suggested that my parents enroll me in a special school, buy me a wheelchair, and make plans for my long-term care. My parents had different dreams, however, and when the doctors introduced them to a young woman suffering with JRA who could not leave her hospital bed, they were even more adamant that I would stay on my feet, go to a regular school, have friends, date, drive a car, and go to college. They were not going to let arthritis get the best of me, and together we fought the disease with a vengeance. Every morning my dad would lift me out of bed and place me in a tub of warm water until my joints loosened up enough for me to move. My mom would get me dressed, and then my dad would take me to school. I didn't know until years later that my dad would go back home and cry before going to work.

Disability affects the whole family. When I got home from school my mom and I would begin a physical therapy routine, an hour of range-of-motion exercises with my mom moving each joint beyond what I could do on my own. It was tough to understand as a child why my mom would want to hurt me, but now I marvel at the love and strength it took to persevere against my tears, hurtful comments, and pleas to stop.

I never considered myself disabled. My parents made me do my share of the jobs around the house, and I considered myself just like the other kids. But I wasn't. I do not remember the name of the boy who walked on my heels all the way home from school, but I do remember how embarrassed I was when his mother made him come over to my house and apologize to me. I remember the principal who grabbed a kid by the neck for calling me names, but I was used to ignoring such scenes. In order to survive I had to forget the children and the adults who stared at me. My mom, however, would ask them if they wanted a picture, my dad would engage them in conversation, and my brother would look prepared to fight. Such incidents contributed to the sense of alienation that disability can produce.

It was in school where I found refuge, a place where I could be successful, a place where I was known for something other than walking funny. It was tough, though, because I felt like a normal kid and wanted to be a normal kid. I loved the teachers who punished me for talking or passing notes and worked much harder for those who didn't appear to notice my disability. In school I could be smart, not handicapped. I became a voracious reader, hungry to live vicariously for a few hours without pain, without feeling awkward or different. I devoured biographies of famous women, convinced I could make a difference some day. I read fantasies, romances, and adventures. I wanted to be Nancy Drew, Cherry Ames, Anne of Green Gables, and Laura Ingalls Wilder. But I was learning more about life not only from books but from hospital visits and surgeries.

I couldn't make it home from the bus stop without my ankles giving out, leaving me stranded in front of a neighbor's home. I couldn't stand in one place very long, and my feet hurt all the time. I wanted so badly to be able to run the track during physical education, sit on the floor with my legs crossed, open my locker easily, and not struggle to get around. I watched my friends doing all the things I wanted to do, and it hurt. As I looked out the hospital room window after visiting hours, I couldn't understand why no one seemed to be hurting as much as I was. The world was going on, seemingly oblivious to the fear and apprehension inside my heart. It didn't take long to find someone with far more serious problems during each of my hospital stays. That knowledge allowed me to feel fortunate—blessed with parents and a brother who loved me. They didn't let me feel disabled. After one of my surgeries, my mom and dad came into the room with a beautiful yellow and white lace dress to wear to my upcoming eighth grade graduation. Such special moments and thoughtful incentives kept me happy and hopeful.

Unfortunately, not everyone took the opportunity to get to know me, to know that I was more than just my physical challenges or some type of inspiration. During a year that I spent in a wheelchair, I discovered that disability can negate any personal qualities. People wouldn't look at me or talk to me. They would talk to whomever was pushing me, admiring the family member or friend who could be so giving and generous. Strangers would ask questions about me as if I wasn't there. Even as an adult, when I wanted to purchase a sweater on my charge card, the salesperson looked at my friend and asked if it was okay. Another time my mom was asked to sign my name. People would begin talking loudly and slowly, as if a physical disability automatically indicates a mental disability. The same impersonal attitude exists in medical facilities. From the moment the identification bracelet went around my wrist, I was a case. I have been a joint replacement candidate, a surgical procedure, an orthopedic patient. Even the language alienates. One doctor wrote on my chart, "Patient seen today. This is a particularly bad Rheumatoid Arthritic who has been through multiple surgeries—triple arthrodesis and revisions, joint replacements of the hips, knees, and hands." I struggle to work beyond those awkward moments, not just with people but also with places. Although there is more awareness now than ever before, the world is not a friendly place for a person with a disability. New places are a source of anxiety. How far will I have to walk? Will there be steps? Handrails? Places to sit? Will I be able to get out of the chairs? Are there curbs? Are the doors heavy? Will I be able to turn the doorknob? Are things too high? Too low?

Meeting people for the first time is difficult. Some people look past me, not at me. Some won't shake my hand, and some people barely touch my hand. I can sense curiosity, pity, and fear. I understand when people are anxious to help, but it makes me uncomfortable and embarrassed. I know someone is thinking of me, not my disability, when they ignore what may be an obstacle or forget that I can't move quickly or easily. Most of my friends have been people I've gone to school with or worked with, people who have taken the time to see beyond my disability and have gotten to know me. It's hard, because I am achingly aware of my disability and yet I don't want others to be.

My identity is intertwined with my disability. The adversities I have faced have contributed to the inner strength I possess even though my disability has also played havoc with my self-esteem. My sense of humor has enabled me to laugh at the innovative ways I have found to accomplish the simplest of tasks and make fun of myself. On rare occasions I wallow, feeling sorry about the things I can't do and the experiences I have missed. Then I think of the children I have seen in rehabilitation centers, their smiles and spirit, and focus on what makes life meaningful and richly rewarding.

EXPERIENCE OF DISABILITY

It has been suggested that approximately 10–15 percent of children face some type of disability or chronic health condition (Hobbs, Perrin, & Ireys 1985). Therefore, all of us can expect to deal with disability in our lives either through personal experience or contact with family or friends. Numerous writers have suggested that reactions to disability may often be viewed as fairly normal responses to an abnormal situation (Vash 1981; Wright 1983). In order to understand this encounter with disability and to better assist students who are disabled or peers of these children, educators and counselors alike must understand the arduous tasks and the myriad emotions that confront them and their families. The purpose of this chapter is to discuss the usefulness of literature in helping students learn the realities of living with a disability. In addition, our goal is to share our reactions, experiences, and knowledge from our different perspectives to help teachers aid those students with disabilities in their classrooms.

As I read the words of my co-author Cynthia Bowman describing her ordeals of growing up, I am again struck by the struggles individuals with disabilities must go through in our society. As she notes, disability is a family experience—a phrase I often repeat to the graduate students in my rehabilitation counseling classes. Due to the attention and care needed to meet the demands of the disabling condition, stress and anxiety are frequently created for both the child and the family. In addition, the sense of loneliness and isolation can be tremendous, as one can sense from the poignant recollections just described. Living with disability means adjusting to loss and debilitation while, it is hoped, finding strength to persevere and succeed. It means dealing with issues of self-esteem, peer relationships, and dating in a society that emphasizes the importance of looks. It often brings disruption to family dynamics, family resources, and family values. Children with disabilities are confronted with worry over present and future plans, while their parents are faced with more responsibility and caregiving duties. Furthermore, parents have to meet this stress while mourning the loss of their own mental picture of a normal child (Ziolko 1991).

Lindgren, Burke, Hainsworth, and Eakes (1992) report that parental responses can be categorized as a *chronic sorrow*, pain associated with loss and long-term sadness and disappointment over the developmental milestones their child may not reach. The sadness felt by Cindy's father is an excellent example. He would help her get ready for school in the morning before driving her there and return home to cry before continuing with his day. Typically, this grief is time-limited, but this type of reaction is not pathological; rather, it is a normal response to a difficult situation (Lindgren et al. 1992). Moreover, these moments of sadness may be episodic, highlighted at some points and waning during times when the illness or disability assumes a secondary role in the family's daily living (Turner-Henson, Holaday, & Swan 1992). Recognizing this sense of grief and loss is crucial as we begin to examine *Izzy, Willy-Nilly* by Cynthia Voigt (1986).

IZZY, WILLY-NILLY

We chose this novel because Cynthia Voigt explores feelings, challenges, and experiences in *Izzy, Willy-Nilly* similar to those we have described. Isobel (Izzy) Lingard wakes up in a hospital with sketchy, blurred memories of the car accident following the party she attended with Marco Griggers. She sees her parents worried, anxious, and exhausted; a nurse is taking her blood pressure, and a doctor is looking at her chart. The impersonal and sterile nature of the hospital belies the very personal tragedy Izzy experiences as she learns that her leg will have to be amputated. Izzy is a popular high school sophomore, a cheerleader, the first of her friends to be asked out by a senior. She didn't even like Marco that much; she did want to go to the party with older and popular students. At the party, there was drinking and drug use, and

Marco was in no condition to drive her home. He insisted, however, and rather than look immature, she went with him.

Izzy needed her friends, and she was counting on them to help her through this tragedy. Unfortunately, one of the hardest lessons she had to learn was that some people do not deal very well with adversity. Her three best friends stayed away. When they called, they didn't know what to say. When they came to the hospital to visit, Lauren stood at the door, Suzy talked incessantly about nothing, and Lisa talked to Lauren and Suzy as if Izzy weren't there. After a while, they no longer called or came by. The reality of her situation hit her all at once. "You don't talk to things. And that's what I was, a thing, a messed-up body" (57).

Body image is important to adolescents, and Izzy had to deal with the reality that her body had been altered by the accident. She worried that no one would want to go out with her. "So I turned the light out early and lay watching the perfect people on TV, with their perfect complexions and perfect bodies acting their parts. It was a color TV, but the grayness had swallowed me up" (63). Izzy thought of the perfect women in the Harlequin novels she read and wondered, "Who would want to go out with a cripple?" (61). Only at night when she was all alone did Izzy cry. All of these feelings are natural, and as Izzy felt sorry for herself she also knew that there were others with more severe health problems. "I didn't care about that, and I knew how mean and selfish that was, but I really didn't care. But I didn't like being so mean and selfish—I was supposed to be nice, that's what I was, a nice girl. Not anymore, that wasn't what I was. Now I was a cripple" (64).

Izzy needed the support of her family, yet her family responded in unusual ways. Her mom and dad made changes to their house without discussing them with Izzy. Rather than addressing the accident in a forthright manner, Izzy had to deal with her younger sister's resentment of all the attention and special consideration she was given as well as her brothers' anger. Even surrounded by her family, Izzy felt alone. "It was so solitary there inside myself. I just wanted someone to reach in there and connect, just for a minute, just so I would know it could be done" (69).

It is Rosamunde who is able to give Izzy the friendship and support she needs, unexpected because Izzy had never taken the time to get to know her even though they were in many of the same classes. Izzy is surprised when Rosamunde comes to the hospital to visit, and doesn't know how to respond to her candid remarks and probing questions. She finds Rosamunde both irritating and exciting, and their emerging friendship allows Izzy the security to face the difficulties of going home after a hospital stay and the fears of returning to school.

Izzy learned that moving around on a walker and negotiating a wheelchair are exhausting. "I never had, though, thought about how it would feel to be so weak that it was hard work, really hard work to get out of bed and into the bathroom" (42). It is discouraging, as Izzy quickly learns. "I didn't want tomorrow to come, because it was going to be a repeat of today" (60). Rosamunde gives her the support to cope with returning home. "Because I was disappointed, and it wasn't anything to do with home and I knew that, but I was still feeling disappointed with home" (144). But Rosamunde is there for her and encourages her to return to school, understanding her fears and finding projects to occupy the empty spaces of her life. Probably the most important lesson Izzy learns is the difficulty and rewards of asking for help.

Three seniors who were at the party made Izzy's life at school more bearable. Tony and Deborah involved her on the newspaper staff, and John Wintersize carried her up the cafeteria steps. Sitting around the newspaper table, feeling like part of a team, helped Izzy adjust to returning to school. "I couldn't break the illusion that we were all just like normal, which was possibly true as long as I didn't roll away from the table" (162). The joy Izzy experiences when Tony forgets to give her her crutches at the end of their newspaper meeting is the pure satisfaction of knowing he was no longer thinking of her as different or disabled.

REACTIONS TO THE BOOK

Izzy, Willy-Nilly is an important contribution to the understanding and acceptance of disability in our society. Through reading this novel, students can begin to identify with someone similar to themselves who becomes physically disabled. Perhaps one of the most difficult realizations for children and adolescents to make is that painful experiences such as the one Izzy goes through can happen to them. First and foremost, this book highlights the horrors and dangers associated with car accidents and substance abuse to a population at risk, with little preachiness or lecturing. Through Izzy's experiences, the reader shares the awareness that one poor decision has changed her life forever and that bad things can indeed happen to good people.

ADJUSTMENT TO DISABILITY

Adapting to a disabling condition requires allowing the individual time to grieve. Having knowledge of the typical grieving process or stage models can assist teachers in understanding the student with a disability, particularly an abrupt physical disability onset such as the one Izzy had. While a number of similar models are cited in the literature along with models specific to traumatic versus gradual onset disability, Livneh (1986) provides a concise overview of the stages addressed in most models and the research pertaining to adjustment.

The first stage, *initial impact*, is the first reaction the person has to the disabling condition. In *Izzy, Willy-Nilly*, it would be when Izzy awakens and realizes she is in the hospital and her leg will be amputated. During this period, Livneh notes two substages as typical—shock and anxiety. Shock is characterized by a numbing of emotion, which is then followed by a more confused and emotional reaction to the event.

The second stage, *defense mobilization*, involves periods of bargaining and denial. Both are normal reactions and help protect the individual from becoming submerged in anxiety and fear. During this period of time, the individual may set unrealistic goals and expectations or minimize the effects of the disability.

The third stage, *initial realization*, is one where the impact of the disability on the individual's life is now becoming evident and real. During this stage, a person experiences a number of emotions such as anger, depression, and grief. We see Izzy reacting in this manner through learning her thoughts in the hospital, her questions about her future—dating, school, extracurricular activities—and her bouts of crying while alone at night. Throughout most of this novel, Izzy appears to be moving back and forth through this stage.

The fourth stage, *retaliation*, is characterized by outward anger and hostility directed at others. This appears to be the stage that Izzy should be moving toward, but there is little discussion in the book of feelings of anger and blame. Since these are normal reactions to this type of injury, it would be unrealistic of teachers to not anticipate this from students who might be returning from a traumatic event. It would be common for Izzy to either blame Marco or feel guilt over her own participation in the accident.

The final stage, *reintegration*, is characterized by three substages: acknowledgment of both the current and future implications of the disability;

acceptance and adjustment to a changed lifestyle; and personal identity. The emotions of the person are more balanced at this point.

The stages of these types of models are not time specific and may be cyclical, but one may question whether three weeks was a realistic time frame for Izzy's return to school. It would help students to know that adjustment is a long-term process. In addition, there appeared to be an implied belief that now that Izzy had a disability, she automatically would know how to use crutches and navigate her environment. In reality, with this type of injury, she would have gone through an extensive rehabilitative process where she would have been taught to walk with crutches, dress herself, work in a kitchen, and return to school. Efforts would have been made to ascertain whether there were steps at school, where her classrooms and lunchroom were located, and what kind of assistance would be needed. The difficulties she experienced in all of these areas were perhaps stressed too much in the novel. Classroom discussion could focus on the realities a newly disabled student might encounter so that students are not left with the impression that everyone who is disabled is also fairly helpless, a view that, unfortunately, could encourage the belief that persons with disabilities are pitiful and unable to be independent, thus fostering the development of negative attitudes.

DISABILITY AND INTERPERSONAL RELATIONSHIPS

One of the major challenges of adolescence is the fostering and building of interpersonal relationships. For all young people, this is a time fraught with excitement and apprehension as they struggle to find their niche in the world. I recall a conversation with a young adolescent who had a significant learning disability that required specialized assistance outside of the regular classroom. He was crying and distraught about his disability, certain that all the other students thought poorly of him and that no girl would ever be interested in a boy with a disability. He was actually a very popular student on campus but, as is typical of many young people his age, could not see it. He was certain that the difficulty he was experiencing was due to his disability. We talked about the realness of his disability, and I listened to his concerns with compassion and caring. At the same time, I began to gently inquire whether he felt that his friends who did not have learning disabilities might have similar concerns. After a time, he began to acknowledge that his peers might be struggling with self-esteem issues of their own. It is important for teachers and counselors to recognize that many issues for children with disabilities are complex, involving the intertwining of disability and developmental stages.

DISABILITY AND DEVELOPMENTAL STAGES

Professionals need to be cautious about ascribing all problems to the disability and to remember that all young people move through developmental periods of struggle and self-doubt. Equally important, though, is an awareness of the unique challenges disability brings. Individuals with disabilities do face considerable difficulty with friendships and dating. As most of us who work or have worked with children know, being accepted by others and fitting in can be a daunting process. Countless stories of damaged self-esteem have been recalled by adults who as children were placed in the lower level reading group or were the last person chosen for the baseball team. Having a disability that separates one from his or her peers in terms of appearance can have a significant impact on self-image. Several good books and videos are available that address a number of self-esteem issues. Steering young people with disabilities to resources that speak of them and to them can be beneficial in helping them recognize that they are not alone. Perhaps what struck me most vividly about Izzy was that others showed little concern about helping her learn about amputation or adaptation. *Withstanding Ovation*, an excellent video listed in the resource section at the end of this chapter, portrays two adolescents who are missing limbs but who are living normal and extremely productive and satisfying lives. It is a wonderful example of the capabilities persons with disabilities possess and provides role models appropriate for those Izzy's age. This video also deals with the issue of not wanting to stand out or be recognized as different. One segment discusses the discomfort one young person feels about associating with other young people with disabilities. While support groups and peer groups may be very helpful for young persons with disabilities, it must be remembered that some may feel stigmatized by being around others with disabilities—a further recognition of their differences. Counselors and teachers need to address these types of issues before assuming that a support group would be beneficial for all students with disabilities. A video such as *Withstanding Ovation* can stimulate a discussion of this issue in a nonthreatening or nonjudgmental manner.

DISABILITY AND IDENTITY

Numerous authors have noted the difficulties young persons with disabilities face in developing a sexual identity and sense of self. It has generally been accepted that society's focus on issues of appearance and functional ability is instrumental in promoting more negative attitudes toward those who deviate from the norm. For both males and females with disabilities, issues regarding dating and social acceptance by the opposite sex are frequent areas of concern. Research by Rousso (1996) suggests that as a group girls who become disabled prior to adolescence subsequently have their first date, first kiss, or steady dating relationship at a much later age than those who become disabled following the adolescent period. Opportunities to develop a positive sense of self as a person and as a potential sexual partner may be hindered by disability. There are steps that both teachers and schools can take to make socialization easier. First, schoolwide diversity training for both faculty and students is helpful. Understanding that differences are okay and that we all differ on a number of dimensions (e.g., race, gender, religion, etc.) helps to put disability issues in perspective. Second, school-sponsored social activities that limit required pairing can aid many adolescents, not just those with disabilities, who struggle in the social arena. Izzy's involvement with the school newspaper is one good example. In addition, role models and peer mentors (e.g., matching popular students with those with disabilities) can be used to demonstrate to others in the school setting the strengths of those with disabilities. Inviting, for example, a successful business man or woman who is disabled to talk to the school population, not about disability but about his or her job, may speak volumes about the capabilities of those with disabilities. As Rousso (1996) notes, women with disabilities who were able to succeed socially during adolescence generally reported "a supportive friend or relative who believed in them socially or a particularly accessible or nonjudgmental community that was receptive to differences among its members" (112) as vital. School personnel have the potential to be that supportive person and to provide the setting that may make all the difference to that particular student with a disability.

QUESTIONS FOR STUDENT DISCUSSION

To facilitate dialogues about disability in general and Izzy's experience in particular, teachers may want to further examine a number of areas with students. The following questions may be posed as journal topics, free-writing activities, and small and large group discussions:

1. How might the reactions of a student who sustains a similar disability at the age of eight differ from Izzy's?
2. Would a boy her age have the same reactions and experiences as Izzy? What are issues specific to gender?
3. Would all Izzy's teachers really have been unable to talk about the accident and disability with her? How might her teachers have handled the situation?
4. Do you think that Izzy and/or her parents should have talked to Marco following the accident about his responsibility? Why or why not? If you had been Izzy, would you have wanted your parents to help you with this decision?
5. What do you think your feelings about being different would be if this accident had happened to you? What personal strengths would help you deal with this situation?
6. Who do you think would be most supportive of you during this time?
7. Imagine that Izzy is one of your best friends at school. How would you help her adjust to her disability and return to school?

Questions such as these can help students process and consider the material in this book in depth. Helping students focus on the strengths both they and Izzy possess can give them a sense of empowerment and allow them to confront a difficult subject with confidence that they could also handle such difficulties. Through this type of discussion, students may also come to appreciate the struggles and hardships their peers with disabilities face and increase their sensitivity to disability issues.

TEACHING STRATEGIES

- I would begin discussing the relationships in the novel by constructing a mural-size diagram of a tree on a classroom wall. On the trunk would be the title of the book, and each branch would have a character's name on it. Small groups would each have the responsibility for one character and would cut out leaves with words or phrases to describe their character. As the groups presented their character's traits, they would attach the leaves to the tree to provide a visual representation for the class.
- We would continue this discussion by brainstorming a list of the qualities a good friend or supportive family member should possess and talk

about how each of the characters did or did not live up to these definitions. This activity could be extended by having students create a list of fun ideas to help encourage and support a friend in the hospital, and perhaps by taking a field trip to the children's ward of a local hospital.

- There are many web sites for adolescents with disabilities and their families. Several contain original poetry or stories written by children in response to a disability, and these children ask for pen pals, or e-mail pals, to correspond and share the feelings and emotions of adolescence. These web sites are included in the list of resources at the end of this chapter.

- Although it is difficult to simulate a disability, I would ask students to keep a log for one day of every activity they do and the potential problems Izzy would face throughout their typical day. The next day students could share their logs and discuss many of the daily activities they take for granted.

- During one class period, I'd have students brainstorm all the ways they are different from each other and what makes them unique. We would put these lists on the board and add ideas the students may have overlooked. The list may contain such items as glasses, hair color, shape, clothing, grades, athletic ability, personality, and so on. I would share some poetry by Sara Holbrook or Sharon Draper and other poets who write about adolescent issues, and would read aloud the poem "Kids Who Are Different" by Digby Wolfe and have each student write his or her own poem about being different.

- Another activity centers around the use of fables. I would read students several fables about differences and discuss the elements of a fable. Once students understand that a fable is a story using animals to teach a moral, they would work in small groups to create their own fable to help others understand about disability. We would word process these fables, and the groups would illustrate them to create a class collection of fables to share with students in the lower grades.

- Izzy finds acceptance on the newspaper staff. Students could create a front page of a newspaper that reflects some of the major ideas of the novel and work in the computer lab to make it look realistic. Sample articles could include:
  - Research statistics on drinking and driving
  - Organization of a SADD (Students Against Drunk Driving) group on campus
  - Research on adolescents with disabilities
  - Interviews with Izzy or Marco about the accident

- Suggestions for the school to make accommodations for students with disabilities
- Creative works such as poetry, short stories, or cartoons.

- I would also have students do an "I-Search" paper (Macrorie 1984) on a disability incorporating the following methods of research: interviews with persons with the disability, letters to agencies dealing with the disability, Internet sources and/or periodicals, and nonfiction resources for children and young adults. I have been interviewed myself for several such research projects, sharing the recollections that began this chapter, and have been fascinated by the thought-provoking and insightful, not to mention candid, questions asked by the students.

- I would develop a WebQuest, an interactive computer-based activity developed by Bernie Dodge, which would require students to make predictions and respond to inference questions as they worked through the text. A sample task might read: "You are responsible for ensuring that Izzy's return to school be as smooth as possible. Who would you need to talk to? What provisions should be made?" How could you make students feel more comfortable around Izzy? Students would be directed to such web sites as the following:

  - The American Disability Association: www.ADANET.SIS-ONLINE.COM
  - The Beach Center on Families and Disability: www.beach.dole.lsi.ukans.edu
  - The National Health Information Center: www.nhicinfo.health.org
  - The National Information Center for Children and Youth with Disabilities: www.nichcy.org

CLOSING THOUGHTS

Adolescence is a time of major adjustments and personal and emotional growth and change. Disability complicates this difficult period, bringing to the forefront issues of identity, self-worth, acceptance, and relationships. *Izzy, Willy-Nilly* is a powerful young adult novel that realistically portrays these struggles. The scene at the lockers when Izzy warns Georgie of the risks of dating Marco and he calls her a bitch resonates with truth and accuracy. Izzy knows, in that instant, that Marco is not seeing her as disabled—he is angry at a fellow teenager. Students and teachers need to understand Izzy's desire to be perceived as an individual, not a disability. Only then can true healing begin.

As we worked on this chapter, we realized that we were just beginning an important conversation that must be continued. The comments and responses of my co-author were significant, in retrospect, to my personal understanding of my feelings and emotions throughout my own adolescence. Doctors told me throughout my life that adolescents with disabilities follow one of two paths—they either choose to develop a talent and strive as a classic overachiever, or they give up, becoming angry, bitter, and disillusioned. As a society we need to eradicate the fear and stigma of disability and promote understanding, awareness, and caring. We need to provide positive role models for our students as well as positive support for those adolescents with disabilities.

RECOMMENDED READINGS

While I was teaching a British literature course at the university lab school, I described this project and asked students to share their perceptions of disability. We attempted to define disability, examine our biases, and openly address issues and concerns. I brought in the texts listed in this portion of the annotated bibliography and asked students to select one to read, write a short abstract, assess grade level, and discuss with the class in a book chat. The annotations are followed by excerpts from the students' abstracts that reveal their responses to these texts.

Disability: Fiction

Bowler, T. (1995). *Midget.* New York: McElderry Books. ISBN: 0–689–80115–7. 159 pp. MS.

Subject to strange fits, fifteen-year-old Midget, who is physically abnormal and psychologically disturbed from the constant torment and abuse of his older brother, finds himself in control of his life for the first time when he gets his own sailboat. *Student Comment*: In one memorable scene, Seb, the older brother, tries to apologize to Midget for hating him all his life. It's about trying to live for the present in spite of the problems of the past. It was nice to see Midget stand tall with the realization of his dream.

Brancato, R. F. (1977). *Winning.* New York: Knopf. ISBN: 0–394–83581–6. 213 pp. MS, HS.

Paralyzed as a result of a football accident, a high school student struggles to accept the reality of his condition and the effect it will have on his friendships and his future. *Student Comment*: This would be an excellent book for high school students and their parents because the story involves a boy whose life is destroyed because of the risks he takes and the lack of trust his parents have in his ability to deal with the truth.

Colman, H. (1980). *Accident*. New York: Morrow. ISBN: 0–688–22238–2. 154 pp. MS.

When a motorcycle accident leaves one of them paralyzed, two young people try to cope with feelings of bitterness and guilt. *Student Comment*: This would be an excellent book for a young girl with a disability to read for inspiration and hope. It might provide parents with an idea of the kinds of things teenagers worry about and help them deal with the disability.

De Angeli, M. (1990). *The door in the wall*. New York: Dell. ISBN: 0–440–40283–2. 120 pp. MS.

In the Middle Ages, a young boy crippled by the plague has an adventurous journey from London to the castle where he becomes a page. (A Newbery Award Winner) *Student Comment*: It is important for people to see their obstacles as challenges to overcome rather than challenges by which to be defeated. The moral of this medieval tale is that one must do what one can and anyone can overcome an adversity if willing to take up the task. All walls do indeed have doors through which one can pass.

Froehlich, M. W. (1983). *Hide Crawford quick*. Boston: Houghton Mifflin. ISBN: 0–395–33884–0. 168 pp. MS.

Gracie and her three sisters are overjoyed when their mother has a baby boy, but the whole family finds itself sharing the burden of a terrible secret when baby Crawford comes home. *Student Comment*: This book shows how disability can tear a family apart and bring it together.

Gorman, C. (1987). *Chelsey and the green-haired kid*. Boston: Houghton Mifflin. ISBN: 0–395–41854–2. 110 pp. MS.

Convinced that the fatal incident she witnessed at the basketball game was not accidental, thirteen-year-old Chelsey, a paraplegic, and her unusual friend Jack team up to prove it was a deliberate murder. *Student Comment*: Chelsey's disability is not a major focus of the novel. It is more a story of drug dealers, attempted murder, kidnapping, and mystery.

Hamilton, D. (1982). *Last one chosen*. Scottsdale, PA: Herald Press. ISBN: 0–836–13306–4. 106 pp. MS.

Because one of his legs is shorter than the other, Scott is never chosen in ball games, but he eventually realizes that some other choices are more important. *Student Comment*: Middle schoolers would love this book because they could relate to the problems Scott faces. His outlook on life is optimistic and powerful, and the book illustrates that people who are "different" are, in reality, just like everyone else.

Johnston, J. (1993). *Hero of lesser causes*. Boston: Joy Street Books. ISBN: 0–316–46988–2. 194 pp. MS.

In 1946, twelve-year-old Keely is devastated when her older brother Patrick is paralyzed by polio, and she starts a campaign to reawaken his interest in life. *Student Comment*: Probably the most significant aspect of this book is the strength of the bond between the siblings. Most people would have given up and left Patrick to wallow in self-pity, but Keely proved to be a hero.

Kingman, L. (1978). *Head over wheels*. Boston: Houghton Mifflin. ISBN: 0–395–27202–5. 186 pp. MS, HS.

After an automobile accident, seventeen-year-old identical twins, Terry and Kerry, must face the fact that Terry will never walk again. *Student Comment*: The most interesting and illuminating message in this book is the way the family has to adjust to taking care of Terry and the extra medical expenses that force them to all take on second jobs.

Konigsburg, E. L. (1996). *The view from Saturday*. New York: Atheneum Books. ISBN: 0–689–80993–X. 163 pp. MS, HS.

Four students, with their own individual stories, develop a special bond and attract the attention of their teacher, a paraplegic, who chooses them to represent their sixth grade in an academic bowl. A Newbery Award Winner. *Student Comment*: This is a book about the importance of kindness, of helping one another, and of knowledge. A continually referenced theme is that of a journey. The children unite under the common purpose of helping their teacher make the journey to overcome her insecurities about teaching from and living in a wheelchair; in return, she leads them on a journey of learning. It is a philosophical journey which makes intelligence and kindness the most worthwhile personal qualities.

Logan, C. (1988). *The power of the Rellard*. New York: McElderry Books. ISBN: 0–689–50445–4. 280 pp. MS.

Lucy, repeating the fourth grade after a malady of the nervous system has left her with a withered arm, finds herself and her siblings in the midst of a power struggle with agents of an ancient evil. *Student Comment*: This is an interesting story about a young girl and her newly found power after being handicapped. The story placed little emphasis on the disability stressing instead the issues of friendship, school, and imagination. Perhaps the power of the Rellard symbolizes the strength Lucy found after her illness.

Metzger, L. (1992). *Barry's sister*. New York: Atheneum Books. ISBN: 0–689–31521–X. 227 pp. MS.

Twelve-year-old Ellen's loathing for her new baby brother Barry, who has cerebral palsy, gradually changes to a fierce, obsessive love, and she must learn to find a balance in her life. *Student Comment*: At first I didn't think Ellen's feelings were realistic, but then I thought of my own sixth grade sister and realized Metzger accurately captured jealousy, guilt, and finally love for a new sibling. This book would be very helpful for brothers or sisters of someone with a disability.

Mikaelsen, B. (1995). *Stranded*. New York: Hyperion Books for Children. ISBN: 0–786–82059–4. 247 pp. MS.

Twelve-year-old Koby, who has lost a foot in an accident, sees a chance to prove her self-reliance to her parents when she tries to rescue two stranded pilot whales near her home in the Florida Keys. *Student Comment*: Koby is dealing with her parents' quarrels and animosity in addition to her inability to find a purpose or joy in life since her accident four years earlier. When her mother decided to move out, Koby felt responsible and found happiness in caring for the whales on Lonesome Key. The community began to see her differently, and she earned the respect of her classmates.

Paulsen, G. (1991). *The monument*. New York: Delacorte Press. ISBN: 0–385–30518–4. 151 pp. MS, HS.

Thirteen-year-old Rocky, self-conscious about the braces on her leg, has her life changed by the remarkable artist who comes to her small Kansas town to design a war memorial. *Student Comment*: Although the book didn't focus on the issues of a typical adolescent Rocky's observations of people and events were really interesting. Rocky seems to study things in a manner that I find myself doing a lot—the inner sight that artists use to see to the truth.

Richmond, S. (1983). *Wheels for walking*. Boston: Atlantic Monthly Press. ISBN: 0–871–13041–6. 195 pp. HS.

After a car accident severs her spinal cord, eighteen-year-old Sally faces a long and painful adjustment to life as a quadriplegic. *Student Comment*: Although this book was attempting to be inspirational, I found it tedious and thought Sally gave people with disabilities a negative perception, as she seemed to complain throughout the story.

Rostkowski, M. I. (1986). *After the dancing days*. New York: Harper and Row. ISBN: 0–060–25077–1. 217 pp. MS, HS.

A forbidden friendship with a badly disfigured soldier in the aftermath of World War I forces thirteen-year-old Annie to redefine the word *hero* and to question conventional ideas of patriotism. *Student Comment*: This book portrays very well how children react to persons with disabilities. They are frightened, scared of weird faces and missing limbs. Even Annie, when she begins making trips to St. John's, is scared of the men there until she falls in love. Although her parents told her to be understanding and accepting, they are not happy when she tells them she has fallen in love with Andrew, who has been severely burned. It offers teens many topics for discussion.

Rue, N. N. (1986). *Row this boat ashore*. Westchester, IL: Crossway Books. ISBN: 0–891–07393–0. 265 pp. HS.

Felix has everything a high school girl could want, but she wonders why she is so miserable until she meets a young man who is both handicapped and religious. *Student Comment*: Although this is a love story, it was touching and worthwhile, as I have friends with disabilities and I have a learning disability myself. I was able to relate to the story and gain a better understanding of the issues of disability. It was also fun to read references to Beowulf, Grendel, and *The Canterbury Tales*.

Sallis, S. (1980). *Only love*. New York: Harper and Row. ISBN: 0–060–25174–3. 250 pp. HS.

When she finds herself the object of a young man's love, a spirited, physically handicapped sixteen-year-old is both touched and frightened, for she knows she may now have to share her painful secret. *Student Comment*: I never would have found this book on my own, and I loved it. Sallis either has a deep empathy for people and situations or she went through personal struggles in her own life which create the tense and deep emotions of the characters.

Strachan, I. (1990). *The flawed glass*. Boston: Little, Brown. ISBN: 0–316–81813–5. 204 pp. MS, HS.

A young girl's life on a remote Scottish island is made difficult by a physical handicap; but when an American businessman buys the island, she has access to a computer and new possibilities open up for her. *Student Comment*: This story displays an altogether too common occurrence—the way people treat others with disabilities. People looked no further than Shona's outward appearance and took it for granted that she was as poor in mind as she was in her physical body. It offers hope that technology can improve the lives of those with disabilities.

Werlin, N. (1994). *Are you alone on purpose?* Boston: Houghton Mifflin. ISBN: 0–395–67350–X. 204 pp. MS, HS.

When two lonely teenagers, one the son of a widowed rabbi and the other the sister of an autistic twin, are drawn together by a tragic accident, they discover that they have more in common than they imagined. *Student Comment*: Fourteen-year-old Alison and Harry were not friends. Harry bullied her for having an autistic brother, and when Harry was injured in an accident Alison struggled with guilt over having wished Harry could know what it was like to have a disability. It was a powerful story of prejudice and exclusion.

Williams, K. L. (1995). *A real Christmas this year*. New York: Clarion Books. ISBN: 0–395–70117–1. 164 pp. MS.

Twelve-year-old Megan's efforts to provide a real Christmas for her multiple handicapped brother and the rest of the family cause problems with her best friend and some other school friends. *Student Comment*: I think this story is good for middle school students to read. It shows how siblings can deal with disabilities at home and creates an awareness of the difficulties of being disabled.

Physical Disability: More Fiction

Calvert, P. (1999). *Picking up the pieces*. New York: Aladdin Paperbacks. ISBN: 0–689–82451–3. 176 pp. MS, HS.

Fourteen-year-old Megan finds her summer vacations changed forever after a spinal cord injury. When she meets Harris, a boy who sees her and not her disability, she begins taking part in activities and meeting the challenges of adolescence and disability.

Covington, D. (1991). *Lizard*. New York: Delacorte Press. ISBN: 0–385–30307–6. 198 pp. MS, HS.

Sent by his guardian to live at a Louisiana school for retarded boys, Lizard, a bright deformed youngster, escapes with the help of a visiting actor who gives him a role in his repertory company's production of *The Tempest*.

Sirof, H. (1993). *Because she's my friend*. New York: Atheneum Books. ISBN: 0–689–31844–8. 184 pp. MS, HS.

When Terri, a fifteen-year-old hospital volunteer, meets Valerie, a teen whose leg has been paralyzed after an accident, the two develop a friendship that inspires, agitates, supports, and hurts.

Voigt, C. (1986). *Izzy, willy-nilly*. New York: Atheneum Books. ISBN: 0–689–31202–4. 258 pp. MS, HS.

This book is discussed in this chapter.

Physical Disability: Nonfiction

Aldape, V. T., and L. S. Kossacoff (1996). *Nicole's story: A book about a girl with juvenile rheumatoid arthritis*. Minneapolis: Lerner Publications. ISBN: 0–822–52578–X. 40 pp. ES, MS.

This is the story of eight-year-old Nicole and how, in spite of her disability, she is more like other children than different from them. She explains her disability and the necessary modifications. Includes information about the Rehabilitation Act of 1973 and the Americans with Disabilities Act.

Behrman, C. H. (1992). *Fiddler to the world: The inspiring life of Itzhak Perlman*. White Hall, VA: Shoe Tree Press (out of print). MS, HS.

Presents the life of the concert violinist whose bout with polio left him disabled but still determined to pursue his love of music and the violin.

Cheney, G. (1995). *Teens with physical disabilities: Real-life stories of meeting the challenges*. Springfield, NJ: Enslow. ISBN: 0–894–90625–9. 112 pp. MS, HS.

Eight teenagers tell their personal stories and the challenges they face living with a disability.

Krementz, J. (1992). *How it feels to live with a physical disability*. New York: Simon and Schuster. ISBN: 0–671–72371–5. 176 pp. MS, HS.

The stories of twelve children who live with physical disabilities including blindness, dwarfism, paralysis, cerebral palsy, and birth anomalies.

Kriegsman, K. H. (1992). *Taking charge*. Rockville, MD: Woodbine House. ISBN: 0–933–14946–8. 164 pp. MS, HS.

A candid conversation among teenagers concerning life with a physical disability. Topics include independence, self-esteem, relationships, and sexuality.

Tada, J. E. (1992). *Joni's story*. N. P. Zondervan Publishing House. ISBN: 0–310–58661–5. 109 pp. MS, HS.

At age seventeen, Joni Eareckson broke her neck in a diving accident. She would never move her arms or legs again. In this autobiography, the author describes how her faith was challenged and her journey from self-pity to service.

FILMS AND OTHER CURRICULAR RESOURCES

Aquarius Productions (1995). *My body is not who I am* [video]. (Available from Aquarius Productions, Inc., 5 Powderhouse Lane, P.O. Box 1159, Sherborn, MA 91770.)

Brodie, J. (1990). *As I am* [video]. (Available from Fanlight Productions, 47 Halifax Street, Boston, MA 02130.) ISBN: 1–57295–058–7.

Human Relations Media (1990). *Just like anyone else: Living with disabilities* [video]. (Available from Human Relations Media, 175 Tompkins Avenue, Pleasantville, NY 10570.)

PBS Series (1995). *People in motion: Changing ideas about physical disability* [video]. (Available from Fanlight Productions, 47 Halifax Street, Boston, MA 02130. Order No. CQ-188; CQ-189; CQ-190.)

Texas Scottish Rite Hospital for Children (1994). *Withstanding ovation* [video]. (Available from Fanlight Productions, 47 Halifax Street, Boston, MA 02130.) ISBN: 1–57295–107–9.

REFERENCES

Hobbs, N., J. Perrin, and H. Ireys (1985). *Chronically ill children and their families*. San Francisco: Jossey-Bass.

Lindgren, C. L., M. L. Burke, M. A. Hainsworth, and G. G. Eakes (1992). "Chronic sorrow: A lifespan concept." *Scholarly Inquiry for Nursing Practice: An International Journal* 6, no. 1: 27–40.

Livneh, H. (1986). "A unified approach to existing models of adaptation to disability: Part I—A model, adaptation." *Journal of Applied Rehabilitation Counseling*, 17, no. 1: 5–16.

Rousso, H. (1996). "Sexuality and a positive sense of self." In D. M. Krotoski, M. A. Nosek, and M. A. Turk, eds. *Women with physical disabilities: Achieving and maintaining health and well-being*. Baltimore: Paul H. Brookes.

Turner-Henson, A., B. Holaday, and J. H. Swan (1992). "When parenting becomes caregiving: Caring for the chronically ill child." *Family Community Health* 15, no. 2: 19–30.

Vash, C. (1981). *The psychology of disability*. New York: Springer.

Wright, B. A. (1983). *Physical disability: A psychosocial approach*. 2nd ed. New York: Harper and Row.

Yuker, H. E. (1988). *Attitudes toward persons with disabilities*. New York: Springer.

Ziolko, M. E. (1991). "Counseling parents of children with disabilities: A review of the literature and implications for practice." *Journal of Rehabilitation* 57, no. 2: 29–34.

CHAPTER 3

Bridging the Alone Space: Fiction for Young People with Sensory Impairments

Kim McCollum-Clark and Kelsey Backels

In the wild, chaotic ferment of childhood and adolescence, many young people experience feelings of isolation and loneliness, as if no one else can understand their feelings and thoughts, as if the gulf between their emerging perceptions and the rest of the indifferent world is far too wide to bridge. This kind of isolation can be particularly difficult for children and adolescents with sensory impairments like blindness and deafness given the importance the non-disabled, mainstream society places on the sensory input gained from seeing and hearing. But to accept that this particular gulf can never be bridged is to accept this isolation and to reject those who attempt to understand. In the following excerpt from *Sees Behind Trees* by Michael Dorris (1996), two Native American boys just entering adulthood discuss how their need for other people has not diminished with their newly won maturity. Three Chances explains that his friend Sees Behind Trees needs people more because his eyes are weak.

> "You get alone faster than other people," Three Chances explains.
> "Your alone space is smaller." He held out both arms and turned around in a circle. "Anything beyond that and to your eyes it might as well not be there."
> "But . . . ," I started to say. "How did he know this about me?" (29)

Children with sensory impairments lack the essential sensory input that non-disabled individuals take for granted. They must compensate for the loss of this input in terms of their mobility and communication, but not in their sense of connection and community with others. Whereas the physical manifestations of their disabilities are readily observable to non-disabled individuals, the particulars of their other, internal conflicts—issues of identity formation, social acceptance, social and intellectual growth, personal autonomy, and self-reliance—are less apparent. And these internal issues are the most important to consider when both mainstream and disabled adults and children attempt to connect as people, not as stereotypes. Three Chances, in the passage described above, understands Sees Behind Trees' visual impairment in terms of the interpersonal "distance" that his friend's impairment imposes. He goes beyond the superficial level to understand and interpret Sees Behind Trees' behavior without judging him.

In this chapter, we hope to help teachers, guidance counselors, and other service providers see beyond the physical limitations to the internal conflicts and resolutions facing children and young adults with sensory impairments, notably blindness and deafness. In describing the protagonists of *Sees Behind Trees* by Michael Dorris and, briefly, *Apple Is My Sign* by Mary Riskind, we want to illustrate how two such children, employing their internal strengths and external resources, successfully confront and resolve the interpersonal and identity issues relating to their impairments. Notable among these challenges is a choice that young people must make between isolation and integration pertaining to themselves and their communities. Can young deaf and blind people learn to accept themselves with the special conditions of their disabilities and add this acceptance to their emerging identity? Will their families offer them acceptance, independence, and support? Will they choose to integrate themselves into the larger, mainstream community? And finally, will the community accept them in return—not as "damaged" members, but as valued individuals with much to contribute?

CHILDREN WITH SENSORY IMPAIRMENTS

Children with visual and auditory impairments are among those groups categorized by the Individuals with Disabilities Education Act of 1997 (IDEA), a federal law that amended Public Law 94–142 promising free, appropriate public education for disabled young people. Public school service providers are expected to create an appropriate and "least restrictive" environment for blind and deaf children and adolescents, following appropriate evaluation and parental and student participation.

Visual impairment is generally defined in terms of the functional loss of vision, ranging from partially-sighted children to those with low vision to those who are totally blind. This sensory impairment in children under the age of eighteen occurs in 12.2 children per 1,000. Severe visual impairment among young people, those defined as legally or totally blind, is more rare and occurs at the rate of .06 per 1,000 (National Information Center for Children and Youth with Disabilities [NICHCY], Visual Impairments Fact Sheet, 1996b).

Typical issues for the blind and visually impaired individual include questions regarding individual competence and independence. According to the degree and nature of the impairment and the circumstances of its occurrence, these issues will vary considerably. Children who encounter visual deficits in later childhood will require different interventions than those who have been blind since birth. All individuals with severe impairments, however, must contend with the common public belief that the blind are helpless and depressed, and should therefore be viewed as objects of pity and targets for assistance in all tasks.

According to the National Information Center for Children and Youth with Disabilities (1996a), approximately 1.3% of all children with disabilities reported to the U.S. Department of Education are categorized as deaf or hearing-impaired. The actual figure is undoubtedly higher, however, because many children are listed under other physical conditions. Children with profound deafness are often educated in schools for the deaf, but many school personnel encounter children with various hearing impairments requiring special services, ranging from amplification devices to sign language interpreters. Because over 90 percent of deaf children are born to hearing parents, the education of parents, teachers, caregivers, and the larger community is essential (NICHCY 1996a).

As with visually impaired children, there is a range in the nature and degrees of impairment for individuals with hearing deficits, but deaf and hearing-impaired individuals often view themselves as one "community" or culture with the mores, expectations, and support inherent in such gatherings of people with similar needs and interests. Many deaf individuals believe that such a united front is necessary for their survival in a hearing world which categorizes them as "disabled." This view is often held by those who define themselves as Deaf with a capital D. These individuals accept American Sign Language (ASL) not as a substitute for spoken or signed English but as a primary language in its own right. They identify themselves as members of the Deaf community, referring to "a particular group of deaf people who share a language—American

Sign Language—and a culture. The members of this group reside in the U.S. and Canada, have inherited their sign language, use it as a primary means of communication among themselves, and hold a set of beliefs about themselves and their connection to the larger society" (Padden & Humphries 1988, 2). The Deaf community stands in contrast to deaf and hearing-impaired individuals who prefer to meet the hearing world on its terms with lip-reading, speech, and signed English, all "oral" traits (Higgins 1980).

Whether deaf or visually impaired, all children with sensory impairments must come to terms with the degree to which they will accept, reject, or negotiate the conditions of the non-disabled, mainstream world around them. Negotiating this distance, surely, is part of the responsibility of all adolescents, but for children with visual and hearing impairments, dealing with these relationships becomes critical. This chapter will describe some of these issues, particularly in highlighting the strengths and resources utilized by the visually impaired and deaf characters in each book. Both Sees Behind Trees and Apple Harry, the protagonist of *Apple Is My Sign*, by Mary Riskind (1993), face challenges which, while unique to their separate impairments, connect forcefully to issues of isolation and integration with those around them. Most of Sees Behind Trees' work is geared toward reaching for maturity in a supportive and loving community which we could describe as inclusive. On the other hand, Harry is pushed by his deaf father to exclude the hearing and their world, although he is, at the same time, encouraged through his own experiences to interact with the hearing. Much of Harry's focus, then, is on coming to terms with this dilemma.

Because literature portraying young people with sensory impairments runs the gamut from stereotyped and hackneyed to complex and detailed, it will be important for adults working with such children to be aware of both kinds of stories and characters. In describing the characters and events in Dorris' *Sees Behind Trees* and, briefly, Riskind's *Apple Is My Sign*, we have selected positive representations of disabled children, one with a severe visual impairment and one who is profoundly deaf.

SEES BEHIND TREES

Sees Behind Trees, published in 1996 by Michael Dorris, places the story of a young man learning to cope with his visual disability in a sixteenth-century Native American tribe. Despite his separation in time from contemporary readers, Sees Behind Trees must confront many of the same choices about self-acceptance and possible isolation from or integration into the "mainstream" community as adolescents today.

Walnut, a young boy in the Powhatan tribe in precolonial Virginia (the Native American tribe that later gave the world Pocahontas), has a serious visual impairment; he can only see things clearly when they are brought close to his face. For most of the tasks of his day-to-day life, Walnut is able to manage, but his differences do not go unnoticed. Walnut, who is about twelve or thirteen, is practicing under his mother's tutelage for a feast in which he and the other boys in the village must pass an archery test to indicate their readiness for adulthood in the community. Walnut dreads these practice sessions before breakfast because he never hits the moss his mother throws into the air; in fact, he has never even seen the moss.

Growing more concerned about his lack of progress at this required skill, Walnut's mother and father come to realize the degree of his impairment, and one morning, the practice sessions change their focus. Tying a sash around his eyes, Walnut's mother takes a new approach.

> "Describe this place to me."
> "But I have never been here before and I can't see."
> "Shh," she said again. "Look with your ears." (6)

With his mother's prompting, Walnut learns to recognize other sensory input—sound, smell, touch, sensitivity to motion—that he has relied upon every day in the absence of his sight. His attention to this input grows steadily, and his mastery over his physical situation grows as well.

Still, some tasks are far beyond his capabilities. The day of the great feast arrives, and Walnut tries to avoid his certain failure by refusing to go. When the family arrives, however, the weroance Otter, the community's "most important person," announces that sometimes the familiar test must be changed. She explains that although hunting is an important skill, the needs of the people are many and diverse. "Sometimes the people need someone to do the impossible. . . . We need someone with the ability to see what can't be seen" (9–10). Walnut is the only boy to pass this new test as he identifies a village elder, Gray Fire, in his silent approach through the forest. Only Walnut has discerned that Gray Fire has his own disability, a limp which he has hidden from the people for many years. In recognition of his triumph, Walnut receives the adult name Sees Behind Trees.

Someone else in the community has taken notice of Sees Behind

Trees' special gift. Gray Fire, whom Sees Behind Trees identified during his test, has a special request. He wants Sees Behind Trees to accompany him on a journey to try to locate a place he had visited in his youth and had never been able to find again, a mysterious "land of waters."

Gray Fire is an enigmatic figure. As the weroance's twin, an artist and craftsman, he occupies a place of respect among the people, but he lives on the outskirts of their community. Sees Behind Trees recognizes that no one knows much about Gray Fire. The mystery deepens as Gray Fire tells Sees Behind Trees a story he had never told anyone—a story of a place of rainbows, mist, and waters where he felt so completely whole that he did not desire to leave. Gray Fire believes that Sees Behind Trees' special gifts will allow him to return to the place he has dreamed of every night since he left it.

Although the notion frightens him as much as it excites him, Sees Behind Trees agrees to go with Gray Fire on his journey. The journey gives Sees Behind Trees many opportunities to confront his own feelings and assumptions about himself, his transitions to adulthood, and his understandings of the world. In the course of this journey, Sees Behind Trees learns that adults do not have all the answers.

Sees Behind Trees finds the land of waters, and it is as glorious as Gray Fire had described, so glorious that Sees Behind Trees does not even feel his disability. He sees things he never imagined. "I had never been anywhere so completely" (80), Sees Behind Trees thinks, absorbed in the richness of the experience. When he finally leaves his reverie, he is alone. Gray Fire has returned to the waters he never wished to leave the first time, placing himself "inside of beauty," never to return to the community. Sees Behind Trees understands that he might make the same choice, to remain in the beautiful land of waters rather than return to his family and his community. He tries to go to Gray Fire's aid, but Gray Fire "was gone, either drowned or reunited with that part of himself that had never gone from this place" (86).

Sees Behind Trees' journey home is even more difficult, for he is now responsible for one even more vulnerable than himself—an infant from another tribe whose parents were attacked or kidnapped. Sees Behind Trees must use all of his new skills—confidence, reasoning, and belief in his abilities—to make the journey back to his community. He can no longer look at his visual impairment as a stumbling block or as a barrier that wishing can remove; it is what it is, and he still must make the right decisions to get home.

Sees Behind Trees and the baby Checha do make it home without

Gray Fire, only to meet Otter, Gray Fire's twin. Her revelation reminds him how much he has yet to learn. His journey complete, Sees Behind Trees marvels at how he has changed since the day of his testing. Even his understanding of his adult name has changed. "The day I received my new name, I had no idea how many trees there were, and how much there was to see behind each of them" (101). Although his visual perception has not been altered, Sees Behind Trees has a new sense of what it means to "see"—to be engaged in the lives of others and to recognize that everyone has hidden places within.

Far from being a simple story about a boy's struggle with his disability, Dorris' *Sees Behind Trees* operates on a number of levels and will satisfy readers of a range of ages and reading interests, whether or not they suffer from sensory impairment. In addition to the focus on Sees Behind Trees' visual impairment, his experiences with his emerging identity will captivate all readers. Younger students will appreciate the exciting and at times humorous plot and the vivid descriptions of life in the Powhatan community. Middle grades and early adolescent readers will identify with Sees Behind Trees' concerns about his changing role in his family and community. The evocative, lyrical style of the book will involve older readers, as will the rich and complex depictions of the two main characters.

Indeed, for older readers, the characters Sees Behind Trees and Gray Fire may present a kind of parallelism or thesis/antithesis structure to explore. Both characters have disabilities that color their perceptions of the world and their relationships, but as they both negotiate their "distance" with the mainstream people in their community, Gray Fire and Sees Behind Trees make different choices that children with visual impairment might consider and discuss. For both characters, "distance" and social isolation are related to their disabilities. Gray Fire imposes his own isolation and distance, choosing to live apart, close only to his sister, in order to hide his disability, the pride that he believes caused it, and the existence of the land of waters. His artistic vision, which culminates in his desire to be "inside" his art, skews his understanding of those around him. He feels that even his twin, with whom he shares a special bond, cannot understand his desires.

For Sees Behind Trees, however, distance is a function of his impairment, giving him, in Three Chances' words, a bigger "alone space." His physical condition might have the effect of holding him literally at arm's length from many social interactions of the community, but because he is surrounded by loving and supportive people, he intuitively understands that he must seek out people with whom to relate. It is the thought of these people that stops him from choosing Gray Fire's way and becoming one with the waters. Although Sees Behind Trees learns much from Gray Fire on their journey, he finally rejects Gray Fire's final lesson, that isolation and self-centeredness are the only choices of those who are different.

As a heroic figure who comes to understand his responsibilities to others in his community, Sees Behind Trees rejects the role of victim that disabled children often find thrust upon them by well-meaning non-disabled adults. He sees himself not as someone for whom the community must always rearrange itself, but as someone who has an integral part to play in the village's life. In a real sense, accommodations are made not only for those with "special needs"; they are made for all individuals daily as a price of living together. Are Sees Behind Trees' needs more "special" than Otter's or Gray Fire's because his needs are manifested physically? In thinking of the archery test, is it appropriate for society to apply a single standard of acceptance to all individuals? Conversely, is it appropriate to make the accommodations that the village makes for Sees Behind Trees? These are just a few of the issues that a reading and discussion of *Sees Behind Trees* might engender. A rich, complex, and lyrically written book, *Sees Behind Trees* is available as a specially recorded four-track cassette from the Library of Congress as part of its lending program for visually impaired readers, the National Library Services for the Blind and Physically Handicapped.

A CLOSER LOOK AT SEES BEHIND TREES

Many of the psychological and developmental issues Sees Behind Trees faces involve the typical concerns of adolescents. However, Sees Behind Trees is also a visually impaired teen, and the issues of visual impairment influence some of the questions he poses and the answers he seeks as he matures in this book. In addition, his parents and the villagers face dual challenges of Sees Behind Trees' adolescence and visual impairment. Accordingly, we should try to understand Sees Behind Trees, the adolescent, as well as Sees Behind Trees, the visually impaired individual, for these challenges are intertwined.

Bear in mind that Sees Behind Trees is often troubled but certainly not disabled by his visual impairment. In fact, according to Sommers' (1944) criteria for adjustment to a visual impairment, Sees Behind Trees exhibits some positive adjustment mechanisms. He illustrates what she labels "compensatory reaction," characterized by recognition and acceptance of limitations and a tendency to focus on "what [one] can do" as opposed to "what [one] cannot do."

Sees Behind Trees is an important character because he models positive choices: he receives and accepts support and encouragement from his family, friends, and the community; and he ultimately decides that his present life with a visual impairment is preferable to an undefined new life without one.

By means of an accommodation to the archery contest, Walnut is given an arena in which to use his adaptive skills of listening and focusing on the environment and is granted his adult name Sees Behind Trees. While the name given him by the village elder indicates the possession of extraordinary abilities, actually Sees Behind Trees has simply learned to compensate for his visual deficits by sharpening his auditory and concentration skills. The villagers, however, believe he can see things that no one else can. A sense of awe develops among the villagers concerning Sees Behind Trees, a not uncommon situation. Willoughby (1979) notes that the accomplishments of the disabled are often thought of as more remarkable than they really are and advises parents and educators to evaluate children objectively.

Walnut's disability is visual, yet it does not truly disable him. He has some vision through which he can distinguish shapes and colors, albeit without clarity. He has compensated by developing excellent hearing skills, learning how to tune out distractions, becoming knowledgeable about his environment in order to discern ordinary and unusual sounds and smells, and asking pertinent questions to gain information. He uses empathy to gauge what others are feeling. He successfully manages the task of becoming at ease with sighted people (Willoughby 1979). Throughout the story, Sees Behind Trees indicates that he is comfortable with his family and with the villagers, and is especially close to his best friend Three Chances. He has lived in the community all of his life, and the villagers have come to accept his limitations.

Blind individuals are often encouraged not to hide their blindness or to feel ashamed about having a visual impairment (Willoughby 1979). While Sees Behind Trees does not appear ashamed of his sight limitations, he is anxious about competing in the shooting contest. In addition, he is not forthcoming with his uncle about what he can and cannot see and makes believe that he is joking about the number of fingers held up by his uncle. Finally, he admits to Gray Fire that he wishes he could just once see as well as the others.

It is obvious that Sees Behind Trees has made important compensations and adjustments to his impairment. In addition, he is fortunate to possess numerous strengths, both internal and external. His internal strengths include acceptance of his limitations, a degree of self-confidence, and the possession of resiliency. His ability to accept his limitations and to focus on the things that he can do is a strength that serves him well. Indeed, he is cognizant of possessing several skills, most of which involve using his senses of hearing, smell, and touch. Sees Behind Trees' knowledge of his limitations and the skills developed in their place are tested as he is expected to return home without Gray Fire.

Another strength evident in Sees Behind Trees is his self-confidence. He is already fairly confident in the skills he possesses, and the accommodations made by his mother (such as altering their practice sessions to strengthen his listening skills) and the villagers (who add a listening component to the contest) increase his self-confidence. These accommodations ensure for Sees Behind Trees a place of respect and usefulness in the village. With a solid place in the community, Sees Behind Trees is able to feel some sense of independence and self-worth (Kastein, Spaulding, & Scharf 1980). He also recognizes the value of his contributions to the community.

Sees Behind Trees also possesses the strength of resiliency. Resiliency is the ability to endure hardship and to continue to grow and develop. Resiliency is composed of protective factors such as self-esteem and a strong sense of identity, is fostered by a supportive network of adults, and, most important, requires a basic trusting relationship with an adult (Gelman 1991). Sees Behind Trees is fortunate to have a trusting relationship not only with his parents and his uncle, but also with the elder villager Gray Fire. The trust he has in Gray Fire enables him to embark on a journey that answers important questions about both his visual impairment and his growth to adulthood. Although Sees Behind Trees' trust in Gray Fire is stretched at one point, his relationship with Gray Fire and their journey together allow him to test himself and ultimately answer a very important question: Will I accept myself as I am?

Sees Behind Trees also possesses external strengths, especially the support and acceptance of his parents and the villagers. Sees Behind Trees finds particular strength in his family. They offer him normalcy, acceptance, and independence. Sees Behind Trees' parents expect him to do his share of work in the family, as evidenced by their expectations that he help his father fix the roof. At this point, Sees Behind Trees feels he is far too extraordinary to engage in such ordinary work! Sees Behind Trees' parents work hard to dispel the village myth that Sees Behind

Trees is somehow special. They manage to deflate his rapidly inflating ego, and he learns a lesson in "greatness." His family sees to it that Sees Behind Trees is treated as normally as possible. They seem to consider him just another child who happens to have poor eyesight. His parents exemplify the preferred parental attitude of "accepting the child and the handicap" (Sommers 1944). Parents embracing this attitude will allow their blind child to assume "a full place in the family with all the privileges and obligations of the other children" (52).

Warren (1994) reports that parents who adjust well to their child's impairment will provide the best setting for the child's social development. Sees Behind Trees' parents have made a good adjustment to his visual impairment and provide a positive setting within which he can thrive. Sees Behind Trees also receives acceptance and support from his siblings in their roles as playmates and family members. In reality, children are often quite affected by a sibling with a disability (Brown, Goodman, & Kupper 1993). His parents also contribute to his independence and his sense of self-worth. Independence has been linked with the development of self-worth in the visually impaired (Kastein, Spaulding, & Scharf 1980). Although Sees Behind Trees does indicate that he wishes he could see as well as the others, he accepts his limitations and doesn't believe that his impairment makes him less worthy or less normal than others in the village. His character illustrates the view that blindness is a characteristic that brings certain limitations and that blind children can be as normal as other children (Willoughby 1979). Willoughby advises parents to help their disabled children learn social skills and to begin this process by giving the child love, support, and encouragement.

The villagers, too, are an important strength for Sees Behind Trees. Their perception of Sees Behind Trees as a valued member of the village and their willingness to validate him help him define himself and accept his visual impairment. The importance of blind children gaining a sense of control over their lives is critical, particularly because they face the public belief that they cannot be independent. Sees Behind Trees, however, is lucky because he does not encounter this belief among the villagers. They give him opportunities to show what he can do and to find his place and purpose among them.

NEEDS OF VISUALLY IMPAIRED CHILDREN

Sees Behind Trees' parents, friends, and the villagers ensure that several important needs are met for him (Lowenfeld 1976). These needs include love and affection; domestication; and opportunities to grow at one's own rate, move, explore, and play. The need for love and affection is supplied in abundance by his parents. Through their practice with the bow and arrow, and later, with listening skills, Sees Behind Trees' parents also assist with the need for domestication, that is, teaching all one needs to know to survive and exist as a normal individual.

Finally, disabled children need the opportunity for play. It is evident that Sees Behind Trees has ample opportunity for play based on his own description of his activities and the close relationship he develops with Three Chances. In addition, his friend Three Chances treats him "normally" by teasing him and roughhousing with him.

GROWTH AND DECISION-MAKING

Perhaps it is Gray Fire who provides the most important opportunity for Sees Behind Trees' growth. Through the story we learn that Gray Fire is also disabled, although he hides it from everyone except his sister. When Gray Fire finally shares his disability with Sees Behind Trees, it gives him a chance to see how Gray Fire has coped with his problem. It also gives the reader the opportunity to compare the ways in which these two characters resolve to live with and deal with their impairments.

Sees Behind Trees is also making decisions common to most adolescents. He often poses the question "Who am I?" in various forms. Sees Behind Trees seems to have integrated his visual impairment into his sense of self and has accepted it. However, it is also important for Sees Behind Trees to compare how he views himself with how significant others expect him to be. This is an integral task in adolescence.

Sees Behind Trees often discusses seeing himself as a reflection of others, which illustrates the young adult's need to check out the reactions of others to his thoughts, feelings, and behaviors. Adolescents often employ different thoughts and behaviors and then choose to keep or discard them. Sees Behind Trees says that "without somebody to be somebody to, it was as though I wasn't somebody myself" (29). As evinced by his decision to leave the land of the water and return home and acknowledge his impairment, Sees Behind Trees eventually decides who he is and that this person is acceptable and has a place in the community.

A WORD ABOUT ACCOMMODATIONS

The term "accommodations" has been used several times throughout this chapter. It refers to a change made in order to aid the disabled individual in accomplishing a task or reaching a goal. It does not indicate a lessening of standards or expectations. Two accommodations are made for Sees Behind Trees. The first is made by his mother as she alters the practice sessions from shooting to listening, after apparently realizing that Sees Behind Trees will likely never be successful with the bow and arrow. More important, she chooses to focus their practice on Sees Behind Trees' existing listening skills. She hopes to strengthen these skills and allow Sees Behind Trees to be known for them.

The second accommodation is made by the villagers in adding the listening component to the name-giving contest. It is implemented in a way that maintains Sees Behind Trees' self-respect without diminishing the self-respect of the other boys. These two changes are good examples of appropriate accommodations because they allow the visually impaired individual to meet his or her goals without lowering existing standards and without diminishing the self-respect of the individuals involved in the accommodation.

USES FOR THIS NOVEL

How can this book be used to help young adolescents with visual impairments and the adults who work with them? Literature is traditionally seen as a reflection of the author and his or her worldview, and literature about children and young adults with disabilities may be used as a starting point for investigating the views about disabled individuals put forward in a given time or culture. This examination is somewhat simplified when the time and culture are not our own, which may be why both Dorris and Riskind chose to place their narratives in the past. Looking at historical depictions, it is simple to give name to what we would consider blatant misrepresentations without having to account for our contemporary prejudices.

Readers of these stories about disabled youth should be prepared for certain pitfalls in saccharine and unrealistic portrayals of blind and deaf characters. In their anthology of literature with deaf characters, for example, Batson and Bergman (1985) point out how individuals with disabilities are often portrayed, particularly by non-disabled authors, as emblems or symbols. The deaf often function in stories as predictable "angels and outcasts," not as complex, dynamic characters. Blind and visually impaired characters often suffer the same fate; a terrible and tragic accident blinds an otherwise "normal" and attractive teenager. Will there be a cure or will the individual learn to deal with the rest of his or her life? According to Batson and Bergman, many stories about the deaf end with a "miraculous" cure, impossible for most of the deaf who suffer from sensorineural damage. Still, unrealistic as many portrayals of this kind may be, they do provide a window into cultural mind-sets about disability. In encountering books of this nature, children may talk about these representations in terms of their own experiences and how they personally are perceived by the hearing and sighted society.

Contemporary views of children's and young adult literature value the response that one brings to the experience of reading a story as much as the viewpoints expressed by the author. For blind or deaf individuals, an encounter with a rich and complex story about a fictional person with similar issues and experiences may give them opportunities to name, explore, and compare their own feelings, perceptions, and understandings of life as a blind or deaf person. Many times, deaf or blind children may have few counterparts with whom to share observations and questions.

Literature may also play a role in strengthening all young adolescents' ability to see the emergence of "gray" within the black and white of childhood. In exposing young people to a diversity of people, cultures, histories, and responses to life's events, wide reading can promote a kind of tolerance for living in a world not created by rule, and right a world inhabited by fallible and complicated people, disabled or not. Through reading and discussing books, children may safely try on a variety of responses to their physical conditions—from rage, defiance, and acquiescence to acceptance, integration, and discovery of their strengths.

Sees Behind Trees may serve as a role model for visually disabled children and adolescents by demonstrating how they can make the choice to accept themselves as they are, including their impairment. Sees Behind Trees views himself as an adolescent first, and a visually impaired individual second. Through him they may learn that he accepts his disability and finds his identity in the same way in which most adolescents do, through experimenting with numerous thoughts, beliefs, feelings, and behaviors. They may find significance in his decision to leave the land of the water, a place where he was visually whole, to return home to the place where he feels complete. Finally, they will see an individual who does many "normal" things, enjoys life, learns from life, and agonizes over life just as nonimpaired individuals do. Sees Behind Trees' parents, the villagers, and even Gray Fire serve as role models for parents and adults working with visually disabled children and teens. The book offers examples of how to make an effective accommodation, how to treat the visually disabled child or teen normally and yet within the limits of the disability, and how to maintain that individual as a viable member of the family and the community. Each of these adults takes an opportunity to provide Sees Behind Trees with self-confidence and self-knowledge, without undue criticism or overprotectiveness.

APPLE IS MY SIGN

Another book with similar themes of coping with decisions about integration and isolations, *Apple Is My Sign*, is suitable for younger readers, late elementary and middle grades. Each chapter relates an episode in the life of Harry, a profoundly deaf child about ten years of age from a deaf family in nineteenth-century rural Pennsylvania. His family's familiar sign for Harry is "Apple" for his great fondness for his father's crop, but in the beginning of the story, Apple Harry is far away from the farm at a school for the deaf in Philadelphia. His loneliness and feelings of isolation quickly subside, though, as he plunges into his new life. His father, who is suspicious and very distrustful of the hearing, has sent Harry to school to learn a trade that will be of assistance to other deaf people.

Harry's view of the world, however, is more expansive than his father's. Harry is curious and open to the world of the hearing, and many of the chapters in *Apple Is My Sign* describe his positive and successful interactions with the mainstream in football matches with hearing boys; exploring the wonders of the city with its shops, churches, and motorcars; and teaching hearing friends some sign language.

Like Sees Behind Trees, Harry has both the inner resources and the supportive community and family to meet the challenges of his disability. On his way home from school during a holiday break, Harry encounters the prejudices of the hearing on the train. He and a friend invite unwelcome attention with their signed language, causing curious stares and whispers. Harry's friend Agnes allows this attention to "silence" her, but, armed with a strong sense of himself and his abilities, Harry demands their positive attention and signs a flamboyant "goodbye" and "Merry Christmas" before he exits the train.

Riskind's book prefigures contemporary issues about isolation and integration of the deaf into mainstream communities. Many deaf people refuse to define themselves in terms of disability, in rejection of the mainstream culture's insistence on oralism—training the deaf in communication strategies emphasizing lip-reading and vocalizing. Early education of the deaf focused on oralism, proposing to equip deaf individuals with the skills the hearing culture required. Harry's nineteenth-century school for the deaf, then, is typical in its attempt to teach Harry to vocalize, an agonizing and tedious process for the young boy. Like Harry's father, contemporary Deaf culture prefers integration mainly within its own ranks, sometimes to the exclusion even of deaf individuals who elect to use "total communication," a combination of speech, lip-reading, and Signed English (Higgins 1980, 64).

As we have seen, well-written fiction about young people with disabilities gives caregivers a chance to help children with sensory impairments describe, explore, and compare their own feelings, perceptions, and assumptions with those of fictional protagonists with similar lives. The vicarious experiences gained in reading may become a sort of stimulus for the child to examine and question his or her experiences. The books can become a starting place for discussions and even therapy in which one may safely discuss one's understandings about living with sensory impairment without beginning in the highly contested and difficult terrain of one's own life.

Similarly, it may be helpful for teachers, counselors, librarians, and other service providers to pair books of this kind for reading and discussion. By juxtaposing two books with similar themes, readers may find much to discover in comparing the experiences of the books' characters. In pairing *Sees Behind Trees* and *Apples Is My Sign*, for example, a reader might notice that both boys have very supportive adults and community structures to strengthen them as they confront conflicts, but Harry alone must make decisions about the degree to which he will engage the non-disabled world. In pairing one of the books described in this chapter with a more stereotyped view of blindness and deafness, readers might expose and discuss cultural views and assumptions about the disabled and how they are perpetuated or overcome.

There is much to be gained from using children's and adolescent literature in helping visually impaired and deaf children understand their impairments. It is our belief, however, that through literature, caregivers, teachers, and other adults are also reminded about the individual journey that every child embarks on in the quest for maturity, recognizing and exploring the developing child within the context of his or her physical abilities and conditions. Recognizing the emerging adult within the child with sensory impairments allows mainstream, non-disabled adults to avoid disabilities of a different kind—ignorance and prejudice.

RECOMMENDED READINGS

Blindness and Visual Impairment

Alexander, S. H. (1990). *Mom can't see me*. Photographs by George Ancona. New York: Macmillam. ISBN: 0–0270–0401–5. ES, MS.

Alexander narrates the story of her active and unconstrained life through the voice of her daughter Leslie, sharing the ordinary and extraordinary aspects of life with a blind parent. Many of Alexander's compensatory devices are depicted in the photographs.

Alexander, S. H. (1994). *Taking hold: My journey into blindness*. New York: Macmillan. ISBN: 0–0270–0402–3. HS.

In a nonfiction memoir, Sally Hobart Alexander describes her life as a young, single schoolteacher in California during the 1970s when she began to lose most of her vision to a rare disease. Left with some perception of light in one eye, Sally begins to learn a new way of living, including a reevaluation of her important relationships.

Dickinson, P. (1974). *Annerton Pit*. Boston: Little, Brown. ISBN: 0–3161–8430–6. 175 pp. HS.

In this complex mystery, Jake, a blind teenager, and his older brother Martin undertake a journey to find their wayfaring grandfather. As a debunker of scientific and paranormal quackery, he was last seen in the coal regions of Great Britain. Jake and Martin fall into the hands of the same people who have trapped their grandfather, and Jake's special acuities prove valuable in his attempt to thwart the villains and rescue his grandfather. Jake's blindness is compellingly and beautifully realized; as a character he is depicted neither as a victim of sentimentality nor as possessing unrealistic "gifts."

Dorris, M. (1996). *Sees Behind Trees*. New York: Hyperion Books for Children. ISBN: 0–786–80224–3. 104 pp. MS.

Ingold, J. (1996). *The window*. San Diego: Harcourt, Brace. ISBN: 0–1520–1264–8. 181 pp. HS.

The victim of a car accident that killed her mother, Mandy goes to live with elderly relatives she never knew she had. As they help her to adjust to her blindness, she is also helped by new friends, including a deaf young man. As Mandy begins to settle into her new life, she discovers that when she looks through the bedroom window, she can "see" events that happened in the past to a young girl named Gwen who used to live in the same house.

Kent, D. (1978). *Belonging*. New York: Dial Press. ISBN: 0–8037–0530–1. 200 pp. MS, HS.

Meg decides to move from a school for the blind to a local public high school. There she faces typical adolescent challenges—will she be liked and included?—and those of one "different" from other young people. Her experiences with her new peers run the gamut from false concern and prejudice to acceptance and friendship.

Martin, B., Jr., and J. Archambault (1997). *Knots on a counting rope*. New York: Henry Holt. ISBN: 0–8050–5479–0. ES.

Boy-with-Strength-of-Blue-Horses copes with his blindness with the help of his wise grandfather, who retells the story of the boy's birth and life with his disability. The retelling of the story and the vivid illustrations emphasize how Boy's self-image is reinforced by the love and support expressed in his grandfather's version of his life and triumphs.

Mathis, S. B. (1990). *Listen for the fig tree*. New York: Puffin Books. ISBN: 0–1403–4364–4. 175 pp. MS, HS.

Marvina "Muffin" Johnson is the mainstay of her household despite her congenital blindness; since her father was killed, her mother's grief has rendered her almost incapable of carrying on, particularly around the winter holidays, the anniversary of her husband's murder. Muffin uses all her coping skills to maintain their life together and even plans to participate in her neighborhood's big Kwanzaa celebration. But can she keep her mother and herself on track?

McDaniel, L. (1996). *I'll be seeing you*. New York: Bantam. ISBN: 0–5535–6718–7. 195 pp. HS.

Carley is hospitalized for an infection when she meets Kyle, who may be permanently blinded in an accident. The teens grow closer as Carley helps Kyle face his disability, but Carley is hiding her own disfiguring condition. Will Kyle's vision return and Carley be exposed? Blindness is used primarily as a romantic plot device in this novel.

McKenzie, E. K. (1990). *Stargone John*. New York: Henry Holt. ISBN: 0–8050–2069–1. 67 pp. ES, MS.

Liza Bain's little brother John has trouble learning to read and to behave in their one room schoolhouse, so the other children tease him as being "star-gone."

Liza struggles without success to help him overcome his difficulties until they visit the town's former schoolmistress, now blind. Miss Mants teaches John to read, and later he is able to reciprocate her kindness and understanding.

Paterson, K. (1978). *The great Gilly Hopkins*. New York: Harper Trophy. ISBN: 0–064–40201–0. 148 pp. MS.

As a child abandoned to the foster care system in Baltimore, Gilly proves to be a hard nut to crack until she finds herself in a new home with people whose problems lead her to use her creativity differently. Among her new "family" members is Mr. Randolph, a blind African American man, who retains his independence with the help of Gilly and her foster mother, Trotter. This novel won the National Book Award for Children's Literature as well as mention as an American Library Association Notable Book and a Newbery Honor Book.

Radin, R. Y. (1990). *Carver*. New York: Macmillan. ISBN: 0–0277–5651–3. 70 pp. ES, MS.

Jon was blinded in an automobile accident that killed his father. Now he and his mother have moved home to the Chesapeake Bay, where he is learning to deal with a new school and new friends. His loneliness lessens when he convinces an irascible neighbor to teach him to carve waterfowl decoys. His relationship with Carver, which brings him closer to the hobby that is Jon's only link to his father, threatens to overwhelm his overprotective and still grieving mother.

Taylor, T. (1995). *The cay*. New York: Flare. ISBN: 0–3800–1003–8. 144 pp. MS.

While fleeing with his mother from German aggression against their Caribbean home, Philip's tanker is torpedoed. During the violence, he is blinded and is rescued by an elderly West Indian sailor named Timothy. The pair make their way to a small cay (island) and, hiding his own fear and ill health, Timothy teaches Philip the skills he will need to survive alone. In the process, Philip questions and discards his previous prejudice and comes to love the old man.

Whelan, G. (1993). *Hannah*. New York: Random House. ISBN: 0–6798–2698–X. 60 pp. ES, MS.

In nineteenth-century Michigan, nine-year-old Hannah's blindness severely limits her world, mainly due to the reactions of her family members. Her life opens up when a new teacher comes to board with Hannah's family, persuading them to allow Hannah to attend school for the blind. This book earned the praise of the National Federation for the Blind for its portrayal of Hannah's experiences and challenges.

Deafness and Hearing Impairment

Addabbom, C. (1998). *Dina the deaf dinosaur*. Stamford, CT: Hannacroix Creek Books. ISBN: 1–8892–6294–8. 32 pp. ES.

Dina, the deaf dinosaur, wants to learn to use sign, but her parents are reluctant to help her. She runs away and encounters other animals who help her to learn it, forming a kind of alternative community for herself.

Andrews, J. F. (1988). *The flying fingers club*. Washington, DC: Kendall Green. ISBN: 0–930323–44–0. 100 pp. ES, MS.

Donald's anger at repeating the third grade and being placed in special classes is lessened through his friendship with Matt, a deaf boy in the same classes. Matt teaches Donald to sign, and they use their communication to solve the mystery of the stolen papers. Further adventures of the club members can be found in *The Secret of the Dorm Attic* (1990), *Hasta Luego, San Diego* (1991), and *The Ghost of Tomahawk Creek* (1993).

Anseltime, L., E. Mueller, and N. Tait (1987). *I'm deaf and it's OK*. Chicago: Albert Whitman. ISBN: 0–8075–3472–2. 40 pp. ES.

A young boy describes his experiences and emotions as a deaf child, including his fears, confusions, and accommodations to everyday life. Because he knows no deaf or hard-of-hearing adults, he expects to put his disability behind him until he meets Bryan, a teenage deaf boy, who explains that it is okay to be deaf and grown up.

Armstrong, J. (1996). *Mary Mehan awake*. New York: Alfred A. Knopf. ISBN: 0–6798–9265–6. 128 pp. HS.

Mary Mehan lost her brother in the American Civil War, and fleeing this pain and her own experiences in a war hospital, the former Irish immigrant accepts a job as a house servant and helper to a photographer in the Midwest. As she gradually grows to accept her past and becomes open to the present, Mary's spiritual journey is paralleled with that of a young man deafened and emotionally scarred in the war himself. Issues of impairment and wholeness are explored in poetic language and an interesting historical setting.

Bunting, E. (1988). *A sudden silence*. New York: Harcourt. ISBN: 0–15–282058–2. 107 pp. HS.

Jesse deals with the guilt he feels after his deaf brother Bryan's death in a hit-and-run accident. He feels he was at fault because when it occurred, he was preoccupied by his feelings for Chloe, the girl Bryan introduced him to that night. The solution of the mystery and Jesse and Chloe's faltering romance make up the main action, but Bry is depicted as a rich and capable character in flash-backs.

Cohen, L. H. (1995). *Train go sorry: Inside a deaf world*. New York: Vintage Books. ISBN: 0–6797–6165–9. 296 pp. HS.

"Train go sorry" is ASL for the metaphoric expression "missing the boat"; this nonfiction book describes one year at the Lexington School for the Deaf in New York City as teachers and administrators endeavor not to miss the boat meeting the needs of their diverse clients. Cohen's family has a long history at the school (her father was superintendent at the time of her reporting), and she narrates both sides of the competing debates within the Deaf community as well as exploring her own insider/outsider status.

Greenberg, J. (1988). *In this sign*. New York: Henry Holt. ISBN: 0–8050–0722–9. HS.

The story of a deaf couple and their struggles communicating and living with their hearing daughter.

Guccione, L. D. (1989). *Tell me how the wind sounds*. New York: Scholastic. ISBN: 0–590–42615–X. 224 pp. MS, HS.

Amanda and Jake meet and create a special relationship during the summer months on a resort island off Massachusetts. At first, Jake's deafness underlines their communication differences, but over time, Amanda learns some sign, and the two become close. Jake's romantic feelings for the young girl are complicated by her overbearing hearing boyfriend, but she comes to appreciate Jake more, and their friendship deepens. The author takes special care to portray Jake's diverse communication strategies in creative ways.

Hodge, L. (1987). *A season of change*. Washington, DC: Kendall Green. ISBN: 0–9303–2327–0. 100 pp. MS, HS.

Biney, a thirteen-year-old girl with a severe hearing impairment, struggles to be a part of life on her own terms despite the conflicts between her wishes and her abilities. Her friends and family encourage her to try hearing aids, speechreading, and other compensatory devices, but Biney is reluctant to draw attention to herself. This book is as much about adolescence as about hearing loss.

Jepson, J., (ed.) (1993). *No walls of stone*. Washington, DC: Gallaudet University Press. ISBN: 1–5636–8019–X. 240 pp. HS.

A collection of short fiction, prose, essays, and poetry by notable Deaf and hard-of-hearing authors.

Kerr, M. E. (1978). *Gentlehands*. New York: Harper and Row. ISBN: 0–0644–7067–9. 183 pp. HS.

Buddy Boyle must balance his allegiance to his suave and cultured grandfather against the charges of a hearing-impaired journalist, Mr. Delucca, who claims that the old man is a notorious Nazi war criminal known as Gentlehands. Appearance and reality—the seemingly perfect versus the seemingly damaged—compete in the protagonist's and the reader's sensibility. Delucca is portrayed as an eccentric but humane person, a foil to Buddy's grandfather's icy perfection.

Martin, A. M. (1988). *Jessi's secret language*. New York: Scholastic. ISBN: 0–5904–1586–7. 145 pp. MS, HS.

Jessi's move to a new town is complicated by the fact that hers is one of the only black families in town, but she soon becomes friends with Matt, a deaf boy. She creates a kind of bridge between some of the hearing children and Matt and his family as she learns and teaches sign language to the children she babysits. Jessi and Matt overcome barriers of race, age, and ability in their friendship.

McCullers, C. (1983). *The heart is a lonely hunter*. New York: Bantam Books. ISBN: 0–5532–6963–1. HS.

This classic novel, first published in 1940, focuses on John Singer, a deaf-mute in the rural South, and his effect on those around him, mostly the outcasts of the town. This novel, McCullers' first, explores the spiritual isolation that all individuals can feel.

Piper, D. (1996). *Jake's the name, sixth grade's the game*. N.p. Royal Fireworks Press. ISBN: 0–8809–2135–8. 62 pp. ES, MS.

Jake moves from a special school for the deaf to a mainstream public school for the first time. He narrates the story of his experiences with humor.

Riskind, M. (1993). *Apple is my sign*. Boston: Houghton Mifflin. ISBN: 0–395–65747–4. 160 pp. MS.

St. George, J. (1992). *Dear Dr. Bell, your friend, Helen Keller*. New York: Beech Tree Books. ISBN: 0–6881–2814–9. 95 pp. MS.

Helen Keller first encountered Alexander Graham Bell, inventor and noted deaf educator, when she was a small child. Eventually, she dedicated her autobiography, *The Story of My Life*, to Bell. Their correspondence and lifelong friendship are recounted in this fictionalized biography of the two notable individuals.

Scott, V. (1986). *Belonging*. Washington, DC: Gallaudet University Press. ISBN: 0–930323–14–9. 200 pp. MS, HS.

After a bout with meningitis, fifteen-year-old Gustie experiences dizziness, problems with balance, and finally, the loss of her hearing. Gustie's challenges with different communication strategies are frustrating and difficult, and she finds some solace in meeting other Deaf people who help her to see her situation as other than a disability. Because Gustie loses her hearing as an adolescent, her experiences are compared with those with congenital deafness.

Shreve, S. R. (1991). *The gift of a girl who couldn't hear*. New York: Tambourine Books. ISBN: 0–6881–1694–9. 79 pp. ES, MS.

Eliza has grown up with her best friend Lucy Bressler, whose congenital deafness has never gotten in her way. A "perfectly ordinary girl in a regular school," Lucy reads lips and speaks, but now she wants a part in the school musical. Can Eliza, a drama and singing buff with her own wishes, help Lucy to make the right decision about auditioning?

Spradley, T. S., and J. P. Spradley (1985). *Deaf like me*. Washington, DC: Gallaudet University Press. ISBN: 0–9303–2311–4. 292 pp. HS.

A memoir of the birth and early life of James Spradley's deaf daughter, Lynn. Over 90 percent of deaf children have hearing parents, and this nonfiction book portrays the reactions, self-education, and adjustments of such parents to their children's experience.

FILMS

Visual Impairment

Butterflies are free (1971). Directed by Milton Katselas. Columbia Pictures. 109 minutes. HS.

Adapted from a stage play about the experiences of a blind law student, this film stars Edward Albert as Dan and Goldie Hawn as the free-spirit girlfriend who helps Dan to deal with his overprotective mother.

Mask (1985). Directed by Peter Bogdanovitch. Universal. 120 minutes. HS.

Rocky Dennis, a young man afflicted with a fatal, disfiguring disease, has an uplifting effect on his wayward mother and a young blind woman who accepts him as he is.

The miracle worker (1962). Directed by Arthur Penn. United Artists. 107 minutes. MS, HS.

The Academy Award winning film adaptation of the play detailing the relationship between the deaf-blind child Helen Keller and her persistent teacher, Annie Sullivan.

Places in the heart (1984). Directed by Rob Benton. Tristar. 113 minutes. HS.

During the Depression, a widow (Sally Field, in an Academy Award winning performance) struggles to keep her family farm afloat with the help of an African American farm worker and a blind boarder. Her family learns lessons of togetherness and tolerance throughout their struggle.

Hearing Impairment

Beethoven lives upstairs (1992). Directed by David Devine. Biography/Children. 52 minutes. HS.

In Vienna, Chris' family takes in a new boarder, Ludwig. Chris becomes friends with the irascible, hard-of-hearing composer.

Children of a lesser god (1986). Directed by Randa Haines. Paramount. 119 minutes. HS.

An adaptation of a Tony Award winning play by Mark Medoff. Jim is a new hearing teacher at a deaf school who provokes the school's conservative administration with his controversial teaching practices and his romantic interest in Sarah, an obstinate former student of the school. Sarah is portrayed by Marlee Matlin, a Deaf actress, who won an Academy Award for her performance.

REFERENCES

Batson, T., and E. Bergman, eds. (1985). *Angels and outcasts: An anthology of deaf characters in literature*. Washington, DC: Gallaudet University Press.

Brown, C., S. Goodman, and L. Kupper (1993). "The unplanned journey: When you learn that your child has a disability." Washington, National Information Center for Children and Youth with Disabilities. Volume 3, no. 1.

Evans, J. W. (1987). "Mental health treatment of hearing impaired adolescents and adults." In B. W. Heller, L. M. Flehr, and L. S. Zegans, eds., *Psychosocial interventions with sensorially disabled persons*. Orlando, FL: Grune and Stratton.

Fichten, C. S., G. Goodrick, R. Amsel, and S. W. McKenzie (1991). "Reactions toward dating peers with visual impairments." *Rehabilitation Psychology* 36, no. 3: 163–178.

Gelman, D. (1991). "The miracle of resiliency." *Newsweek* 117, no. 26: 44–48.

Higgins, P. C. (1980). *Outsiders in a hearing world: A sociology of deafness*. Beverly Hills, CA: Sage Publications.

Holbrook, M. C. (1996). *Children with visual impairments: A parent's guide*. Bethesda, MD: Woodbine House.

Hollins, M. (1989). *Understanding blindness: An integrative approach*. Hillsdale, NJ: Lawrence Erlbaum.

Johnson, C. L., and J. A. Johnson (1991). "Using short-term group counseling with visually impaired adolescents." *Journal of Visual Impairment and Blindness* 85, no. 4: 166–170.

Kastein, S., I. Spaulding, and B. Scharf (1980). *Raising the young blind child*. New York: Human Sciences Press.

Lowenfeld, B. (1976). *Our blind children*. Springfield, IL: Charles C Thomas.

Luterman, D. (1979). *Counseling parents of hearing impaired children*. Boston: Little, Brown.

National Information Center for Children and Youth with Disabilities (1996a). Deafness fact sheet. Washington, DC: NICHCY. *www.nichcy.org*.

National Information Center for Children and Youth with Disabilities (1996b). Visual impairments fact sheet. Washington, DC: NICHCY. *www.nichcy.org*.

Padden, C., and T. Humphries (1988). *Deaf in America: Voices from a culture.* Cambridge, MA: Harvard University Press.

Schirmer, B. R. (1994). *Language and literacy development in children who are deaf.* New York: Merrill.

Sommers, V. S. (1944). *The influence of parental attitudes and social environment on the personality development of the adolescent blind.* New York: American Foundation for the Blind.

Warren, D. H. (1994). *Blindness and children: An individual differences approach.* Cambridge: Cambridge University Press.

Webster, E. J. (1977). *Counseling parents of handicapped children.* Orlando, FL: Grune and Stratton.

Willoughby, D. M. (1979). *A resource guide for parents and educators of blind children.* Baltimore: National Federation of the Blind.

CHAPTER 4

Tracking Adolescent Responses to Cancer

Jim Powell and Nancy Lafferty

Literature is a powerful force for changing the way the reader sees his or her world. The best adolescent authors recognize this and strive to create realistic, imaginative stories that help young readers come to grips with problems they are encountering, often for the first time. Although these novels are labeled "high-interest," that does not negate the fact that they cover very important issues that early and young adolescents have to tackle. Having acquired the social, emotional, and physical knowledge required to negotiate their way through daily life, adults often forget just how unsettling it can be to try to understand and respond to unfamiliar and previously inexperienced social situations.

Chronic illness and death are two of these social situations, and often the most troubling. Cancer and leukemia are realities that adolescents must face. Whether attacking a parent, relative, close friend, or the adolescent, cancer will affect the lives, directly or indirectly, of most adolescents. Leukemia, which is more commonly found in children and young adolescents, engages the entire school and community in support and understanding. Two texts, *Tracker* by Gary Paulsen and *Hunter in the Dark* by Monica Hughes (both published in 1984), deal with these two issues; studied together, they can serve as a powerful bridge that ties together the social and emotional development of the adolescent while allowing for a full range of literary discussion.

The ability to understand and cope with serious illness and the possibility of death is not innate. It is learned behavior, and most adolescents must learn how to deal with these issues at a time when their social support structure is least able to give them adequate assistance. When families, schools, and communities are struggling to deal with an illness or grieving over a loss, they do not have the time to recognize that young adolescents need to be guided through the process. These two texts have the ability to educate adolescents about chronic illness and death, and therefore make the events surrounding the illness less frightening and traumatic.

When we first considered these texts, it was with the idea that the two books could be used simultaneously. We viewed *Tracker* as a high-interest text for students who are reluctant or struggling readers, with *Hunter in the Dark* as an alternative text for the more advanced students. But as we continued to discuss the works, it became apparent that they would work best in tandem. There are too many common themes running through the works that would be missed by using them separately.

These choices, however, lead to several critical issues that we must address—language, gender, and subject matter. *Hunter in the Dark* is currently under fire from those who believe the book should be excluded from libraries and classrooms because of objectionable language, and the appropriateness of some of Gary Paulsen's novels has also been questioned. Therefore, teachers may find themselves having to defend their choice of either of these works. The National Council of Teachers of English (NCTE) guidelines on censorship offer practical suggestions for teachers as well as procedures to follow when selecting texts.

These texts are also male-oriented. In each case the females in the books serve as minor characters, and in *Hunter in the Dark* the mother and the girlfriend are portrayed in seemingly negative ways. This issue can and should be addressed in a discussion of the characters. Both texts can serve as entry into a larger discussion of gender, and several activities will be suggested to assist in developing this theme.

Both books are focused around the theme of hunting. Hunting is viewed by many as primarily a male activity. However, gender is not the greatest issue faced when dealing with hunting. Both hunting and fishing, sports that involve the killing of animals, are viewed very negatively by many Americans today. While one hundred years ago most Americans either hunted for sustenance or accepted hunting as a viable outdoor activity, today those who hunt or accept hunting as a legitimate form of recreation are definitely in the minority. In fact, hunting has so many negative connotations that it can overshadow the primary purpose in using either of these texts. As with the issue of language, teachers will have to evaluate their classes carefully to ensure that the stigma against hunting will not interfere with discussions and activities. As with the gender issue, several activities are suggested that students can engage in before and while reading the books that will help them and their families wrestle with the issue of hunting as a sport.

TRACKER

Tracker revolves around John, the thirteen-year-old main character, and his struggle to come to grips with his grandfather's imminent death. John has been living with his grandparents, Clay and Agatha Borne, since his parents' death when he was very young. Emil, John's best friend at school, enters into the story only once and serves as a foil for John's public announcement of his grandfather's illness. As with most Paulsen novels, this story takes place in the north woods region of Minnesota. The entire book is set in the kitchen, the barn, and the woods. School is mentioned only in passing and gets little description, but the other three settings are rich in detail. John's pursuit of the doe is a physical embodiment of his attempt to overtake and overcome death. The story opens with John refusing to accept his grandfather's cancer, seeing no changes in his grandfather's physical condition or daily behavior. But things are changing; established routines are being altered by the disease. Deer season is coming, and John and his grandfather have always hunted together. This year they won't, and John begins to get angry about the illness that is now affecting his life.

John and Clay do not view hunting as a sport; they call it "making meat." The taking of a deer is a necessary part of obtaining food for the winter. To emphasize this point, Paulsen includes a flashback in which John remembers Clay's refusing to let sportsmen hunt on their land because they did not respect this process. It was not a game for the Bornes; they believed hunting to be the act of turning a material resource into valuable food.

Through the opening sections, Paulsen uses the chores and family conversations to establish the conflict. Everything seems normal, but underlying it is the dark specter of his grandfather's illness. As with most Paulsen novels, the action is told from a third-person omniscient point of view and deals heavily with how the protagonist constructs his world around the problem. The deer, a small doe, is introduced through an unusual sighting by John while he is doing his chores. John's reaction to the doe serves to foreshadow the coming conflict. Paulsen, apparently drawing on personal experience, does an excellent job of capturing the process and thinking of a person prior to and during a deer hunt. He details the discussions and preparations before taking the field, and his rich description of the pre-hunt breakfast captures the emotions of the characters and the atmosphere surrounding opening morning.

Once in the field, John has to leave the world behind and concentrate solely on hunting. He jumps a deer and begins the tracking process required to kill it. After seeing the deer twice and missing several potential opportunities to kill it, John begins to believe he is following the doe he had seen earlier and that there is some special significance in his tracking her. As John goes further into the forest he turns from the task of "making meat." Instead he hangs his gun in a tree and seeks to walk the deer down. He now views his quest to be the defeat of death itself. Following the doe throughout the first day and night, John catches up with her late in the second day. Both are completely exhausted by this time, and John collapses upon touching the deer. Having succeeded, John then returns home feeling that he has conquered death. Once he begins to relate the story to his grandparents, he comes to realize that he has not won and that nothing can stop the inevitable circle of life and death. This is the message that Clay, his grandfather, has been trying to convey throughout the story. John accepts this universal truth not only for his grandfather, but for himself as well.

HUNTER IN THE DARK

Mike Rankin, the fifteen-year-old main character in *Hunter in the Dark*, is busily engaged in all the activities that occupy the life of a typical teenager. He has had some success on the basketball team and has recently begun dating a popular girl in his class. He lives with his parents in a large, well-maintained home. His father is a highly successful businessman, and his mother is active in a number of worthwhile charities. His best friend, Doug O'Reilly, shares his love of shooting and hunting, and Doug's father provides both boys with the opportunities and information they need to become hunters.

Mike's trouble begins when he experiences a blackout during a basketball game. After extensive testing, Mike's parents tell him that he is ill, but never reveal that he has leukemia. Due to the level of medical information provided by television, it is possible that at least a few readers will diagnose the exact nature of Mike's illness before it is exposed in the book. They might even question how Mike and his friends could not know what was happening. To compound the problem, George Rankin, Mike's father, has a somewhat distant relationship with his son. He loves him, but is unable to demonstrate it openly and physically. This is evidenced in his providing Mike with appropriate and expensive gifts while denying him the emotional support he needs throughout his crisis. His mother, Anita Rankin, loves Mike but is unable to face his illness openly and emotionally. Doug's parents serve as a contrast to Mike's parents. They are seen as warm and nurturing, and in Doug's family emotions are dealt with honestly and shared openly.

Gloria, Mike's girlfriend, is not told the truth about Mike's illness and assumes that his actions throughout the book reflect his lack of interest in her. This leads her to break off their relationship when Mike becomes too sick to attend school and take part in everyday activities. Particular care should be taken to discuss how realistically the author develops this character.

Mike is under the care of a specialist who takes over when the diagnosis of leukemia is confirmed. A caring person, he is locked into silence by Mike's parents. He seems relieved when Mike finally figures out what is wrong, telling him the truth about his illness and his chances of recovery.

The action shifts back and forth between the woods and the city through the use of flashbacks. Mike relives the events of the last two years that lead up to the deer hunt that is the climax of the book. The scenes in the woods are well constructed, and Mike's establishing camp at the beginning of the book is highly reminiscent of Nick Adams' actions in Ernest Hemingway's "Big Two-Hearted River." There is also a series of events that lead Mike to set up a survival shelter later in the book that can be compared with Jack London's "To Light a Fire."

This story opens with a rather mysterious journey. Mike is clearly trying to get somewhere and must avoid the police. The reader is not certain what he has done or why he is trying to avoid recognition until after he sets up camp and has his first flashback involving the events leading up to his diagnosis and initial treatment for leukemia. The reader discovers throughout the book that Mike has not had a full night's sleep for over two years due to his repeated nightmares about the hospital. From this point in the novel, the action moves back and forth from the present, Mike's hunt, to his past, his battle with leukemia. Each flashback and recollection is reanalyzed based on his recently acquired knowledge of his illness.

The hunt, as in *Tracker*, requires Mike's total concentration. When he is in the woods he is able to leave his memories behind, but when he stops to rest or returns to camp, the story is relived in either daydreams or nightmares. Mike has run away from home for the weekend to fulfill his dream of shooting a large buck. Unlike John, he must rely only on what he has read or heard about hunting. He fails in the first attempt to shoot a buck and gets caught in a violent snowstorm. This is the climax of the story; for as he struggles to stay alive and questions his desire to live, Mike comes to the realization that life is too important to toss away. Returning to camp, he sleeps untroubled throughout the night for the first time since becoming ill. The resolution of the story deals with Mike's locating the deer and having the chance to fulfill his dream of bagging a trophy. When Mike finally has the opportunity to take his deer, he chooses not to shoot and makes plans to go home and help his parents face the issue of his illness. Hughes does not give the reader any assurance that Mike's remission will continue; however, it is clear that Mike has now gained control over the disease and will face it on his own terms.

Hughes does a superb job of building a parallel between the hunt and Mike's illness. First, both Mike and his doctor must locate the object of their hunt. Mike's doctor must identify the source of Mike's illness, and Mike must establish where the deer are feeding, traveling, and bedding. Once these tasks are accomplished, both Mike and the doctor need to devise a strategy that will allow them to achieve their respective goals of killing the buck and killing the disease.

UNDERSTANDING DISEASE AND DEATH

These two texts, *Tracker* and *Hunter in the Dark*, represent an excellent medium through which to analyze and discuss our individual perceptions of disease and death. More important, they offer a meaningful way to talk about cancer and leukemia. At one time, both diseases were considered to be almost always fatal; with advances in prevention, early identification, and treatment technology, the prognosis for both cancer and leukemia is much more positive. It is important to remember that culture and religion strongly impact the manner in which the ill and deceased are viewed (Berger 1998). Throughout most of history, chronic illness and death were accepted, familiar events that were dealt with at home (Aries 1981). Family members of all ages had intimate contact with the problems associated with disease, childbirth, infections, accidents, and the consequences of old age. In general, family members were the caregivers and, ultimately, the funeral directors.

In mid-twentieth-century Western Europe and particularly in North America, with the ascendancy of modern medicine, most illnesses were no longer life-threatening and were not viewed as critical events. The act of dying, except through accident, was withdrawn from everyday life and generally occurred in hospitals away from the immediate notice of most of the family. To make the situation even worse, doctors and nurses routinely resisted telling terminally ill patients the truth about their condition. This allowed doctors and patients' families to avoid dealing with the possibility of dying. Before the end of biological life, the dying, in effect, experienced a "social death," a kind of institutionalized isolation in which they found themselves shunned by their medical caregivers and constricted in their intimacy with family and friends by hospital procedures and protocol (Kastenbaum 1992).

Elisabeth Kubler-Ross, a pioneer in the understanding of the process of death, dying, and grief, discovered how important it is to inform patients of their condition. She discovered that doctors sometimes fully informed a patient's immediate family about the nature and prognosis of the patient's illness and then explicitly instructed them to keep the facts from the patient in order to avoid an emotional outburst. In many cases the patients were unable to talk about their feelings because family and staff continued to pretend that all would be well. The result of this "conspiracy of silence" was increased isolation and sorrow for both the patients and their families (Moller 1996). This is demonstrated clearly in *Hunter in the Dark*, and the consequences of withholding the truth need to be a central part of class discussion.

Kubler-Ross's research (1969, 1975) led her to propose that, when told the truth by an empathetic listener, patients will go through five emotional stages in confronting the disease. The first is denial, in which they refuse to accept the outcome of their condition. Typically, they convince themselves that their laboratory tests were inaccurate or that the disease will have an unexpected remission. The second stage is anger—at everyone else for not caring enough or for caring too much, or simply for being healthy. The third stage is bargaining, in which a person tries to negotiate away the potential outcome, promising God or fate that they will do more or pray more or live a better life. When bargaining appears to have failed, depression sets in, causing the patient to mourn his or her own unfortunate circumstances and to be unwilling to make any plans or to take an interest in medical treatment. Finally, acceptance can occur. Adolescents respond similarly to chronic illness, and these books can be used to discuss the following points:

- Why it is important to discuss the illness with the child as soon as possible
- What types of changes in daily routine are going to be experienced
- How to let the child know he or she is not responsible for the illness
- How to include the child in the treatment and recovery process
- How changes in behavior can serve as clues to how the patient is feeling.

Adolescents focus not on the distant future but on the quality of their present life. Thus, to seriously ill adolescents, the effect of their condition on their appearance and social relationships may be of primary importance. For the young adult, coping with the effects of the illness or the possibility of death often produces great rage and depression at the idea that just as life is about to begin in earnest it must be delayed or denied (Berger 1998). Therefore, these two books, *Tracker* and *Hunter in the Dark*, are excellent novels with which to address the issues of disease and death for the adolescent.

ISSUES FOR THE THERAPIST

In *Tracker*, John is knowledgeable about his grandfather's condition from the opening of the book. He is certainly in denial about the seriousness of the disease, but at least he is aware that a problem exists. In this case he knows as much as his grandmother about the illness and the condition of his grandfather. John's shock and denial are highlighted throughout the initial seventeen pages of the text.

In direct contrast, in *Hunter in the Dark*, Mike is completely ignorant about his illness. He knows he feels weak and that he passed out while playing basketball. The doctors tell him only that he has a severe case of anemia. Mike is subjected to multiple and sometimes painful tests and treatments, but never told what is actually going on—even the doctors dodge his questions and make excuses to exit the room hastily, thus the symbolism of the title *Hunter in the Dark*.

After observing behaviors in his family and friends that do not seem to make sense to him, Mike investigates his symptoms and treatment. Searching through the medical reference books at the local library, he discovers that he has leukemia. In *Tracker*, John is able to progress through his relationships with his family in a healthier manner than Mike. In fact, Mike's family in *Hunter* exhibits many signs of pathology and dysfunction.

INTERPERSONAL RELATIONSHIPS

The way those around Mike and John behave differs greatly. Because John is privy to the information concerning his grandfather's disease, he is allowed to see his grandparents react to the news of Clay's prognosis. Emotions are allowed to be expressed in *Tracker*. John's grandmother cries and his grandfather gets angry. In direct contrast, in *Hunter in the Dark*, Mike's parents do everything possible not to let him see their emotional distress at his illness. They continually project a sense of false bravado. Hughes draws a clear distinction between the differences in Mike's and Doug's homes. Doug's parents are involved and communicative. Mike's parents are deceptive and protective. Ultimately, it is the lies and denial of his parents that drive Mike to two brave acts of independence—seeking out the truth and hunting a deer. He later realizes that his parents' behaviors were born of love and protection and that he will have to confront them upon his return home.

ACTIVITIES

These texts were selected to support student discussion through analysis of adolescent characters with interests and concerns typical of middle and high school students, yet different enough to provide a safe distance for open and honest responses and questions. Many of the activities described in this section suggest the use of group work. This teaching method tends to be very effective in constructing lessons on controversial subjects and parallels the use of group counseling strategies a therapist would employ. Working with peers encourages students to take into consideration the views and beliefs of others, and it forces them to defend or modify their own position on many of these issues. In addition, groups can provide a much safer—and thus more open—environment for students who are exploring these emotional issues for the first time.

The Gender Issue

Before reading the books, the students should engage in a discussion about gender issues and literature. I would highlight the fact that Hughes, a female author, is writing about hunting, a typically male activity. The students can discuss whether the gender of these two authors made for any significant differences in these two books.

- Take the students to the library and have them do a survey of fiction by male and female authors. How do the numbers compare? Are there clear differences in the topics of their works? Finally, ask each student to do a quick review of two books to see if the main character is of the same gender as the author. Have the students write a short story in which the gender of the main character is opposite of theirs and then have the boys trade papers with the girls to evaluate how "correctly" the main character was portrayed. This should lead to some lively discussions not only about gender, but also about the difficulty in creating realistic, living characters.

The second issue concerns gender and hunting. Why do more men than women hunt? Why is it more socially acceptable for men to hunt and to carry guns or other weapons?

- After reading the books it might be highly beneficial to revisit the gender issue and discuss how the stories could be told if the protagonists were female. Would the stories be the same? Could the female characters hunt? Could something else be substituted for the hunting activity for females? What might be the equivalent of a hunting trophy for a female? Discussions and writing activities would be beneficial so that female students do not feel overlooked or undervalued during this unit.

Magazine Reviews

Magazines can provide a rich context within which to set these two stories. They are usually easily obtainable, and if they are discards from students and friends they can be used to create collages and other visual projects. Magazines demonstrate visually, as well as verbally, society's values and mores, both in the stories they carry and the ads they accept.

- Divide students into groups and give them a series of articles that cover as many aspects of hunting as possible. To find suitable articles, locate a number of different magazines that deal with the outdoors and the sport of hunting. The obvious place to begin would be with such publications as *Outdoor Life, Field and Stream*, and *Sports Afield*, three of the major national magazines that cover hunting and shooting sports. The best issues to locate are those published in late summer and fall when deer hunting is covered most frequently. Besides the how-to articles that are sure to be found, they each have columns on the ethics of hunting and conservation. To balance out these publications, bring in

Audubon, National Wildlife, and *Outdoors.* This will probably entail searching through several years' worth of issues to find ones that contain specific mention of hunting, but they will provide a good counterpoint to the earlier magazines. Another magazine worth reviewing would be *Mother Earth News,* which tends to treat hunting not as a sport, but as a way of bringing food to the table. This is very similar to the viewpoint that John and Clay have about hunting. Articles based on this philosophical view of hunting can then be compared and contrasted to the articles in the earlier magazines. Finally, to cover the two extremes of this issue, locate magazines such as *Whitetail Hunter* and contact the organization Bucks Unlimited. This will provide a very aggressive pro-hunting stance. People for the Ethical Treatment of Animals (PETA) should also be contacted since they are sure to have an equally viable anti-hunting stance. It pays to be cautious, however, since these organizations distrust each other.

The purpose of the magazine activity is threefold. First, it will allow the students to make comparisons between the ideas about hunting held by both John and Mike and those held by hunters and nonhunters in America today. The goal for this unit is not to promote hunting or anti-hunting sentiments, but to demonstrate the wide range of viewpoints on hunting and to give students the tools to make informed decisions about this issue. Second, it will supply some basic information about hunting that the students will need to make judgments about the authenticity of the two novels. Finally, the magazines provide different perspectives from which the students can analyze this issue.

- As they read the articles selected to best exemplify the issue of hunting, students should keep an individual journal about their interpretations of each of them. In this exercise the students should be comparing and contrasting their philosophy of hunting to that presented in the articles. Again be sure that the students are addressing the political, social, and emotional issues raised in the articles.

- Have the students write a collective response on the issue and present it to the class. Emphasize that the group is not expected to come to total agreement on the issue, but that each member must be able to support the response the group presents. In addition, the group should be able to recognize the debate points by supporters on both sides of the issue. This is critical to helping students understand that, as with any number of current emotional issues facing America today, there is no clear-cut answer on the issue of hunting. As they mature they must understand that there is seldom a right and wrong answer that can apply to everyone, and that they will have to live with this ambiguity.

- The students' individual journal responses and the group position paper will provide a background against which to measure the actions of John and Mike. Periodically ask the students to review their earlier statements and compare them to the position being espoused by the two main characters. Then ask them to describe if and how their beliefs about this issue have changed over the course of the readings.

- Have the students outline the articles to detail factual information on finding, tracking, and shooting deer. During this exercise the groups can create powerpoint demonstrations, poster projects, and maps, since both books talk about how John and Mike have to find their way in the woods.

Journal Writing

Journal writing will give students the means to reflect on a number of issues raised in the two works. Topics suggested as writing activities include the following:

- Have the students discuss how treatment for leukemia and cancer has changed in the last fifteen years. Then have the students write journal entries about how the stories might be written today, when there is a much more positive prognosis for these diseases.

- *Euphemisms*—Begin by explaining that the two texts deal with the issue of disease and potentially terminal illnesses. As the students go through the two novels, have them collect euphemisms that are used to discuss these issues. Explain the process by discussing some of the common ones, such as "not feeling well," "under the weather," "caught something," and finally "passing on," "going to one's eternal rest," and "kicking the bucket." Some of them are gentle, some are humorous, and often they can be cruel, but the point to be made is that they provide an easier way for people to talk about a very difficult subject. This activity should help students become more attuned to how we manipulate language to achieve specific ends.

- Students can keep a journal from the perspective of different characters as they read the novels. One way to do this would be to divide the class into groups for each character. Have the groups meet frequently to compare their perceptions of what the characters would be recording in their journals. Then have the groups share and compare how the different characters are responding to the same events.

- Students might also project themselves into the role of the protagonist in each story and write a letter to a family member detailing how he would like to be treated. Students could then take the role of the family members in the books and respond to the letters written by replying to the protagonists—this steps outside the boundaries of the books and allows students to be more concerned, empathetic, and compassionate than the characters were. Students might also do the same letter-writing activity with the friends of the protagonists, Emil, Doug, and Gloria.

- Rituals and sports can also be the subject for journal writing. Have the students record in their journals the actions that John goes through as he gets ready for the deer hunt. The gun cleaning, discussion of conditions before the hunt, breakfast, and so on, are all well-documented aspects of pre–deer hunting behavior that most hunters have experienced. They could compare John's actions to some of the articles they have read on different types of prehunt ritual actions. Discuss this type of behavior in class and identify how these actions are seen not only in hunting, but also in a number of other situations, for example before and during performances by professional actors and sports figures. Have the group research their favorite star or athlete and report on what superstitions they exhibit. Also have them interview a family member to see if they can find similar types of behavior. Then have the students write about any rituals they might have discovered lurking in their family's activities, and how they think the ritual helps or hinders their family.

Literary Styles

Hunter in the Dark provides two excellent opportunities to compare the literary styles of several authors. As stated earlier, Mike's setting up of camp can easily be compared to Nick Adams' actions in Hemingway's "Big Two-Hearted River."

- Have the students do stream-of-consciousness writing about what they are reading. Begin with a discussion about Hemingway's experiences and how he was able to capture the outdoor experience in his writing. Then have them try to write a journal entry about some activity with which they are very familiar. The students would then pair up and share their entries. Their partners would focus on whether they were able to follow the sequence of the events and construct a clear picture of the activity.

- Have the students begin by noting the similarities between the two works. Then have them find the differences between the two scenes.

How do the authors make use of language, especially adjectives and adverbs, to convey the experience to the reader? Is it possible in either work for a reader unfamiliar with wilderness or camping to understand what the characters are experiencing? Finally, have the students, working individually, take a personal experience and try to describe it in the style of either of these authors.

- Another possibility would be to have the students do a descriptive essay about some outdoor activity. Begin by having them draw a picture. Then have them write a description of their picture. They would then select background music to accompany the reading of their essay. Finally, have the students watch a Discovery Channel documentary or National Geographic video and compare how they use pictures and words to highlight nature.

A second work that lends itself to this exercise is "To Build a Fire" by Jack London. Have the students read about Mike's struggle first. Then stop and have them read the London story.

- Again, they would get into their groups to compare and contrast the two stories. Then have the students locate information on hypothermia and analyze how well the two stories deal with what we know about the process of freezing to death. Have the students write about which story is most accurate. Finally, have them prepare a safety pamphlet on what one should do to prepare for and how to behave during such an emergency.

Tracking Exercise

Tracking is a dying craft. In the past, there were outdoorsmen who were masters at following any animal through any type of cover. Today, however, tracking is less important, and many outdoorsmen cannot even backtrack themselves, let alone a game animal. Since both books deal with the art of tracking, have the students do several activities based on this skill.

First, determine what types of animals it might be possible to track in your area. Even the largest of cities should provide some examples of animals to track (squirrels, dogs, cats, birds). Begin by talking about the fact that all animals leave tracks, even birds when they land on the ground. Next get a fieldbook on tracking from the library and have the students study several common animal tracks. These are a few possible activities:

- Find out what wild animals (such as raccoons, rabbits, and squirrels) live near the school and set up a bait station. To do this mark off one square yard of ground and prepare the soil as if you were going to plant. Then lightly sift flour over the soil and place dog or cat food and rabbit pellets in the center of the square. Each morning check to see what has visited the station. The flour will clearly show the tracks of any visiting animals. By doing this exercise as they read the books, the students should begin to recognize differences in the size and species of animals that visit the station.

- It is also possible to have the students begin to track each other. We all leave tracks, but most of us do not recognize the signs we leave behind. Begin by having the same student walk, run, and jump across soft soil. Examine his or her tracks. How are they different? Can you tell what the student was doing by the tracks left behind? Have the student walk forward through the soft soil and then have the same student walk backwards right next to the original tracks, a trick that was used to fool trackers in the past. The students should be able to see that although the tracks look like they are going in the same direction, it is possible to determine what really happened. By looking closely they will also see that the tracks do not look the same, because the way the weight is distributed differs depending on direction of travel.

Literary Concepts

One obvious aspect of the books to be considered is the use of literary terms and conventions. Plot, setting, motivation, conflict, climax, resolution, and symbolism are important aspects of the novels that need to be discussed and analyzed. However, utilizing Howard Gardner's (1983) theory about various intelligences might give the students opportunities to become engaged in ways that the writing exercises cannot.

- Have the students create a soundtrack of songs that captures the events and emotions of the novel. Have them compose their own song or lyrics for a theme song for the book.

- Maps would provide a good visual reference for what was happening in the book.

- Have students draw storyboards and design collages as a means of describing how these literary concepts are evidenced within the story. Two items that should receive special attention are symbolism and metaphor. The deer in both stories are symbols of the life/death struggle everything goes through. The hunt in *Hunter in the Dark* is a metaphor for Mike's illness and treatment. The use of these literary techniques should be highlighted several times in each book. Have the students keep a running journal on where and how they find them used, and how they think their use affects the story.

We believe that these novels and activities can provide a safe space within which to share, discuss, debate, and understand a disease that is touching the lives of so many adolescents and their families in ever-increasing numbers.

RECOMMENDED READINGS

Cancer: Fiction

Bunting, E. (1987). *Will you be my posslq?* San Diego: Harcourt Brace. ISBN: 0–152–97399–0. HS.

Jamie, the narrator and cancer success story, agrees to share an apartment with Kyle, an archeology major. Jamie is trying to overcome her fear about the recurrence of her cancer. As Jamie comes to realize that the current living arrangement will make it difficult to maintain her moral standards, she chooses to change the way she is living. In the end she is able to retain her virtue and keep Kyle as a friend. The story tells of the hopes and dreads of having cancer, and of the successes and failures that come with the disease.

Christainsen, C. B. (1988). *A small pleasure.* New York: Atheneum. ISBN: 0–689–31369–1. 137 pp. MS, HS.

This is a story about how a teenager named Wray Jean Child deals with life's important issues, including her father's cancer. A typical teenager, Wray Jean is always tying to improve herself to become the best person she can be. A part of her hectic life is dealing with her father's illness when his cancer, which had been in remission, returns. When her father dies Wray Jean has to learn to deal with the reality that her father is gone. She discovers that only she can make herself happy, and that her father will always be with her in her memories.

Coerr, E. (1977). *Sadako and the thousand paper cranes.* New York: Putnam. ISBN: 0–399–20520–9. 64 pp. MS.

This classic was reissued with a different illustrator by Putnam in 1993. The story is the same in both the old and the new version (ISBN: 0–399–21771–1). Sadako, an atom bomb survivor, gets leukemia, one of the diseases associated with the radiation poisoning from the bomb. She tries to fold one thousand paper cranes and verify the legend that by doing so a sick person will become healthy. Although she dies, her story lives on and continues to be a powerful message even today.

Ferris, J. (1994). *Invincible summer.* New York: Farrar, Straus and Giroux. ISBN: 0–374–43608–8. MS, HS.

This is the love story of two leukemia patients. Robin, the seventeen-year-old main character, falls in love with a boy who also has the disease. The book details how they attempt to survive their ordeal and carry on with their lives as normally as possible. A good, easy story that most middle school girls will enjoy.

Grant, C. D. (1991). *Phoenix rising, or how to survive your life.* New York: Atheneum. ISBN: 0–689–31458–2. MS, HS.

Half of the book is told from the first-person perspective of Jessie Castle, the main character. The second half includes excerpts from the diary of Helen Castle, Jessie's sister, who died of cancer. The book does a good job of showing how the whole family has to cope with death and that everyone comes up with his or her own strategy. In the end, Jessie starts the process of learning to deal with the loss of her sister and begins to come out of her shell and live again.

Greenberg, J. (1983). *No dragons to slay.* New York: Farrar, Straus and Giroux. ISBN: 0–374–35528–2. MS.

Thomas, the main character, gets cancer. The story does an excellent job of showing how people react to the patient. Thomas' father escapes to his office and is embarrassed when Thomas loses his hair. His mother constantly talks on the phone with comforting friends, buys him presents, and takes him to his treatments in the hospital. Thomas at first thinks that having cancer is like a test, or having a dragon to slay. He thought he would be a hero, but finds himself shunned by friends because they felt threatened by the disease. It made him feel depressed and vulnerable. In the end, Thomas learns that miracles do happen and that you have to be ready to grab them when they come.

Guernsey, J. (1983). *Five summers.* New York: Clarion Books. ISBN: 0–899–19147–9. MS, HS.

This novel deals with the trials and tribulations of a farm family over a five-year period. The main character, Amanda Smetana, grows up, going from twelve to seventeen over the course of the book. One of the issues that Amanda has to deal with is her mother's breast cancer. The cancer and its recurrence covers the last three years of the story. The book does an excellent job of showing how the family dealt with a number of different problems and managed to continue despite the hardships and kept their farm going. It is also good to see how Amanda's ability to deal with problems changes as she grows older, an important issue to demonstrate to young adolescents.

Hermes, P. (1982). *You shouldn't have to say goodbye.* San Diego: Harcourt Brace. ISBN: 0–152–99944–2. MS, HS.

An excellent book to help students understand the four stages of grief that people move through in dealing with cancer and death. Sarah, the main character, has to deal with her mother's illness and death from cancer. She is helped through the process by a journal her mother, who knew she was dying, kept for Sarah. The journal was her mother's way of communicating with Sarah. Sarah begins to keep her own journal, which also helps her learn to deal with the loss of her mother. An excellent work to get across the concept of journaling.

Hughes, M. (1984). *Hunter in the dark.* New York: Atheneum. ISBN: 0–689–30959–7. MS, HS.

This novel is discussed in this chapter.

Hurwin, D. (1995). *A time for dancing: A novel.* Boston: Little, Brown. ISBN: 0–316–38351–1. 272 pp. HS.

Julie (Jules) and Samantha (Sam) are best friends. They met while they were dancing and have danced together for years. In their junior year in high school, Julie gets cancer. Chemotherapy helps, but does not get rid of the cancer. Julie eventually dies. A great book that helps students understand the hardships that go with cancer and the realities that are so hard to face.

Johnson, A. (1993). *Toning the sweep.* New York: Orchard Books. ISBN: 0–531–05476–4. 103 pp. MS.

This book begins as fourteen-year-old Emily and her mother arrive at her grandmother's house in the California desert. Grandmother, dying of cancer, is going to go back to Ohio with them. The book centers around Emily's struggle to come to grips with her grandmother's illness. Her mother, describing how she had to deal with her father's death, helps Emily begin to accept her grandmother's death. This book is an excellent example of the effect that family stories can have on us.

Kehret, P. (1990). *Sisters long ago.* New York: Cobblehill Books. ISBN: 0–525–65021–0. MS.

Willow Paige, the main character, has visions of a "past life" when she almost drowns. This causes her to begin to explore the possibility of reincarnation. The subject is important to her since she uses it to give hope and strength to her sister, who has leukemia. An interesting book that students who like fantasy novels should enjoy.

L'Engle, M. (1980). *A ring of endless light*. New York: Farrar, Straus and Giroux. ISBN: 0–374–36299–8. 324 pp. MS, HS.

This is the story of fifteen-year-old Vicky Austin. She is faced with death for the first time when her grandfather is diagnosed with leukemia. When Vicky starts working on a scientific project about communicating with dolphins, she begins to understand that there is more to life than death. She develops a telepathic communication with the dolphins and finds comfort spending time with them. Through them she is able to see that life is made up not only of death, but more important of love, joy, and silent understandings. She learns not to bear the crosses of others and that life can be more magical than it sometimes appears to be on the surface. An excellent book for all students.

Little, J. (1984). *Mama's going to buy you a mockingbird*. Ontario: Puffin Books. ISBN: 0–140–31737–6. MS, HS.

Another story of two young people, Jeremy and Sarah, who learn to cope with their father's battle with cancer. In addition to learning to cope with their grief over their father, the children must also deal with what happens to the family as a result of his illness. Their mother has to sell their house and go back to school full time to be able to provide for them in the future. An excellent text to help students realize how cancer changes everything in the lives of those it touches.

McDaniel, L. (1995). *Don't die, my love*. New York: Bantam Books. ISBN: 0–553–56715–2. 256 pp. MS, HS.

Luke has liked Julie since elementary school. They started dating and became a steady couple in high school. In their junior year, Luke is diagnosed with Hodgkin's lymphoma. He goes through chemotherapy and is in remission for a short time. Luke eventually dies, but leaves a reminder for Julie that is a great ending for the book. This will definitely appeal to middle school girls.

Paulsen, G. (1984). *Tracker*. New York: Scholastic. ISBN: 0–590–44098–5. MS.

This text is highlighted in the analysis of cancer in this chapter.

Polikoff, B. G. (1992). *Life's a funny proposition, Horatio*. New York: Holt. ISBN: 0–805–01972–3. 103 pp. MS.

This book deals with how Horatio works to adjust to the death of his father. At the same time, his grandfather, O.P., is trying to deal with the death of his dog.

It is an excellent text to help students begin to understand the ways in which we come to accept the death of a loved one, and that even pets must be mourned.

Wenderli, S. (1996). *The heartbeat of halftime*. New York: Holt. ISBN: 0–805–04713–1. 128 pp. MS.

In this story, a thirteen-year-old boy, Wing, dreams about winning the championship football game before his father dies of cancer. It is a high-interest, easily read story that should appeal to middle school students with an interest in sports.

Cancer: Nonfiction

Landau, E. (1994). *Cancer*. New York: Century Books. ISBN: 0–805–02990–7. MS, HS.

This is a great nonfiction book that will help students understand the causes and effects of cancer. It also tells the stories of some cancer patients who have overcome the disease.

REFERENCES

Aries, P. (1981). *The hour of our death*. New York: Knopf.
Berger, K. S. (1998). *The developing person through the life span*. 4th ed. New York: Worth.
Gardner, H. (1983). *Frames of mind*. New York: Basic Books.
Kastenbaum, R. J. (1992). *The psychology of death*. New York: Springer-Verlag.
Kubler-Ross, E. (1969). *On death and dying*. New York: Macmillan.
Kubler-Ross, E. (1975). *Death: The final stage of growth*. Englewood Cliffs, NJ: Prentice-Hall.
Moller, D. W. (1996). *Confronting death: Values, institutions, and human mortality*. New York: Oxford University Press.
Stillion, J. M. (1995). "Death in the lives of adults: Responding to the tolling of the bell." In H. Wass and R. A. Neimeyer, eds., *Dying: Facing the facts*. Washington, DC: Taylor and Francis.
Wass, H. (1995). "Death in the lives of children and adolescents." In H. Wass and R. A. Neimeyer, eds., *Dying: Facing the facts*. Washington, DC: Taylor and Francis.

CHAPTER 5

Normalcy Was All She Wanted: Learning to Live with Diabetes

Sue F. Johnson and Claire J. Dandeneau

Knowing that diabetes is one of the most prevalent health issues facing adolescents and their families, we began to seek out young adult literature that had protagonists with diabetes and that showed adolescents dealing with the disease and/or gave some positive information on how to cope with diabetes. According to the American Diabetes Association, the risk of developing insulin-dependent diabetes or juvenile diabetes is higher than that for virtually all other severe chronic diseases of childhood. About 18 out of 100,000 people under the age of twenty will develop diabetes. The peak onset of the illness is around ten to twelve years old for girls and twelve to fourteen years old for boys. It is not often discovered in the early stages because the initial symptoms of diabetes can mimic the flu in most children.

Finding information about the disease was easy; finding just one good young adult novel with a diabetic teen as the protagonist was almost impossible. Both of us were stymied at every turn. We discovered that very few adolescent authors have dealt with this illness. Ultimately, we did find a few books, but only four really fit the criteria for an adolescent reader, and all four tended to be girl-oriented. The novel that presented the world of an adolescent with juvenile diabetes most accurately and appropriately, in our estimation, was Lurlene McDaniel's *All the Days of Her Life*. McDaniel was able to depict the world of an adolescent with diabetes so well because her son was diagnosed with juvenile diabetes. "I saw firsthand how chronic illness affects every aspect of a person's life," she has said. "I want kids to know that while people don't get to choose what life gives to them, they do get to choose how they respond."

ALL THE DAYS OF HER LIFE

At no time in our lives is the need to belong as strong as it is during adolescence. Consequently, the one theme with which all adolescents will readily identify is that of belonging, of feeling a part of the world in which they live. This theme of finding acceptance, of belonging, is central to *All the Days of Her Life*.

Lacey Duval, a typical teenage girl, is looking for acceptance by her peers, looking for a boyfriend, and looking to be like the other kids in her school. Above all else, she just wants to be normal. She believes that if she is normal, she will be accepted by her peers. She defines normal as perfect and healthy. But Lacey has juvenile diabetes; she is not healthy and not normal. Because of her diabetes, she must watch her weight, keep close track of her blood sugar levels, watch what she eats and drinks very carefully, and give herself insulin injections twice every day. Pigging out with her girlfriends, eating burgers and fries, staying up all night, devouring chocolate, and maybe having a beer are not in her personal regimen. Lacey believes that she must conceal her illness from her school friends so that she can fit in.

For most teenage girls, fitting in requires not only being healthy, but being thin, especially to be noticed by the man of one's dreams. These two criteria, fitting in and being thin, focus most of Lacey's energies throughout the story. She refuses to tell anyone at school about her diabetes, even Terri, who is becoming a good friend. She hides taking her insulin, so that no one will suspect. She is even willing to miss an injection if it means she might get caught. When she thinks she is gaining weight, she begins to manipulate her insulin dosages and juggle her diet to lose weight. The more attention Todd, a popular boy, pays to her, the more she juggles her insulin and diet. She also learns about vomiting to lose weight from Monet, the campus beauty, who models and is her rival for Todd's attention.

Another common theme teens can identify with that flows through the text and adds to that of belonging is family relationships. Lacey believes she is the only teen in her group who has divorced parents. She thinks that to be normal, her parents need to be together. The fact that her parents are divorced complicates Lacey's ability to take care of her diabetes properly; both parents, because of their feelings of guilt—guilt for the divorce, guilt for "causing" Lacey's illness—find it difficult to take responsibility to help Lacey come to terms with her situation. Therefore, Lacey becomes totally in charge of controlling and taking care of her diabetes herself from about age twelve. As a result she also develops feelings of isolation, feeling very alone in the world.

To make things more difficult for Lacey, Uncle Nelson is her doctor. Because he is her mother's brother, he is careful to trust Lacey and follow her mother's wishes, which makes it easier for Lacey to avoid her office checkups and to control her disease. Lacey's ability to manipulate her family through her diabetes becomes the way she attempts to punish them and herself. She almost succeeds.

Throughout the novel Lacey is learning about friendship and who her real friends are. In the beginning Lacey divides her friends into two groups. In the first group are her ill friends, Katie and Jeff, whom she met at Jenny House, a camp for severely ill kids, during the summer and who know about her illness. Katie has had a heart transplant and Jeff is a hemophiliac. Her relationship with these two is up and down throughout the novel as they try to be her real friends and help her come to terms with her illness and control it.

Her friendship with Jeff is complicated in that at Jenny House, the relationship had begun to be romantic, and Jeff still has strong feelings for Lacey. Lacey returns his feelings, but works very hard to conceal them and repress them because she does not want a boyfriend who is sick. When she finally becomes aware of how important these two friends are to her, it is almost too late. She has a huge fight with Katie and hurts Jeff. Her relationship with Katie gets back on track, but she will have to work hard and it will take time to become close to Jeff again.

Her other friends are those from school who do not know anything about her illness. They are Terri, who sticks close to Lacey through thick and thin, and Todd, who really likes to party, hangs out with Monet, and develops a "thing" for Lacey directly related to and parallel to Lacey's losing weight and willingness to party.

When Lacey is in crisis, Terri comes through for her and shows Lacey another type of friendship she did not believe possible. When Terri learns what is wrong with Lacey, she seeks out information about diabetes so that she can be a better friend. She gives Lacey a genuine, unconditional friendship that Lacey had not thought possible from someone who was not sick. Terri also informs Lacey's other healthy friends and creates an accepting environment for Lacey.

Finally, although the text represents many of the common issues reflected in the life of an adolescent, the issue that we see as being at the heart of learning to live with diabetes and growing up is that of making choices. Lacey has a difficult time making good choices because of her secrets and various relationships and her strong desire to belong at any cost, a desire that almost costs her her life.

Throughout the story, McDaniel consistently and accurately integrates facts about diabetes and issues on how to live with the illness. The information she presents is thoroughly researched and current according to the information we received from the American Diabetes Association and is presented in a way that student readers can easily grasp.

Although some may be critical of this text because it may be perceived as too melodramatic, it is a very accessible text for adolescents. Both criteria used to select this novel—the way it deals specifically with diabetes and its exploration of themes significant to most adolescents—are met with skill and knowledge.

POSSIBLE ACTIVITIES

One thing we did notice about this text and the others we reviewed is that the authors often pay particular attention to presenting accurate medical facts and neglect the counseling issues. In this novel no counseling is initiated for, nor is the school informed about, either the disease or the divorce. Whatever emotional support Lacey receives comes from her peers; the adults are distanced from her world until there is a crisis.

One critical need is for professionals to work together and possibly team teach some of the important issues suggested by or left out of these texts. Part of the school counselor's job is to provide classroom guidance, for example by presenting workshops on making choices, friendships, and self-esteem. The school health professional can share information about common illnesses and where to get help and information. If the school has a health class, the English teacher and the health teacher can collaborate to create some units using adolescent literature to support the issues being discussed in health class. The school dietician and the physical education teacher could also be included in such a unit. The key point is to model for students how these professionals work together to support students and how students can support each other in positive ways.

The following questions could be possible writing prompts:

- Remember a time when you felt either out of place or alone and needed to belong. Explain the situation and describe how you felt.
- What does being responsible mean to you? Are you responsible? Why or why not?
- Remember a time when you had to make a difficult choice or choices. What was the choice and why was it difficult? How did you feel about the situation? What choice did you make and why?
- How does it feel to be left out? Have you ever felt alienated or isolated from your friends? Different from them? Have you ever gone to extremes to belong—to be like everyone else? Lied? What were the consequences? Was it worth the effort?

Also, the school counselor might conduct a session on risk and risk management. Students would be asked to define what risks are, to role play a situation that involves risk-taking, and then to brainstorm the types of risks adolescents take and possible outcomes.

Depending on the focus of the unit or individual readings, students can develop responses to the following types of questions as they read *All the Days of Her Life*:

- How is Lacey like other teenagers? How is she different? What characteristics does she share with most teenage girls? Which are different?
- Using scenes from the text, explore the choices you might make in that situation. Would you have made the same choice Lacey did, or would you do something different? Why or why not? Be honest.
- Who are Lacey's real friends? Why? Define what/who friends are.
- What other types of illnesses might make someone feel different or alienated? How would you react if you had that illness? How would you be a friend to that person?
- If you were Lacey's friend, what advice might you give to her? Select a scene from the text and role play what happens with a different ending.
- Copy a provocative/interesting/important/enjoyable passage and comment on it.
- Explain why you would or would not have a particular character as a friend.
- What other characters besides Lacey make choices and change during the course of the novel? Explain the changes.
- As you read this novel keep a record of what you learn about diabetes.
- What feelings/emotions does the novel evoke in you?

The following activities could be done by individual students or in small groups:

- Research local resources available for diabetes patients. Who would you go to for assistance if you had a serious illness?
- Create a powerpoint presentation that shares what you have learned about diabetes.
- Write a skit with dialogue that reflects the internal dialogue of one of the characters externally.
- What is your decision-making process? Create a diagram that depicts Lacey's decision-making processes.
- Develop a talk show with Lacey, Dr. Rosenberg, Terri, Katie, and Monet as guests.
- Role play a counseling session that Lacey and her family might have attended.
- Debate the issues of sharing or being private about yourself in new situations.

FROM THE COUNSELOR'S PERSPECTIVE

The main character, Lacey Duval, a sixteen-year-old female with juvenile onset diabetes, "presents" with several issues that warrant further exploration with a professional counselor. They include developmental issues associated with her age, environmental issues, and issues that result from her adjustment to and management of her disease.

Developmental issues arise due to an individual's adjustment to normal changes that occur as a result of growing up. Lacey faces these issues as any other teenager might. Lacey struggles with the need for peer acceptance, to define her own identity within her peer groups, and to fit in and be liked by all. She especially just wants to belong and be normal.

Lacey's relationships with Jeff and Todd clearly indicate that she is working through and learning to understand key issues with respect to developing relationships with the opposite sex. She questions herself, she examines her choices, and she explores her own values, particularly with respect to the importance of her boyfriends' personality characteristics and status within the peer group.

Underage drinking is only a minor issue for Lacey. In one instance, she is able to deflect the peer pressure to drink; yet, on another occasion, while on a date with Todd, she succumbs to peer pressure and drinks a beer, knowing it will complicate her disease.

Like many other young women her age, Lacey struggles with her self-image with respect to her weight and body image. As she strives to meet an ideal image, she takes dramatic steps—changing her insulin dosage and vomiting—to control her weight and to become more attractive to herself and others. This is consistent with evidence that young non-obese girls with diabetes are more likely to develop eating disorders than girls without diabetes. (Vila, Robert, Nollet-Clememcon, Vera, et al. 1995).

Her developmental issues are made more complex because of her parents' divorce. Their divorce represents an environmental issue—one occurring within one of her main social environments, her family. The divorce disrupted Lacey's family and her life. In the transition from her family to the separated family, she has to adjust to the difference in her relationships with her parents. In addition to the adjustments, she questions whether she is to blame for the problems in her parents' marriage and the resulting divorce; she becomes a pawn between her parents. As a result of the divorce and her parents' relational problems, Lacey feels alone and frightened.

In addition to these issues, Lacey struggles with her disease. In many ways, she chooses to deny her diabetes. She feels ashamed for not being normal. She has learned to inject herself with insulin, to make adult decisions about her diet and eating habits/patterns, and to manage her diabetes with minimal assistance from her parents. Simply put, her diabetes impacts all aspects of her life, especially her self-image.

In the course of the story, Lacey is connected with a psychologist, Dr. Rosenberg. He helps her deal with her diabetes and also works to facilitate an understanding between her parents as to how their behaviors impact Lacey and, more important, her management of her diabetes. Unfortunately, Lacey's relationship with Dr. Rosenberg is not fully developed and represented within the story. Counseling for Lacey seems almost an afterthought.

It is true that defining and delineating counseling treatment is not an easy task. This is typically done within a particular theoretical orientation and in concert with the philosophical ideology of the counselor and the professional training of the counselor. A delineation of counseling theory is beyond the scope of this chapter. It is, however, possible to examine the various factors or issues present for the client and how they could be addressed within a counseling setting and to suggest the type of counseling that would be appropriate for a child like Lacey.

The first and perhaps the most important aspect of all counseling is the referral. Somehow, and in some way, a client must present himself or herself for counseling. A referral can be made either by a second party, in this case Uncle Nelson, Lacey's doctor, or it can be initiated by the client himself/herself. The referral in essence starts the counseling, healing, and growth process. In this story, the protagonist is referred to counseling only after a life-threatening crisis has occurred. It is never made clear why Lacey is never referred to a counselor earlier.

It is as if both doctor and patient are operating from stereotypical beliefs about counseling. Clearly, these beliefs will impact the client's acceptance of the referral and potential willingness to engage in the counseling process. Any and all individuals making referrals for counseling should understand that counseling is a natural part of the healing and growing process. Seen as such, counseling can be viewed as a normal extension of other forms of treatment that produce similar healing, and not as an afterthought or a response to crisis.

The client, Lacey, would need to understand and fully appreciate that counseling is a form of helping that is designed to assist individuals, groups, or families make changes in their lives and grow. If it is okay to heal one's body, it is okay to heal one's heart and soul.

Given Lacey's acceptance of counseling as a helping process, the next step for the counselor would be to assess the type of counseling that would best suit the therapeutic needs of the client. Various forms of counseling could be made available for Lacey: individual, family, and group counseling. Since Lacey's needs are in several areas, one or more of these counseling options could be helpful in her healing and growing process.

Since a majority of the issues Lacey is coping with are developmental ones, the best treatment approach would be group counseling (Worzbyt & O'Rourke 1997) with other teenagers who are facing similar adjustments, situations, and/or difficulties. Lacey could benefit greatly from participation in group counseling. The advantages of group counseling are numerous, and there are several curative factors associated with it (Yalom 1995) that would help Lacey. Lacey could begin to understand that she is not alone and that other teenagers are experiencing similar situations and issues. Her self-esteem could also be enhanced as she would become a contributing member in the group, and the group could give her feedback on her value and worth—both as a person and a group member.

Additionally, she could learn new interpersonal and communication skills and practice them in the safety of the group experience. Peer support (La Greca et al. 1995) is the critical social support for adolescents dealing with their diabetes (Varni et al. 1989). A group setting can be an excellent vehicle for developing and providing that support, and group dynamics facilitate the development of emotional support as well.

The counselor's role in this process is to work in conjunction with the group so that appropriate norms are established that will allow the group to communicate genuinely and openly. Creating a safe and supportive environment in the group allows members to openly share, building bonds between members. Along with the sharing, the counselor helps the group develop a manner whereby members can challenge each other, support each other, and encourage each other to make changes toward their goals. For example, Lacey might have felt safe enough in the group to share her confusion about dating. She might not have chosen initially to discuss the issue of dating someone with an illness; however, she might have begun to discuss dating someone for prestige and for acceptance; a peer group could understand her motivations and help her evaluate her choices and decisions. Group counseling could have been highly beneficial in assisting Lacey with her developmental issues. Also, as the group developed and Lacey felt more comfortable within it, she could possibly have begun to address issues related to her parents' divorce and her disease.

In addition to the group work, it would be critical to provide Lacey with individual counseling, creating a safe place, an environment and a relationship where she could share all her thoughts and feelings, a place where she could say what she wants and needs without fear of being judged, disrespected, and devalued.

The counselor would have to initiate Lacey to counseling. The counseling process would then allow Lacey to share her feelings and be acknowledged and heard. The foundation of this process is the counselor's ability to fully enter and truly experience Lacey's world. This empathy would help Lacey feel valued and heard and also allow her to fully hear herself, and as a result come to a greater understanding of her needs, wants, and desire for change.

For Lacey, this counseling would be critical. She needs a place where she can express her anger at her diabetes, verbalize all of her feelings about her parents' divorce, share her feelings about herself, acknowledge her uncertainties about her relationships, explore the meaning of friendship and the importance of these relationships in her life, and confront the decision to control her weight by manipulating her insulin and vomiting. She might also need to address her issues of uniqueness, mourn the loss of health, and examine what may now seem to be a flawed identity (Chigier 1992).

Lacey would be helped to see all the areas in her life that are causing her stress. She would be helped to understand how the behaviors she chooses contribute to that stress. Providing some stress management training might be highly beneficial (Boardway et al. 1993). For example, when she admits to Jeff that she has made a mess of her life, the counselor would have her examine what she has been choosing to do that has contributed to her problems. The focus of counseling then could be to assist Lacey in understanding what she truly needs and wants and help her begin to make decisions that will facilitate the fulfillment of them.

Both individual and group counseling are important for Lacey's growth and mental health; however, the importance of family issues in Lacey's treatment is critical and should not be underestimated. Her family is undergoing some dramatic changes, and although they are saying that "this is all for the best," several underlying family issues still exist for Lacey. The book illustrates the powerful changes that can occur when family issues are addressed and when each member is challenged to examine his/her role in the family. Research also indicates that children will demonstrate better glycemic control when there is greater emotional involvement by their parents (Stevenson, Sensky, & Petty 1991) and that family support (La Greca 1991; Hanson et al. 1987) and parent-child conflict (Miller-Johnson 1994) can be related to treatment adherence.

There is evidence, although it is presented in a cursory way, that Lacey is subconsciously using her diabetes to control several areas of her life, including her family situation. The focus of the family counseling would be to address the changes occurring in the family, the subsequent emotions related to the changes, and the family's response to Lacey's disease. It would be helpful for them to work through the process of adjusting to all these changes.

In the case of her diabetes, both her mother and her father admit to relinquishing control of the treatment for the disease to Lacey. Very soon after the diagnosis there apparently is little or no parental involvement in her treatment. Evidence suggests that parents will give greater control of the management of the diabetes as the child ages (Drotar & Ievers 1994); however, in Lacey's case she is given control very early, at the age of eleven or twelve. Lacey is charged with the adult responsibility of managing the disease. There is some indication that she is developmentally ready to take on this responsibility, but there are also indications that she takes on sole responsibility because neither her father nor her mother really wants to be involved. It is as if they collude in the process of hiding the disease and, in effect, abandon their child.

Never is she assisted in telling anyone about her disease or confronting the social issues related to her disease. It would be helpful if she and her family developed plans to assist her in this social process (Solomon 1993). In many ways her family has left her alone with the diabetes and related decisions. Every time one of her parents tries to be more involved, Lacey simply shuts the discussion down by asserting her independence and her ability to handle her treatment. No adult in her life surfaces to help her until crisis occurs.

It should be noted that in the story, Dr. Rosenberg never elects to see the family together as a unit. Many family counselors would have preferred to engage the family all at one time and then facilitate the discussion of change and adjustments among all family members. This ensures that all the relevant issues are raised and addressed with all parties.

Counseling could have provided the very help the family needed, if only the family, the school, and the medical community believed counseling to be part of the healing and adjustment process and not just a last resort.

RECOMMENDED READINGS

Classroom Resources for Diabetes

Beatty, M. D. (1997). *My sister Rose has diabetes*. Santa Fe, NM: Health Press. ISBN: 0–929–17327–9. MS.

Presenting the point of view of other children in the family, James tells about his ten-year-old sister, Rose, who has diabetes. James is afraid that he too will catch diabetes. Rose tells her story as well, about staying in the hospital, learning to care for her diabetes, and what it means to have diabetes.

Betschart, J., and S. Thom (1995). *In control: A guide for teens with diabetes*. Minneapolis: Chronimed Publishing. ISBN: 1–56561–061–X. 116 pp. MS, HS.

Life with diabetes is a challenge for anyone. Life as a teenager with diabetes is a tremendous adversity. This book clearly addresses *all* the concerns and issues of teens with diabetes, including alcohol use, drugs, and sexuality, because knowledge is what is needed to manage diabetes successfully.

Carter, A. R. (1995). *Between a rock and a hard place*. New York: Scholastic. ISBN: 0–590–48684–5. 213 pp. HS.

Fifteen-year-old Mark Severenson and his diabetic cousin, Randy, are really not looking forward to their family's traditional rite-of-passage canoe trip, but they must go. After a rocky start, they begin to enjoy themselves as they make their way through Minnesota's many waterways and get to know each other. Diabetes presents itself here as a social problem for both Mark and Randy. This novel is a really good outdoor adventure story.

Children with Diabetes. *http://www.childrenwithdiabetes.com*

A wonderful web site with many connections to other web pages of importance to children and parents, including chat rooms for families dealing with diabetes, camps for kids with diabetes, and much more.

Christopher, M. (1995). *Shoot for the hoop*. Boston: Little, Brown. ISBN: 0–316–14125–9. 129 pp. MS.

When Rusty Young is diagnosed with diabetes, his parents want him to quit basketball, but Rusty is determined to play, especially in the new summer league. This is a good sports novel for young men with a minimum of information about dealing with diabetes.

Giff, P. R. (1982). *The gift of the Pirate Queen*. New York: Bantam Doubleday. ISBN: 0–440–43046–1. MS.

When her mother dies, Grace must grow up quickly, taking charge of the household and making sure her sister Amy takes proper care of her diabetes. When an Irish cousin comes to take care of them, Grace learns about an Irish legend— Grania (Grace) the Pirate Queen and her special courage. Through the legend Grace learns that honesty is the best policy.

Haines, S. (1994). *Donnie makes a difference*. Boise, ID: Writers' Press Service. ISBN: 1–88–510106–6. MS.

After trying out for the football team, Donnie is diagnosed with diabetes. He is quite upset that, until his blood sugars stabilize, he has to stop playing football with the team. His family, friends, and coaches help Donnie realize that he can make a big difference by being an assistant coach since he knows so much about football.

Loski, D. (1995). *Zack attacks*. Boise, ID: Writers' Press Service. ISBN: 1–885101–10–4. 107 pp. MS, HS.

Teenager Zack struggles to come to terms with the accidental death of his father, with his diabetes, and with acceptance by the kids at his new school. When challenged by a group of boys who are into drinking and stealing, Zack has the strength to say no.

Mazur, M. L., P. Banks, and A. Keegan (1995). *The dinosaur tamer and other stories for children with diabetes.* Alexandria, VA: American Diabetes Association. ISBN: 0–9454–4858–9. 186 pp. MS, HS.

The Dinosaur Tamer is a collection of twenty-five stories about children/adolescents with diabetes. The stories contain examples of some of the challenges that adolescents and teens with diabetes face every day and how they manage to overcome these challenges and live life to the fullest.

McDaniel, L. (1994). *All the days of her life.* New York: Bantam Books. ISBN: 0–553–56264–9. 153 pp. MS, HS.

This book is featured in this chapter.

Miller, J. (1988). *Grilled cheese at four o'clock in the morning.* Alexandria, VA: American Diabetes Association. ISBN: 0–9454–4802–3. 90 pp. MS.

Sixth grade soccer player Scott develops diabetes and learns how to deal with his condition, including what to do when his blood sugar is low at night—eat a grilled cheese sandwich.

Taylor, T. (1994). *Sweet Friday Island.* New York: Harcourt, Brace. ISBN: 0–15–200012–7. 173 pp. MS, HS.

Peg Toland and her dad often go on adventures together, and their camping trip to the island in the Sea of Cortez seemed to be the perfect place. However, their vacation quickly becomes dangerous and deadly and is complicated when her father goes into insulin shock. A great adventure/mystery with a female heroine. Although the teenager does not have diabetes, her knowledge of how to help her dad is critical.

REFERENCES

Boardway, R., A. Delamater, J. Tomakowsky, and J. Gutai (1993). "Stress management training for adolescents with diabetes." *Journal of Pediatric Psychology* 18: 29–45.

Bowman, V., and J. DeLucia (1993). "Preparation for group therapy: The effects of preparer and modality on group process and individual functioning." *Journal for Specialists in Group Work* 18: 67–79.

Chigier, E. (1992). "Compliance in adolescents with epilepsy or diabetes." Fifth Congress of the International Association for Adolescent Health. *Journal of Adolescent Health* 13: 375–379.

Corey, G. (1990). *Theory and practice of group counseling.* 3rd ed. Pacific Grove: Brooks/Cole.

Drotar, D., and C. Levers (1994). "Age differences in parent and child responsibilities for management for cystic fibrosis and insulin-dependent diabetes mellitus." *Journal of Developmental and Behavioral Pediatrics* 15: 265–272.

Hanson, C. et al. (1987). "Social competence and parental support as mediators of the link between stress and metabolic control in adolescents with insulin-dependent diabetes mellitus." *Journal of Consulting and Clinical Psychology* 55: 529–533.

LaGreca, A. (1991). "The role of families in childhood diabetes." *Family Psychologist* 7: 12–14.

LaGreca, A., W. Auslander, P. Greco, D. Spetter, et al. (1995). "I get by with a little help from my family and friends: Adolescents' support for diabetes care." *Journal of Pediatric Psychology* 20: 449–476.

Miller-Johnson, S. (1994). "Parent-child relationships and the management of insulin-dependent diabetes mellitus." *Journal of Consulting and Clinical Psychology* 62: 603–610.

Solomon, M. (1993). "How to ease your concerns about your teen at parties." *Diabetes in the News* 12: 24.

Stevenson, K., T. Sensky, and R. Petty (1991). "Glycaemic control in adolescents with Type I diabetes and parental expressed emotions." Eighteenth European Conference on Psychosomatic Research. *Psychotherapy and Psychosomatics* 55:170–175.

Varni, J. et al. (1989). "Social support and self-esteem effects on psychological adjustment in children and adolescents with insulin-dependent diabetes mellitus." *Child and Family Behavior Therapy* 11: 1–17.

Vila, G., J. Robert, C. Nollet-Clemencon, L. Vera, et al. (1995). "Eating and emotional disorders in adolescent obese girls with insulin-dependent diabetes mellitus." *European Child and Adolescent Psychiatry* 4: 270–279.

Worzbyt, J., and K. O'Rourke (1997). *Elementary school counseling: A blueprint for today and tomorrow.* Muncie, IN: Accelerated Development.

Yalom, I. (1995). *The theory and practice of group psychotherapy.* 4th ed. New York: Basic Books.

CHAPTER 6

Focusing Our Attention: Reading about ADHD

A. Lee Williams and Albert Scott

While both of us focus much of our professional work on children, our different fields (one of us a reading teacher and the other a clinical psychologist) give us two different perspectives on both the meaning of attention deficit hyperactivity disorder (ADHD) itself and the meaning of having the disorder or living with someone who has it. Understanding children in the classroom is different from understanding children in a clinical setting; helping parents understand the implications of their child's behavior at school is different from helping them understand the implications (and reasons for) behaviors in the entirety of the child's life. However, both of us need to work with ADHD children and with parents who may still be coming to terms with what it means to have an ADHD child.

Al's research began during the early days of his graduate education and his private practice, as he looked at the clinical studies defining symptoms, causes, and treatments for ADHD. His interest began as he considered the needs of his own sons, his young clients, and their families. What did the most current research explain about the disorder? What kinds of treatment options made sense for him and his clients? How did family interactions impact these children? What support could and should teachers provide for ADHD children?

As a teacher, Lee needed to understand ADHD in terms of students and classrooms. Her questions were classroom focused. Who has ADHD, and who is just normally active and impulsive? How are hyperactivity and inattentiveness related in attention problems? What (if anything) can be believed that is reported in the popular media? How can parents be helped to understand their children so that the child can be more successful in school? What makes it possible for a classroom with one or more children with ADHD to remain productive and happy?

We spent many hours sharing our takes on children with ADHD. We read, discussed, explained, and questioned. In coming to consensus and writing this chapter, we needed to align our lenses and bring into focus our separate points of view. Please note that one choice we made is our use of the acronym ADHD to represent the types of the disorder recognized in the current diagnosis criteria of the Diagnostic and Statistical Manual of Mental Disorders (DSM-IV). We don't use the acronym ADD to represent the disorder, since it is no longer current; however, it is still used in books, on the Internet, and in the popular press. We learned during the writing process from each other, and having done so, hope to make both ADHD and appropriate books and resources more accessible for school personnel, for parents, and for teachers who work with and need to reach the children and young adults whose lives it affects. We begin with two stories of children who could very well be in our lives as student or client.

KATIE'S STORY

Katie was a pleasant, pretty toddler and child. She didn't adjust well to change—in her diet, her schedule, or her daily activities. But as an only child, her parents thought she was fine—just a little fussy. As she got older, she never seemed to really listen to what her parents asked of her. They would send her to get her sweater, and she would come back with a book she had found along the way. They would send her up to her room to straighten it and find her sitting in the midst of a pile of clothes, playing with her dolls. In elementary school, friends liked her— she loved to talk and socialize. Katie was fun to be with, even if she didn't seem to be interested in anything for too long. However, she was mostly invisible to her teachers. She didn't cause trouble in class, unless she was chatting with someone when she should have been working. On the whole, she did average academic work, although sometimes it was done extremely well and other times quite poorly, with careless errors or sloppy presentation that lowered her grade significantly. Teachers told Katie and her parents the same story every year. "Katie needs to try harder. She knows what to do, but she needs to actually do it! She seems bright enough if she's doing what she wants to do. Her problem is she is disorganized and unmotivated."

Katie did indeed know what she was supposed to do, but found it impossible to organize herself and maintain a focus long enough to make the kind of progress everyone seemed to expect of her. While the teacher would give directions, she would find watching the children outside on the playground irresistible. While the class was completing seatwork, she would be thinking of the way the sunlight shone through the window and danced on the walls, and noticing how the pencils sounded as the other kids wrote on their papers. She knew everything that was going on except for the things the teacher seemed to value. She never could tell exactly what to do or how to do it.

But Katie did well enough that no one thought of her as anything other than an average student who was a little lazy. It was hard for Katie's parents to believe anything was really wrong. She was basically such a good kid. That is, until middle school, when assignments were given a week in advance, and she either forgot about them until the teacher asked for them, or started them too late to do a good job. The teachers expected students to take lecture notes, and Katie had trouble listening and writing quickly. When directions were complex and multi-stepped, Katie was soon lost. The teachers seemed to expect the students to just do all the things that Katie struggled with, and most did. As the work became harder and harder for her, Katie became more and more surly and developed a "why try?" attitude. She focused more on her relationships with her peers and the older boys in the school who really seemed to like her.

By eighth grade Katie's average grades became failing grades. Her parents, at their wits' end, were tired of her promises to do better that never seemed to result in any change in her behavior. When they tried to correct her, Katie just burst into tears and stormed away. She blamed her subjects for failing to interest her, her teachers for not teaching, and her parents for not understanding.

Her parents were worried about Katie's school performance, her choice of friends, and their deteriorating relationship with their daughter. If this was what it was like to raise an adolescent daughter, they certainly weren't prepared for it. Even as she got older, she never seemed to be able to learn how to focus and carry through on demands made on her. But wasn't this what a normal teenager was like?

Unknown to her parents, Katie had begun to experiment with drinking and abusing street drugs. Mixed in with the other trauma of Katie's behaviors, they never noticed her growing use of alcohol to escape the pain of her family and school problems. Sometimes Katie thought it would be easier to die than to feel like such a failure at controlling herself. Her parents finally brought her for counseling when one of Katie's friends confided to them that Katie was drinking before school and hinting to friends about a specific suicide plan.

JASON'S STORY

Jason was in Katie's grade in school, although they had never been assigned the same teacher. Jason's parents, unlike Katie's, had found their child to be a handful ever since he was born. He had boundless energy, never napped, and threw himself—literally—at everything he did. He was reckless and clumsy, yet scrapes and scratches didn't seem to teach him any lessons about being careful. He went through more toys in fifteen minutes than most kids played with in a day. After a change in routine, Jason was especially excited, and large groups and lots of novelty seemed to render him uncontrollable.

In school, Jason yelled out answers, jumped up from his seat, and lost his crayons and pencils, his coat, his books, and his milk money. He paid no heed to repeated teacher warnings and spent more and more instructional time removed from the other kids at a separate desk in the back of the room. Sitting there he played with little toys, his shoelaces, or a pencil while the rest of the class listened to the teacher. He never quite heard what she was saying, and what he did hear he never seemed to remember.

When Jason exhibited difficulty in attending to print and showed signs of a reading disability, his teacher and his parents met to discuss his school behavior and his lack of academic success. Jason's uncle had had similar trouble in school, and his parents were concerned. Suspecting attention deficit hyperactivity disorder, the adults arranged for Jason to have a thorough evaluation, and the psychologist determined that he met the criteria for ADHD. With a combination of drug therapy, structured school expectations that provided him with predictable routines and meaningful work choices, and cognitive psychotherapy and treatment where Jason learned strategies for coping with his distractibility and his learning struggles, he was able to feel success at school.

He started doing the kinds of things the other children did without thinking—paying attention to the activities that counted, listening and remembering directions to tasks, and making better decisions about time and behavior. Direct instruction and modeling helped him to compensate for distractions by learning some strategies that would help him focus, remember, and organize what he learned. As he got a bit older, he started playing on the community soccer team, where his boundless energy found an outlet. While school was never a breeze for Jason, neither was it a place of dread. And as he learned to control the soccer ball and work as a team member with a nurturing yet firm coach, he actually gained status with his peers as an athlete, an accomplishment that carried over into his social relationships at school. As Jason got older, with continued drug therapy, he found order in his life and choices got easier.

UNDERSTANDING ATTENTION DEFICIT HYPERACTIVITY DISORDER

Both Katie and Jason have ADHD, although only one was lucky enough to be diagnosed early and treated as such. Attention is the ability to concentrate on one aspect of the stimuli available to us in our environment. As you read this, you are probably not aware of the texture of the chair you are sitting in, what others around you are doing, or noise generated by appliances or fixtures in your surroundings. But if you stop reading, shifting your attention, you will no longer be aware of the words on the page but of the sights, sounds, and smells around you. You may hear parts of a conversation in another room, and yet choose to ignore it, knowing that this reading needs your attention now. It is our capacity to focus attention that allows us to respond to or ignore stimuli, and we have flexibility in choosing to attend or to ignore. We can choose to pay attention carefully, or we can choose to divide our attention. We decide what is important and what we will act on in our surroundings.

However, that is not the case for the person with ADHD. This disorder means that a person will be uniformly aroused by environmental and internal stimuli and easily distracted. Attention may be focused on irrelevant stimuli while important stimuli are ignored. Things attended to may not be remembered. Children and adults with ADHD are fidgety, impulsive, and seem to shift from uncompleted activity to uncompleted activity. Sitting still, remembering, and following directions are difficult. We all have times when we are distracted and inattentive, but for persons with ADHD, distraction is a way of life.

Five subtypes of ADHD are described in the DSM-IV. Katie and Jason are different types. A child may not be capable of remaining focused and attentive and still not meet the criteria for hyperactivity and extreme impulsiveness that are linked to other ADHD types. While teachers often over-recognize difficult boys, many of whom do not have ADHD but are developmentally immature, quiet girls with ADHD-I who cause no trouble and yet remain unfocused and fall behind academically can easily slip through the diagnostic cracks.

Although symptoms of ADHD should be evident before age seven, the change in expectations that accompanies school attendance often makes symptoms suddenly apparent. All small children have shorter attention spans than do older children, and differentiating immaturity and ADHD is important. Gifted ADHD children often compensate for their lack of ability to focus attention with their intelligence during their elementary years, finally reaching a point in middle school or high school where changed expectations for student behavior and more complex tasks mean that their disability catches up with them. It is then that behaviors associated with the disorder keep them from functioning appropriately in school or with their peers.

Recent research studies, especially neuropsychological research on the brain functions that contribute to the ability to focus attention, have helped us understand that ADHD is not a moral defect, a failure of will, or an emotional maladjustment. It is instead a failure of the neurotransmitters in the area of the brain that controls and supervises attention functions. The brain operates in most people to screen the competing stimuli in the environment so that only the critical signals are attended to. However, in ADHD children, this attention focusing capacity is diminished. Brain scan studies of persons with and without the symptoms of ADHD show lower levels of brain activity in areas of the brain associated with functions such as attention, concentration, planning, and organization in the ADHD groups when compared to the control groups. Drugs such as Ritalin, Adderal, and Dexedrine act to stimulate these underused brain areas, helping children choose what portions of the environment to attend to in order to focus on relevant tasks. Ritalin and other stimulant drugs help ADHD children perceive the world in a more usual and less fragmented manner. Knowing about the biological etiology of ADHD helps children and parents understand why and how appropriate medication works and reassures them that medication is not a sign of failure, but an often necessary first step in treating ADHD.

TEACHERS, PHYSICIANS, THERAPISTS, AND ADHD

Teachers don't always understand ADHD. Much of the current re-search is more biological and less social than it was when many of today's classroom teachers were undergraduates. Children with ADHD are frustratingly normal in appearance and intelligence and seem able to focus when they "want to," such as when playing computer video games. Some teachers are reluctant to encourage the medication of children, believing that if the child tried harder or that if the learning situation were inviting enough, that would be sufficient for children to focus and do what is expected. Given the false negative reports about Ritalin and overprescription of medication in the popular press, teachers may not want to be part of advocating drug therapy.

Other teachers may expect every child to sit quietly for long stretches, or they may structure classes with lectures and worksheets, even for young students. When children are unable or unwilling to do such work, teachers may believe ADHD is responsible, when in fact the child's development level or the structure of the instruction may contribute to the child's wandering attention as much or more than a tendency toward ADHD. Failure to attend can be related to boredom (as when a gifted child is not appropriately challenged), to childhood depression, to learn-ing disabilities, to poor nutrition or lack of sleep, or to immaturity and a slower psychological development. These causes might not merit drug therapy with stimulant medication, but the symptoms the child exhibited would be similar to those of a child with ADHD.

Psychologists play an invaluable role as partners with educators, ther-apists, and physicians in diagnosing children who exhibit the kinds of behaviors associated with ADHD. Compounding diagnostic difficulty is the close co-occurrence of depression, learning disabilities, reading dis-abilities, and oppositional defiant disorder with ADHD. Many children are diagnosed as having ADHD when in fact they suffer from a bipolar illness.

While traditional therapies like play therapy or talk therapy have not proven to be effective in treating ADHD, therapy can be useful in teach-ing children how to cope with their disorder. Family therapy and edu-cation can be beneficial interventions. Cognitive behavioral therapy can also have a positive long-term impact. Learning changes the brain, and such changes may, in the long run, alter brain functioning and reduce symptoms.

In addition, counseling is useful to help a child rebuild self-esteem damaged as the result of living with the effects of ADHD. Counseling can also help parents learn to cope with the demands of the ADHD child on family life by suggesting household routines and expectations that nurture the child and support his or her needs.

WORKING TOGETHER TO SUPPORT KIDS WITH ADHD

A team approach to diagnosis and treatment is especially important for the ADHD child, who can exhibit behaviors easily confused with or co-occurring with other causes. Teachers may be asked to respond to questionnaires important in the diagnostic process. Since the child spends much of his time in school, medication often needs to be partially evaluated at school. The classroom teacher, especially, will need to evaluate treatment plans in action. Also, teachers are often the adults in the best position to see that children remember to take medication, and their sensitivity can help self-conscious students take prescribed drugs without embarrassment and in accordance with school policy. Providing children with books on the subject may help students understand ADHD; why having the disorder is not the same as being bad or stupid; and why taking medication is often an appropriate treatment, not a sign of failure or a punishment. When psychologists, physicians, therapists, and teachers work together focusing on what is best for the ADHD child, teachers often have a heightened sense of efficacy.

Creating routines and predictable structures and teaching children how to make productive choices within the structure is beneficial for all children, but essential for ADHD children. Teachers may understand classic behavior modification (punishment and reward) programs. Perhaps more useful is the cognitive-behavioral approach, which helps children learn problem-solving and self-monitoring strategies so that they can assume responsibility for their own behavior over time. Psychologists may work with families to help create appropriate home settings; teachers need to develop cooperative relationships with parents as well. Children who are ready to give up on themselves in frustration can be helped by caring and consistent support from adults.

By understanding the nature of the disorder, creating appropriate classroom structures, teaching children strategies for coping with classroom tasks, and seeing that needful children receive the appropriate treatment, classroom order can return from the precipice of disaster created when one or several ADHD children are assigned to a class. Understanding that children with ADHD can't pay attention rather than won't pay attention minimizes emotional responses from teachers frustrated with the impulsivity and failure to learn from mistakes that characterize the ADHD child. Teachers who understand why Ritalin (or another drug) works are less likely to feel guilty that a child in their room is taking it and will recognize that if it doesn't seem to work, another cause for attention problems is probably responsible.

Combining proper medication (if needed to allow children to focus attention) with teaching children to take responsibility for their behavior choices and teaching them coping strategies for their different learning needs is essential. Rather than requiring children to do what they are unable to, it is also important to organize classroom structure and activities so that they can engage in meaningful tasks they are able to do. These accommodations give ADHD children a chance at the success they are ultimately capable of achieving. When teachers are able to treat children with ADHD appropriately and matter-of-factly, they model a dynamic for caring and responsible community-building with all members of the class.

READING ABOUT ADHD IN *FALLING IN LOVE IS NO SNAP*

Adolescents enjoy reading about people they admire and about people with whom they can identify. They are drawn to characters that they see as like themselves—facing the same challenges, sharing the same goals. Given the importance to young readers of finding characters they can identify with, and given the number of children who probably have ADHD (studies project 3–10 percent of the population) and the number of classrooms that could be expected to have an ADHD child in them, one would expect to find a number of books dealing with the subject. Yet finding a fictional book at a young adult level with an ADHD character (even if not the main character!) is not so easy.

Falling in Love Is No Snap by Jane Foley (1989) is one of the few novels with an ADHD character written for a young adult audience. Foley's book is delightful and useful in thinking about ADHD even though the character with ADHD plays a minor (albeit significant) role. Unfortunately, the book is out of print. However, it is available in many libraries, and if your library has an interlibrary loan system, it should not be difficult to locate a copy; Internet and local booksellers offer book-finding services as well. The book is of interest and is accessible to middle school readers in general and older students who either struggle with reading or who would like an entertaining yet engaging quick read. It is a love story told from a young woman's point of view—and as such may be a tough sell to male readers, many of whom are quick to dismiss "chick books." Teachers and librarians can often influence such readers, however, to give a book like this a try.

Alexandra Susskind, from whose point of view the story is told, has moved with her single mother to New York City after her parent's divorce. Her mother values the private school education that she works so hard to afford for her daughter, hoping Alexandra will become a whiz in the corporate world after attending Harvard Business School. But Alexandra has other ideas—she wants to be a photographer. As she roams the neighborhood taking pictures, she discovers a handsome young man, Heracles Damaskinakis, working at the local delicatessen. She falls in love at first sight and manages to get herself a job at the deli, which turns out to be owned by Heracles' father. Heracles and Alexandra spend time together, finding that they talk easily and feel good in each other's company. After a kiss, Alexandra is convinced that she is in love, until Heracles tells her that he already has a girlfriend. To save face, she invents a boyfriend for herself, pointing out a boy from her school the students call Tweed, but whom she claims is a college man.

The two continue to share a friendship and discover that they each have goals for themselves different from what their parents want for them. Alexandra does not want to go to Harvard Business School but since she does not spend much time with her workaholic mother she doesn't spend the time they do have together discussing what she fears may be an unpleasant subject. Heracles wants to study science at Stanford, not run the deli, as his father expects. But his father is uncommunicative and will not talk about his wife's, Heracles' mother's, death, or the problems with his younger son, eleven-year-old Theo, who is a whirling dervish, running into and out of the deli as Alex puzzles about what it all means.

While Heracles and Alex each think the other should confide in their parent the truth about their ambitions, neither is able to do so. Heracles wants to support Alex's photography and commissions her to take a portrait of his brother as a gift for his father. Alex is upstairs taking Theo's picture when Heracles must take over the deli when his father suddenly becomes ill. Alex decides to help out by bringing Theo home with her. Theo is a handful, but Alex discovers he likes art and draws well. But Theo's unrelenting energy is ultimately too much for her to handle—he never stops moving and never stops resisting—that is, until Alexandra's mother comes home. She has had experience with students with ADHD and knows strategies for dealing with the child. She sends for Theo's medicine, which his father does not insist he take, sets clear boundaries for him, helps him to focus his energy, and reads him a story. Theo responds warmly to the structure and positive attention.

Alexandra sees her mother in a new way and admits to her that she wants a career in photography. Mr. Damaskinakis agrees to follow up with Theo's medicine more carefully and to monitor his behavior more closely. Heracles, seeing that Theo can help out in the delicatessen, decides to go to Stanford to study science and breaks up with his girlfriend, who is not happy with this new plan. Alexandra admits that she has no real boyfriend, and she and Heracles end up together.

Foley's portrayal of Theo is dramatic, but realistic. Mrs. Susskind recognizes that Theo needs structure and needs to take his medicine routinely. Alexandra discovers Theo's creative side and his artistic talent. Mr. Damaskinakis clearly adores his son, although he indulges Theo's disruptive and unproductive choices. Seemingly a simple adolescent love story on the surface, the novel introduces complex threads of social class expectations (Heracles' family as first-generation working class; Alexandra and her mother as upwardly mobile middle class; and Tweed as upper class); parental expectations versus children's aspirations; and single parenting (Alexandra's mother and father are divorced; Heracles' mother has died). Additionally, Theo's ADHD is treated realistically— as a real issue in the family dynamics, but one that can be successfully (if not always straightforwardly) addressed. Theo is portrayed as a difficult, but not impossible, child who has special needs but also special talents. Because this book deals with sophisticated subject matter (family dynamics and expectations, falling in love, social and cultural differences, and planning for life after high school) it has appeal for older readers, but its first-person format and easy reading make it appropriate as well for students who may struggle with reading or learning disabilities. Both readers who themselves have ADHD and readers who have siblings, friends, or classmates who have ADHD would undoubtedly enjoy Theo's characterization in this book. Either way, the sympathetic treatment of Theo would allow for discussion of the impact of the disability on the person who suffers from it as well as those around him. That Theo's artistic talent was partially hidden because of his disruptive behaviors could also spark discussion about any person's hidden skills and talents that may not be given an opportunity to show or to grow because of lack of opportunity or lack of interest by significant others. Teachers or librarians could also make use of this book in a theme-related study dealing with family, disabilities, or constraints of class, circumstance, or health on life choices.

One specific activity that could be used in conjunction with this book would be to have students select a character from the story and one decision that character might have to make. Ask the students to make the decision for the character, writing down their decision and the rationale behind it on notecards. Collect the notecards and discuss the decisions in small groups, then have one student from each group share in the whole class discussion. This activity could be followed by creating a consequence tree or web guided by such questions as, What effect would this decision have on others? What would be some possible alternatives? How would this decision be influenced by others?

THERAPY FOR THEO

An appropriate diagnosis is the first step in deciding on a treatment plan for any client, but especially when ADHD is suspected. Inattention and impulsivity are manifested in many childhood situations, including times when these behaviors are developmentally appropriate, and the diagnosis is sometimes misapplied to a variety of childhood disorders having elements associated with ADHD.

Although Foley's description of Theo suggests attention deficit hyperactivity disorder, a thorough evaluation would be made before a course of treatment would be outlined. Foley also suggests that Theo has a learning disability, although not all ADHD children or adults do. Ruling out bipolar disorder (or determining if it co-occurs) is also necessary. Behavioral symptoms are similar, yet medication and treatment are different. Often co-occurring or confused with ADHD are conduct disorder and oppositional defiant disorder. Again, a careful evaluation is necessary to determine an appropriate diagnosis and a beneficial course of treatment. A medical evaluation should rule out physiological/medical causes for hyperactivity or inattentiveness—hyperthyroidism, sleep apnea, iron deficiency anemia, or medication toxicity. Nonremedial cases of ADHD due to lead poisoning or brain injury should also be ruled out. Foley suggests that Theo should be on a special diet; however, research suggests that diet does not significantly contribute to ADHD.

Data from parent interviews and questionnaires, teacher reports, direct observation of the child in a school setting, and clinical measures of focused attention along with intelligence tests and measures of neuro-psychological status are aspects of the procedure for diagnosing ADHD in children. Observing the child's behavior in terms of focus, level of attentiveness and distractibility, and alertness during assessment provides additional insight into the child's attentional functions. The focus of assessment is on the variance of the individual child's behavior compared with that of others of the same age, intelligence, and gender, and behaviors must be evidenced for at least six months.

Six or more of the following symptoms of inattention need to be present for a diagnosis of ADHD:

- Is inattentive to close details and careless mistakes
- Finds sustaining close attention difficult
- Does not seem to listen when spoken to directly
- Fails to follow through on instructions
- Has trouble organizing tasks
- Resists engagement in tasks requiring sustained mental engagement
- Loses necessary items
- Is easily distracted by stimuli in the environment
- Is forgetful in daily activities

Foley writes, "[T]he doctor said he was *hyperactive*. Now the school says he has some kind of learning disability. Five years ago when he started school the teachers called him hyperactive. Now they say he has . . . an *attention deficit disorder*" (46). This is evidence of long-term symptoms, as well as teacher assessments. Additionally, Foley has given Theo many of the symptoms of ADHD that are apparent in his behaviors. Theo's impulsivity, his intrusions into others' space, and his disruptive, inappropriate, negative behavior are evidenced when he pushes Alex so hard she hits her head against a wall, when he skateboards into the store, and when he knocks over the candy display. He is unable to sit still as Alex prepares to take his photo, crossing his eyes when he finally manages six quiet seconds. Heracles tells Alex that "everything excites him. He gets out of control" (46). Bored and then angry when accompanying Heracles and Alex on a walk, he recklessly runs ahead, not paying attention to the inherent dangers of a New York City street. When Alex takes Theo home, her requests to him seem to fall on deaf ears. Opening her drawers, scattering her clothes, wearing her bra on his head, jumping on her bed, and crawling on the floor and roaring like a lion in a matter of minutes, Theo reduces Alex to tears when he finally ends up biting her hand as she struggles to restrain him. When Mrs. Susskind comes in to see what is happening, she asks Theo about taking his medicine, and he admits, "I forgot . . . I always forget" (113). Theo's distractibility and short attention span are evidenced in each scene in which he appears.

A TREATMENT PLAN

Three areas of Theo's life need to be addressed for him to benefit—school, medical/psychological, and home. At school, Theo will require moderate amounts of teacher supervision and considerable teacher direction, especially as he begins to learn what is expected. His work needs to be assigned based on what he is capable of—his measured abilities, rather than age-normative standards. Instruction should be multisensory. Theo will need to listen, watch, and participate actively. At least a half-hour should be spent each day on individual, creative exploration time. Sitting still should not be a prerequisite for learning. Classroom interactions and teaching methods need to be structured, predictable, and routine. Procedures for classroom routines as well as for study and school performance need to be explicitly taught, modeled, and practiced, one step at a time. Multi-stepped directions are overly confusing for a child with ADHD.

Theo's teachers will also need to work constantly on his self-esteem, as this will be the key to engaging and motivating him. Social and organizational skills should be explicitly taught. All teachers of ADHD children need to avoid frustrating them, while teaching them independence and protecting them from their impulsive and potentially dangerous behavior.

In Foley's book, Mrs. Susskind asks Theo to sit still, and he insists, "I can't" (116). But Mrs. Susskind helps him make choices, using a timer to show how long he must sit before a break. Both parents and teachers need to set limits and maintain them. Phelan's model for child management, *"1–2–3" Magic: Training Your Preschoolers and Preteens to Do What You Want* (1995) works for parents as well as in the classroom. Based on adult no-emotion response to misbehavior and time out if children do not choose on their own to stop the offending behavior, *"1–2–3" Magic* helps children know that they have behaved inappropriately and will be held responsible for their misbehavior. This system avoids a power struggle between adult and child and keeps counterproductive

adult responses out of the situation, preventing the escalation of misbe-
haviors. It is essential that teachers monitor Theo so that they can intervene before inappropriate thoughts, feelings, and behaviors have become
disruptive misbehavior.

In all, Theo's teachers will need to be caring, fair, patient, and consistent. Recognizing positive behavior and attitudes (even marginal ones)
will encourage children with ADHD to continue those behaviors, and
helping them to keep track of them (by using a chart or sticker program)
may also be helpful. Ignoring negative attention-seeking behaviors if
they are not overly interruptive is useful. Using prearranged signals to
help children notice and self-correct misbehavior helps—and Theo and
his teachers should work out such a system.

During psychotherapy, several outcomes are desirable. One is to educate parents and siblings. They need to understand the disorder—why
children behave as they do, what they are capable of and what they find
difficult, and how medication and school and family structure impact the
child's behavior. A family with an ADHD member often needs support
to understand and to identify ways to cope positively with a "live wire"
in the family.

Helping parents learn how to provide a structure for the child to ensure
success helps children learn to make, and to be responsible for, good
choices. Using timers, calendars, charts, notebooks, and school assignment books to help the child focus on what chores, homework, and
general behavior need to be done, when, and how—and then to monitor
progress in completing tasks—increases children's on-task behavior. Parents should be helped to develop routines for household procedures and
the child's school and household responsibilities.

It is often useful for parents to learn specifically how to give ADHD
children directions—by getting their attention, making one request at a
time, having the child repeat the request—and how to establish clear
rules and boundaries for the child. Parents usually find that participating
in a support group for ADHD is useful.

Another desirable outcome is for Theo himself. Children also benefit
from learning about ADHD. It is comforting for children to know that
their behavior is a result of a disorder, not a failure of will or some kind
of inherent "badness." Bibliotherapy can be helpful in giving children
(and parents) a means to understand and think about the disorder. Specific issues can be addressed: What is it like to have ADHD? What
strengths and weaknesses do children and adults with ADHD have? What
coping strategies can be used? In addition, emotional growth can be

fostered with the use of children's and young adult literature. Tolerance of and empathy with children with differences can be encouraged in ADHD children themselves as well as in the children who live with them at home and in classrooms. Hoagland (1972) notes three stages for social/emotional growth using literature: identification, catharsis, and insight. Useful books for understanding ADHD are listed below.

RECOMMENDED READINGS

Attention Deficit Hyperactivity Disorder: Fiction

Foley, J. (1989). *Falling in love is no snap*. New York: Laureleaf. ISBN: 0–4402034–9. 139 pp. MS, HS.

Complete commentary on this young adult novel with an ADHD character is found in this chapter.

Janover, C. (1997). *Zipper, the kid with ADHD*. Bethesda, MD: Woodbine. ISBN: 0–9331–4995–6. 108 pp. ES, MS.

Zipper, a bright fifth grader with classic ADHD problems—blurting out rude comments, annoying peers, forgetting homework and the big game—needs to manage his behavior if he is going to be successful at his new goal—jamming on the drums with his new friend Pete.

Nielsen, S. (1987). *Autograph, please, Victoria*. N. p. David C. Cook/Cahriot Books. ISBN: 1–55513–216–2. 126 pp. MS.

Victoria Mahoney is an eighth grader with a younger brother who acts out and has a learning disability. When she wins a national writing contest, she looks anew at her brother's problems. Helpful to those children with a sibling or classmate whose ADHD requires adjustments and emotional understanding.

Parker, H. C., R. N. Parker, and R. Di Matteo (1992). *Making the grade: An adolescent's struggle with ADHD*. Plantation, FL: Specialty Press. ISBN: 0–9621–6291–4. 47 pp. Spanish Edition: *Como Pasar de Grado*. MS, HS.

The story of Jim Jerome's transition from elementary school to middle school and the impact of a diagnosis of ADHD.

Parker, R. N. (1996). *Slam dunk: A young boy's struggle with ADHD*. Plantation, FL: Specialty Press. ISBN: 0–9216–2949. ES, MS.

The story of a fifth grader's life with ADHD—classroom adaptations, medication, and behavioral interventions. This book ends with a question and answer section about ADHD.

Attention Deficit Hyperactivity Disorder: Nonfiction

Deephaven School's Learning Lab Students and M. H. Dinneen (1992). *If they can do it, we can too!* N.p. Fairview Press. ISBN: 0–92519–061–6. 87 pp. ES, MS.

Students with special learning needs reveal that successful adults may have had learning problems as well. Student-written with commentary by their teacher.

Gehret, J. (1996). *I'm somebody too.* Reprint. Fairport, NY: Verbal Images Press. ISBN: 1–884–28112–5. 170 pp. MS.

Told from the point of view of Ben, a boy with ADHD, this book focuses on the social and emotional needs of children with the disorder and provides practical strategies for dealing with these issues.

Gehret, J. (1996). *Eagle eyes: A child's guide to paying attention.* 3rd ed., revised. Fairport, NY: Verbal Images Press. ISBN: 1–88428–111–7. 40 pp. ES, MS.

Told from twelve-year-old Emily's point of view about her brother, Ben. At first Ben's behavior causes her worry, but after her parents seek professional help for him and he begins taking medication and learning to structure his behavior, Emily finds she is jealous, angry, and guilty over Ben's changing family role.

Gordon, M. (1992a). *I would if I could: A teenager's guide to ADHD/hyperactivity.* DeWitt, NY: GSI Publications. ISBN: 0–9627–7013–2. MS, HS.

A light-hearted examination of the effect of ADHD on school, family, and social relationships from an adolescent's point of view.

Gordon, M. (1992b). *My brother's a world class pain: A sibling's guide to ADHD.* DeWitt, NY: GSI Publications. ISBN: 0–962–77012–4. 40 pp. ES, MS.

A book that explores some of the issues that siblings face when a brother or sister has ADHD.

Ingersoll, B. (1997). *Distant drums, different drummers: A guide for young people with ADHD*. ISBN: 0–9648–5480–5. 48 pp. MS.

Ingersoll examines deficit, disability, and difference and puts a positive spin on ADHD so that young people can understand difference without becoming overwhelmed by challenge.

Moser, A. (1991a). *Don't feed the monster on Tuesdays! The children's self-esteem book*. Kansas City, MO: Landmark Editions. ISBN: 0–93384–938–9. 55 pp. ES, MS.

Low self-esteem often accompanies ADHD in children. This book provides practical ways for children to understand and improve self-esteem.

Moser, A. (1991b). *Don't rant and rave on Wednesdays! The children's anger-control book*. Kansas City, MO: Landmark Editions. ISBN: 0–933–84954–0. 61 pp. ES, MS.

Again, controlling angry emotions is often difficult for ADHD children. This book helps children understand and cope with anger in a practical way.

Nadeau, K., and E. Dixon (1997). *Learning to slow down and pay attention: A book for kids about ADHD*. Washington, DC: American Psychological Association. ISBN: 0–9453–5479–7. 64 pp. ES, MS.

Written for children, this book presents ways to manage the effects of ADHD—disorganization, emotional distress, and inability to focus attention. Discusses the roles of adults in treatment.

Nadeau, K. G. (1994). *Survival guide for college students with ADD or LD*. New York: Magination Press. ISBN: 0–945354–63–0. HS, College.

The study suggestions in this book would benefit high school students as well, but advice about finding and using support services, scheduling classes, and creating optimum study conditions is college and university specific.

Quinn, P. O., and J. M. Stern (1991). *Putting on the brakes: A child's guide to understanding and gaining control over attention deficit hyperactivity disorder*. New York: Magination Press. ISBN: 0–945354–32–0. ES, MS.

This book provides ADHD readers with a sense of efficacy and community in regard to their problems.

Westridge Young Writers Workshop (1994). *Kids explore the gifts of children with special needs*. Santa Fe, NM: John Muir Publications. ISBN: 1–56261–156–9. 112 pp. ES, MS.

Written by peers of children with special needs, and with a section written by individual children, this is a child's view of living with a disability and living in the proximity of the disability. Includes a chapter about Lance Petrillo, a young person with ADHD.

SUPPORT ORGANIZATIONS

Attention Deficit Information Network (Ad-IN)
57 Hillside Avenue
Needham, Massachusetts 02194

Center for Mental Health Services (a component of the U.S. Public Health Service)
Office of Consumer, Family, and Public Information
5600 Fishers Lane, Room 15–105
Rockville, Maryland 20857

Children and Adults with Attention Deficit Disorders (CH.A.D.D.)
499 NW 70th Avenue, Suite 109
Plantation, Florida 33317

National Attention Deficit Disorder Association
9930 Johnnycake Ridge Road, Suite 3E
Mentor, Ohio 44060

INTERNET RESOURCES

Note: Internet servers change rapidly! Addresses may no longer be current. A search engine is useful in finding other sites that provide links to still others.

A.D.D. Warehouse: *http://addwarehouse.com*

Online catalog of resources—books, videos, newsletters, assessments, games—that can be purchased online or ordered by phone or mail. For teachers, parents, children and adults.

ADHD Owner's Manual: *http://ourworld.compuserve.com*

Information about ADHD includes references to related articles in scholarly sources.

ASK about ADD: *http://azstarnet.com~ask*

"Adults Seeking Knowledge" with information for and from children and adults with ADHD.

Children and Adults with Attention Deficit Disorder: *http://www.chadd.org*

Information about ADHD and C.H.A.D.D. Includes online issues of *Attention!* Magazine. The spring 1998 issue focused on the topic "Helping Teens Succeed."

Pursuit: *http://pursuit.rehab.uiuc.edu*

Disability information—education, accommodation, and resources—and careers in science, engineering, and mathematics for persons with disabilities, including ADHD.

REFERENCES

Alexander-Roberts, C. (1994). *The ADHD parenting handbook: Practical advice for parents from parents*. Dallas: Taylor Publications. ISBN: 0–87833–862–4. 176 pp.

Tips from parents, educators, and professionals on managing the day-to-day routines of life with a child who has ADHD.

Brawell, L., and M. Bloomquist (1991). *Cognitive-behavioral therapy with ADHD children*. New York: Guilford Press. ISBN: 0–89042–061–0. 391 pp.

Written for practitioners. When coupled with appropriate medication, cognitive-behavioral therapy seems to produce better results than behavioral therapy alone since it helps those with ADHD take responsibility for self-monitoring their behaviors.

Children with ADD: A shared responsibility. Based on a report of the Council of Exceptional Children with Attention Deficit Disorder (1992). Reston, VA: Council for Exceptional Children, 1920 Association Drive, Reston, VA. Order No. P385.

Useful for understanding implications of the federal law including the Individuals with Disabilities Act and school responsibility for failing to provide special education services for ADHD students.

Fisher, B. C. (1998). *Attention deficit disorder misdiagnosis: Approaching ADD from a brain-behavior/neuropsychological perspective for assessment and treatment*. CPR Press. ISBN: 1–574–44097–7. 300 pp.

A thorough and current examination of recent research on brain functions and attention. Written for practitioners, it offers a complete guide to treatment for ADHD and highlights co-morbid conditions.

Fouse, B., and S. Brians (1993). *A primer on attention deficit disorder*. Bloomington, IN: Phi Delta Kappa Educational Foundation. ISBN: 0–87367–354–9. 43 pp.

Written for educators, this short book provides a balanced overview of ADHD including symptoms, treatment, and educational accommodations.

Golden, G. S. (1992). "Attention deficit hyperactivity disorder." In D. M. Kaufmann, G. E. Solomon, and C. R. Pfeffer, eds., *Child and adolescent neurology for psychiatrists*. Baltimore: Williams and Wilkins, 43–55.

Goldstein, S., and M. Goldstein (1993). *Managing attention disorders in children: A guide for practitioners*. New York: John Wiley and Sons. ISBN: 0–471–61137–9.

Hallowell, E., and J. J. Ratey (1995). *Driven to distraction*. New York: Simon and Schuster. ISBN: 0–684–80128–0. 319 pp.

Written by a doctor who himself has ADHD, this book is balanced and reasonable. While it is still accessible to general readers, it is more academic than the book *Answers to Distraction*.

Hallowell, E., and J. J. Ratey (1996). *Answers to distraction*. New York: Bantam Books. ISBN: 0–5533–7821–X.

Also available in audiocassette, a media appreciated by those with ADHD or who struggle with reading. Written in a question/answer format, it is less complex than *Driven to Distraction*, by the same authors, providing information and solutions.

Hoagland, J. (1972). "Bibliotherapy: Aiding children in personality development." *Elementary English* 49, 390–394.

Outlines the use of books to aid emotional growth in children.

Ingersoll, B. D. (1997). *Daredevils and daydreamers: New perspectives on attention deficit hyperactivity disorder.* New York: Doubleday. ISBN: 0–38548–757–6. 224 pp.

Updated information from the last decade of research on ADHD. Ingersoll discusses family issues and clarifies symptoms and treatments for children and adults with ADHD.

Jongsma, A. E., Jr., L. M. Peterson, and W. P. McInnis (1996). *The child and adolescent psychotherapy treatment planner.* New York: John Wiley and Sons. ISBN: 0–471–15647–7.

Shows the relationship of behaviors to diagnosis and treatment options. Since ADHD may co-occur with other issues such as Oppositional Defiant Disorder (ODD), bipolar illness, and learning disabilities, a careful examination of evaluative data is a key in planning treatment.

Phelan, T. W. (1995). *"1-2-3 magic": Training your preschoolers and preteens to do what you want.* Glen Ellyn, IL: Child Management. (Also available in color video—120 minutes). ISBN: 0–963–38619–0. 175 pp.

A step-by-step plan for organizing a structure that will enable children to understand limits and for providing parents and teachers with nonemotional responses to unacceptable behaviors.

Purvis, K. L., and R. Tannock (1997). "Language abilities in children with attention deficit hyperactivity disorder, reading disabilities, and normal controls." *Journal of Abnormal Child Psychology* 25, no. 2: 133–145.

A research study showing that not all ADHD children also have reading disabilities; however, those who do have more severe language deficits.

Sears, W., and L. Thompson (1998). *The A.D.D. book: New understandings, new approaches to parenting your child.* New York: Little, Brown. ISBN: 0–31677–873–7.

While this book focuses on the positive side of ADHD and offers parents both support and insight for dealing with their ADHD child, it suggests treatment options that have not been shown effective. However, this book does offer resources and information parents may find useful.

Weaver, C. (1992). *Understanding and educating attention-deficit hyperactive students: Towards a systems-theory and whole language perspective*. Eric Document Reproduction Service. ED 344 376, EC 301 103.

Weaver, C., ed. (1994). *Success at last! Helping students with attention deficit (hyperactivity) achieve their potential*. Portsmouth, NH: Heinemann. ISBN: 0–435–08808–4. 290 pp.

Stories from students and teachers about learning and living with ADHD. Argues for support and freedom within structure so that students with ADHD can become active and successful learners. Classroom stories focus on literacy across the curriculum.

Webb, J. T., and D. Latimer (1993). *ADHD and children who are gifted*. ERIC Digest #522. Eric Clearinghouse on Disabilities and Education. ED 358 673.

CHAPTER 7

The Friends: Promoting Adolescent Mental Health Through Awareness and Literature

Karen L. Ford and Charlene Alexander

I remember the chain of events like it was yesterday. I had waited for weeks to see my dad, who had been in the hospital with a series of heart attacks. Now he was home, and as a special treat my mom fixed a TV tray dinner so that I could eat in his bedroom with him. We were laughing and watching the small black and white TV when he started to choke and make a horrible throaty sound. Things happened so quickly. My brother, who was studying to be a doctor, pushed me out of the room, and my mother and sister knocked the milk over on the kitchen table as they rushed into the room. And then we were at the funeral home. My sister insisted that I kiss my dad good-bye. What a horrible feeling, so cold and stiff, not at all like my dad. *I can't ever forget that coldness!*

And then my mother had to go away for a while. I went to stay with my grandma, who finally told me that my mother had gone to the hospital for a while. I remember being so excited on the day she was to come home. Finally, I'd get to go home to my own room and my mom. I walked home with the intent of surprising her, but when I saw her on the porch I couldn't even go over to her. For some reason I was scared. I ran instead to my grandma's house and, after much coaxing, she convinced me it was time to go home.

I remember that life at home was a little different. My mom had to take a lot of pills, and she always set them out on the kitchen counter so she wouldn't forget them. She let me come home for lunch, and one day when I came home I couldn't find her. Sometimes we'd play this hide-n-seek game and I thought she was hiding, so I looked around the rooms for her . . . nowhere to be found. I did notice that her pills had not been taken and that my lunch wasn't on the table as it usually was. It was then that I noticed the weird smell in the house. It smelled like gas, so I went downstairs to the basement to see if something was wrong. I found my mom in the garage bent over on her hands and knees and holding my raincoat to her chest. I remember yelling to her and touching her, but she wouldn't move. The car was running and it smelled awful in the garage. I thought something was wrong with the car, so I ran to my friend's house to get her sister to come and help. We called the police. I remember telling them that I thought the engine or something had exploded and that my mom was in there with it.

It was really hectic after that call to the police. I went to the other next door neighbor's to wait until my brother could get there from his practice in another city. He called me on the phone and said that everything would be all right. I felt so alone, and I worried about insignificant things, like paying for the umbrella that my mom had bought me with her new Elder Beerman's charge. I remember the doctor there and then lying down to take a nap. When I woke up my brother was there, and he told me we were going back to the house to get my things and I would stay at my aunt's house for a while. I asked about Mom and all he said was, "Mother's gone." I knew what that meant. It was a circus at my house. There were police asking questions, people taking pictures, and grandma sitting on the porch crying. I remember my brother telling me that I didn't have to talk to anyone, and I didn't. He made a path for me through the maze of people, past grandma, and into the house. I got my things together, and as we left I noticed that my mom's pills were still on the kitchen counter.

That night at my aunt's house I dreamed that my mom came into my bedroom and told me everything was going to be all right. I woke up scared, but I believed what she had told me. After all, she was my mom. The next afternoon as I walked my aunt's dog, one of my aunt's neighbors stopped me and said, "Oh, you're the little girl from the Residence Park suicide. . . ." Someone else talked to me saying, "Oh yes, you're the one from that killing on the west side." I remember what they said, but I really didn't connect with what they were actually saying.

Then there was the funeral. Lots of people were saying "poor little girl" or "poor little Karen." I was standing by my brother, and my sister was saying, "Don't you want to kiss Mommy good-bye?" In that instant I remembered how my dad had felt and I said, "No!" I remember going back to the house with my brother and sister after the funeral. I walked into my mom's room for some reason and then I went to the kitchen to look for her pills. They were gone. We stayed at the house for a couple of weeks; I went back to school for those two weeks and everyone was really nice to me. We even had my ninth birthday party—the one my mom *had been planning—and it was fun. I remember hearing my brother and sister talking or arguing about some other things and me after I was in bed, but whenever I was around they were always happy.*

And then I moved in with my brother, his wife, and their baby daughter. I started a new school and the teachers were really supportive and understanding, but kids were always asking me about my mom. Everyone always said, "I'm so sorry." I remember being sick of hearing that. I made some friends at school, but always felt uncomfortable at home. I guess it was like I didn't really belong to this family. I felt better when I was alone with my brother, but I had some real struggles with my sister-in-law. He wanted me to kiss her goodnight, like I had done to my mom and, for some reason, I hated doing that. Whenever she told me to do something or to come home at a certain time, I would do what I wanted to, come home when I wanted to, and have a tremendous yelling match with her— telling her there were other places I could go to live. I always sort of knew that my brother would side with me about things and that was the only thing that seemed to make living there bearable.

And then I got sick. It was in the winter, somewhere close to Christmas or just after. I started having stomachaches all of the time and only felt comfortable when I was in bed. I couldn't go to school and I didn't play anymore. I know I lost a lot of weight because my brother made me stand on the scale every night after I refused to eat supper. I remember him talking to me about being there, but only part of the conversation, although I have a sense that he talked to me quite a lot. All I really remember is something about me not having to kiss my sister-in-law anymore unless I wanted to and that things would be different if I got better.

In reflecting on my childhood and adolescence, I am amazed at the variety of events and situations and the impact they have had on me—then and now. I can't help but think that the experiences of my early life have helped me in dealing with adolescents as an educator. Unfortunately, many people are not fully aware that adolescents continually face a barrage of seemingly insignificant events that have the potential of turning their world upside down and impacting their mental well-being. Being the new kid in school, the biggest student in class, the one who talks differently than everyone else, or the one who is a different color from the the rest of the students—are all situations that can promote stress and contribute to the deterioration of the adolescent's mental health.

The issue of mental health is frequently overshadowed by the condition of mental illness and often carries with it a negative connotation.

Our society has typically focused more on helping the mentally ill get better than on helping the mentally healthy stay that way. Nowhere is this more evident than in dealing with adolescents, a population of individuals struggling to move from the freedoms of childhood to the responsibilities of adulthood. A children's mental health report recently indicated that approximately "20 percent of all children from birth through seventeen years of age suffer from a diagnosable mental, emotional, or behavioral disorder." (Mental Health Net-SAMHSA 1999). These disorders can include "depression, anxiety, attention-deficit/hyperactivity disorder conduct, and eating disorders," all of which can disrupt the individual's functioning at home, in the school, or in the community (Elsen et al. 1995).

In the period of flux known as adolescence, individuals may fall victim, as I did, to situations they clearly do not know how to deal with. What may then result is a manifestation of this uncertainty into feelings and behaviors that are perceived as indicative of emotional problems or, even worse, mental illness. A recent comment by Michael Faenza, president and CEO of the National Mental Health Association, reiterates the reality that millions of children in our country suffer from mental health disorders that are "unrecognized, misdiagnosed, and undertreated" (Mental Health Net 1999). He suggests that all individuals dealing with adolescents must realize that "mental health issues are as important as physical health issues in the total well-being of a child" (Mental Health Net 1999).

Like many of today's adolescents, I was totally unprepared to deal with the events surrounding my parents' deaths and the subsequent move to live with my brother's family. Even more significant, the adults charged with my care were equally unprepared to identify or handle the fallout from these devastating circumstances. As a result, all parties struggled, and the end result was not as good as my mother had predicted when she visited me in that dream the night of her death.

A chance reading of *The Friends* by Rosa Guy (1996) and a few of the other novels listed at the end of this chapter prompted some intense reflection on my adolescence, and I made a startling discovery. A book like one of these might have made a difference in how I dealt with my situation. Like most adolescents, I was starved for something I could relate to—something that would help me make sense of things. Seeing how someone else had handled situations or just that someone else had struggled with some of the same circumstances might have made my experiences less arduous. With that in mind we chose to write about *The

Friends. Through sharing our personal stories and reactions to the book, we hope to promote discussion of how literature can be used to help adolescents cope with the realities of their lives.

THE FRIENDS

The Friends by Rosa Guy is an American Library Association Notable Book and the first segment of a trilogy about three young black women growing up in Harlem during the early seventies. *The Friends* represents an insider's view of three adolescents from different cultures dealing with the everyday pressures of their age group, pressures that, to varying degrees, impact their mental health.

The novel begins as Phyllisia Cathy, a West Indian girl who has recently moved with her family to New York, finds life in this big city more difficult than she had expected. Life at school is not fun. She is mocked for her peculiar mannerisms; students mimic her foreign accent and ridicule her intelligence. The only person who seems genuinely interested in being her friend is Edith, another loner who "always came to school with her clothes unpressed, her stockings bagging about her legs with big holes" (5) and who seemed intent upon disrupting the class every time she entered the room. This is not someone Phyllisia wants to have as her friend, and yet, somehow, the two strike up a friendship, as Phyllisia finds herself in need of assistance when she is threatened and eventually beaten up by the class bully, Beulah.

Phyllisia's family does not seem to face the acculturation difficulties that she does. Her father, Calvin, has come to New York to make his fortune as a restaurant owner. Supported by his nearby family members and friends, he has relocated his wife and two daughters from Trinidad to Harlem. Ruby, Phyllisia's older sister, is quite the beauty and, in Phyllisia's eyes, the favorite of her father. Ruby has made the most of her looks and has done practically anything to fit in with the rest of the kids at school—a compromise Phyllisia refuses to make. Phyllisia considers her mother, Ramona, quite beautiful, almost like "a queen out of a fairy story" (25); she represents a tie to the other life that Phyllisia desperately misses and also serves as a buffer for Calvin's continual ranting and raving.

Desperate for a companion, and feeling somewhat guilty about being mean to the only person who has befriended her, Phyllisia allows her friendship with Edith to deepen. She lets Edith show her a side of life and a city that she has never known. Together they experience Phyllisia's first subway ride, take a trip to the zoo, and tour one of the largest cities in the world. When Edith shoplifts and encourages Phyllisia to do the same, something snaps, Phyllisia runs from Edith, her only thought being "that nasty little thief" (50). In her haste to escape from the lifestyle she thinks Edith represents, she ignores Edith's calls and finds herself in the middle of a riot, where she unfortunately runs into Calvin. In the nick of time Edith comes to the rescue and whisks Phyllisia home with her. Once again Phyllisia is troubled by life in this city as she sees the way Edith and her motherless family live.

The second part of the novel begins with Edith and Phyllisia as very good friends. The closeness of this friendship, however, has both good and bad elements. While the girls share many wonderful experiences as they grow up together, they also begin to face difficult moments as their friendship allows some painful introspection into their personalities and family situations.

The friendship with Edith has helped Phyllisia become more satisfied with her life. As time passes, however, Phyllisia faces an ongoing confrontation with Calvin's demands to stop associating with "those kinds" of people. He perceives his family to be of a higher status than what Edith represents. This confrontation poses a real challenge to Phyllisia, who appears to see beyond Calvin's social-climbing behavior. Eventually the pressure from Calvin and changing situations with Edith's home life combine to distance the friends. Phyllisia reluctantly turns elsewhere for companionship.

As Phyllisia struggles with the unraveling of her friendship with Edith, she is also forced to deal with her mother's illness and subsequent death. This proves to be too much for her, and part three of the novel begins with Phyllisia suffering from the nightmares and depressed behaviors that accompany uncontrolled grief. Throughout this low period in her life, Phyllisia receives support from her sister, Ruby, who has now assumed many of the roles her mother used to fill. Calvin seems oblivious to his daughters' struggles and continues to react to his wife's death with anger and by abusing his children.

Somehow, during her "illness" Phyllisia begins to realize that she really misses Edith; she desperately wants to see her, but she resists the impulse to follow through. She continually fills the void of Edith's absence by hanging out with her new companions. At one point she begins skipping school to meet a boy, but when she refuses to have sex, the affair ends and she is forced to face Calvin's outrage at her behavior.

Toward the end of the novel, Phyllisia seems to mature and seeks out her old friend. To her shock, she finds Edith alone at home. She discovers that Edith's youngest sister has died from an illness, her older brother has been shot to death by the police, and her other siblings have been placed in an orphanage by the welfare department. Edith is waiting for the welfare people to come and take her to the orphanage, where she has been given the option of caring for her brother and sister while still working to support herself. The two girls promise to maintain their friendship through visits and letters.

Phyllisia returns home to find a raging father who is insistent upon sending both daughters away. The pain of losing his wife and having to raise two adolescent daughters appears uncontrollable. Forced to face her father, Phyllisia finally manages to communicate her feelings and, through a series of negotiations, the situation is resolved and a bond between father and daughters begins to form.

REACTION TO THE NOVEL

In reading the novel, my task was to get a feeling for how well the character of Phyllisia Cathy represented normal adolescent development. Since our purpose was to provide literature that adolescents could relate to in their efforts to make sense of events in their daily lives, we wanted to make sure that at least the primary characters in our novel actually portrayed many aspects of normal adolescent development. The American Academy of Child and Adolescent Psychiatry (AACAP) has identified a number of developmental issues that most individuals face during the adolescent years. These issues are grouped into four areas: (1) movement toward independence; (2) future interests and cognitive changes; (3) sexuality; and (4) morals, values, and self-direction (March 1999). We were fortunate in our choice of *The Friends* because Phyllisia Cathy's character does manifest characteristics of a number of these developmental issues.

Phyllisia has a major struggle with the issue of her movement toward independence. Early in the novel she faces a tremendous challenge as she deals with her struggle for identity and the strangeness that she presents to the other students in her class. She speaks differently, looks somewhat different, and conducts herself differently from the rest of her classmates. Her recent immigration and the way her family, particularly her father, view their position in this new environment distances her even farther from her classmates. Her father's preconceived negative attitudes toward African Americans also create a conflict that Phyllisia must deal with daily. The ongoing conflicts with her father push Phyllisia toward a focus on her father's faults. As the novel progresses she intensifies this focus on his failings, becoming increasingly rebellious toward him and the life he wants his family to have.

The rebellion that Phyllisia presents is also indicative of the issue of morals, values, and self-direction. The changes Phyllisia is forced to make in her life create internal struggles that seem to erupt in the rebellious attitude she maintains throughout much of the novel. Part of this rebellion manifests itself in a testing of the rules and limits her father has set for her. Going places she knows he won't permit, maintaining friendships he doesn't like, and doing things that would embarrass him are all part of her struggle for self-direction. Another component of this issue relates to the development of conscience; although subtly presented, a significant aspect of the novel and Phyllisia's character is this development of conscience. It is present in her relationship with her father; she really knows what he expects of her, and worries about not doing it. She feels guilt over Edith's repeated attempts to befriend her, and she really struggles with the relationship after it has been ended.

Phyllisia also struggles with the issue of sexuality. Being forced to move from a home she loved, forced to make friends with people she really doesn't like, and forced to give up her mother, her only link with her previous life, all contribute to a struggle with changing relationships. In fact, Edith, whom Phyllisia initially dislikes, is the only stable element in her life at this point, yet she eventually rejects Edith's friendship. While this stems partly from her father's repeated insistence on "getting away from people like that," a large part of the rejection is really Phyllisia's doing. Throughout the novel she worries about being normal, something that she appears not to be, but something her sister constantly encourages her to become. Many of the moves Phyllisia makes with her friendships revolve around this issue of wanting to be normal.

Phyllisia needed support in dealing with her feelings of alienation and isolation. It was apparent that her father was not capable of identifying and discussing her needs; her sister was dealing with similar adjustments in totally different ways; her mother attempted to help her until her death; and Edith was, like Phyllisia, struggling through difficult situations. The friendship between the two girls is a result of their inability to find stability and security during tumultuous times as well as a recognition of their mutual needs. There would be many rewards in working with Phyllisia in therapy. Opportunities to express her sense of loss and displacement and to be truly heard would provide an outlet for her emotions. Reassurances that she is experiencing universal adolescent issues might boost her self-confidence and allow her to focus on her strengths (Rutter 1995). I would involve Phyllisia in group therapy with other adolescents not only to discuss issues of adjustment and family pressures but also to provide social opportunities with professional guidance and support. In addition to group therapy, I would also counsel Phyllisia individually through empathetic listening and discussion, journaling, an artistic medium, and novels, films, and short stories dealing with loss and alienation. As my co-author pointed out, young adult novels and caring teachers can make a tremendous difference in the lives of troubled adolescents.

USING THE NOVEL

I would enjoy using this novel (and others like it) in a class of middle or high school students because it is so flexible and real—quite different from some of the stories found in district mandated literature anthologies. This novel and many of those listed in the reference section readily lend themselves to thematic units and teaching. A history or social studies class, for instance, could be studying Harlem or Trinidad and their histories while the students are reading the novel in their English or language arts class. An art or music class could support this approach by studying the art and music of Trinidad or the corresponding time period in Harlem. This type of immersion in a novel really promotes thorough learning of the work and its corresponding elements. It does, however, demand more time and energy than addressing various elements of the novel in the English or language arts class.

Before having them read *The Friends*, I would have my class focus on some of the peripheral elements of the novel in a pre-reading or setting-the-stage mode. For instance, we would explore the Internet and library resources to find information about Trinidad and Harlem during the 1970s. The most effective use of time would be to present this component of the novel's study through a WebQuest (online reference) which defines web sites where students can find required information. We might also watch some video clips that depict scenes from Trinidad and Harlem during the seventies.

Then we would read the novel. While I might use basic comprehension questions to ensure that students identify important elements of the novel, much of our work would fall in the reader-response category. Students would be guided to make regular journal entries in response to what they have read and prompts that I have identified. These prompts would follow the story line, so they would vary somewhat; however, certain prompts could be used throughout the novel. For instance, early in the novel, students might be asked to write about what Phyllisia is feeling in her new school or how Edith feels as she tries to make friends with Phyllisia. Recurring prompts might revolve around how the students think Phyllisia is changing as we proceed through the novel or why her father is constantly angry with his family. The class would be involved in considerable discussion as we try to understand what Phyllisia and the other characters are going through.

In addition to the journal writing I would also engage the students in other activities designed to support and extend their understanding of the novel. One such activity would be to design a postcard for Phyllisia to send to a friend in Trinidad. With this assignment the students could illustrate their understanding of where Phyllisia is currently living by designing a postcard from Harlem or New York, or they might choose another approach and design the card from another perspective that more closely matches Phyllisia's mood or feeling. In addition to designing the postcard, the students would be required to write a message they think Phyllisia might send to this person.

Another activity to support the journal writing would be to have the students identify or write a theme song for one of the main characters in the novel. This activity is similar to writing a biopoem about a character, but it allows for more flexibility. I would keep the biopoem in reserve for students who seem to need more support than the theme song task provides. An activity that might take the place of the theme song would be a prescribed series of activities where groups of students choose a character that they are familiar with and eventually design a compact disk (songs, biography, and cover) around this individual.

A final but important aspect of teaching this novel would involve the students in responding to Phyllisia as a friend. Periodically throughout our reading of the novel I would ask the students to either e-mail or write a note to Phyllisia as her friend. Although I would like to prescribe the focus of the message, I feel more comfortable in letting the students decide what to say. Before writing the message, however, our class discussion would focus on the problems or issues confronting her and how we might help her. Another aspect of responding to Phyllisia as a friend would involve using the Internet to select sites that might be helpful to

Phyllisia in her struggles with friends and family issues. Again, an effective use of time would involve pre-identifying certain sites that would be suitable for this activity and then letting the students work among those sites. Once the students have chosen a site or sites, they would give Phyllisia the information in an e-mail or note.

CONCLUSION

Everyday struggles can readily impact an adolescent's mental health, leading to more serious mental problems and physical manifestations. The adolescents in our classrooms are experiencing more issues than we can possibly fathom, and many are dealing with them with little or no support. Teaching today's troubled teens requires the type of collaboration proposed in this series to meet the needs of our students and create young adults who can grow mentally, physically, and socially.

Forty years and hours of adult therapy later I'm beginning to believe what my mother said in my dream the night of her death . . . everything will be all right. Still, I can't help but wonder if my life could have been different. If I would have found something more to relate to, something more to think about, or someone else to talk to, would things have been different? Would I have had to wait this long to believe if only someone had put a book like this in my hands?

RECOMMENDED READINGS

Mental Health: Fiction

Alder, C. S. (1983). *The shell lady's daughter.* New York: Coward-McCann. ISBN: 0–698–20580–4. 140 pp. MS, HS.

When fourteen-year-old Kelly is sent off to Florida after her mother's nervous breakdown to stay with her rigid grandparents, she learns the meaning of love and support.

Calvert, P. (1989). *When morning comes.* New York: C. Scribner's Sons. ISBN: 0–684–19105–9. 153 pp. HS.

Fifteen-year-old Cat Kincaid, having failed to fit into a series of foster homes and finding herself stuck on a farm with an elderly female beekeeper, secretly longs for a place to be herself, not somebody she has invented.

Crutcher, C. (1983). *Running loose*. New York: Greenwillow Books. ISBN: 0–688–02002–X. 190 pp. HS.

Louie, a high school senior in a small Idaho town, learns about sportsmanship, love, and death as he matures into manhood.

Crutcher, C. (1987). *The crazy horse electric game*. New York: Greenwillow Books. ISBN: 0–688–06683–6. 215 pp. HS.

A high school athlete, frustrated at being handicapped after an accident, runs away from home and is helped back to mental and physical health by a black benefactor and the people in a special school where he enrolls.

Dessen, S. (1998). *Someone like you*. New York: Viking. ISBN: 0–670–87778–6. 281 pp. HS.

Halley's junior year of high school includes the death of her best friend Scarlett's boyfriend, the discovery that Scarlett is pregnant, and Halley's own first serious relationship.

Franklin, K. L. (1996). *Nerd no more*. Cambridge, MA: Candlewick Press. ISBN: 1–564–02674–4. 143 pp. MS.

Wiggie Carter gets himself into real trouble because he tries desperately to be a cool kid instead of a nerd with a mom who hosts a TV science show.

Grant, C. D. (1989). *Phoenix rising, or how to survive your life*. New York: Atheneum. ISBN: 0–689–31458–2. 148 pp. MS, HS.

Helen's death at eighteen from cancer shatters the lives of her parents and siblings, especially younger sister Jessie, who tries to cope with her feelings of pain and confusion by reading pages from Helen's diary.

Grant, S. D. (1992). *Shadow man*. New York: Atheneum. ISBN: 0–689–31772–7. 149 pp. HS.

Gabriel McCloud was eighteen when he died as his pickup crashed into a tree. This first-person novel portrays the effect of his death on his community.

Guy, R. (1996). *The friends*. New York: Bantam. ISBN: 0–440–22667–8. 185 pp. MS, HS.

Phyllisia Cathy realizes the role that her mother's death and her father's tyrannical behavior play in creating a rift between her and her best friend.

Hayden, T. L. (1984). *The sunflower forest.* New York: Putnam. ISBN: 0–399–12946–4. 344 pp. HS.

Torn between an intimate reality that is insane and the worldly pressures of her coming of age, seventeen-year-old Lesley musters her strength to stand firm in the face of cataclysm.

Hesse, K. (1994). *Phoenix rising.* New York: Holt. ISBN: 0–805–03108–1. 182 pp. MS, HS.

Thirteen-year-old Nyle learns about relationships and death when fifteen-year-old Ezra, who was exposed to radiation leaked from a nearby nuclear plant, comes to stay at her grandmother's Vermont farmhouse.

Hesser, T. S. (1998). *Kissing doorknobs.* New York: Delacorte. ISBN: 0–385–32329–8. 176 pp. HS.

Fourteen-year-old Tara Sullivan has obsessive-compulsive behavior disorder. This novel explores how this situation begins to control Tara's life and how she deals with it.

Johnson, A. (1998). *Gone from home: Short takes.* New York: DK Ink. ISBN: 0–789–42499–1. 112 pp. HS.

This collection of short stories identifies young people who are helping other individuals find positive answers to life's problems.

Johnson, A. (1995). *Humming whispers.* New York: Orchard Books. ISBN: 0–531–06898–6. 121 pp. HS.

When fourteen-year-old Sophy believes she is schizophrenic like her older sister, she turns to her Aunt Shirley and others for help.

Koertge, R. (1996). *Confess-O-Rama.* New York: Orchard Books. ISBN: 0–531–09515–0. 165 pp. HS.

While his mother grieves the death of her fourth husband, Tony vents his feelings to the Confess-O-Rama, never suspecting who's on the other end of the line.

Mazer, N. F. (1997). *When she was good.* New York: Arthur Levine Books. ISBN: 0–590–31990–6. 228 pp. HS.

The death of her abusive, manipulative older sister prompts seventeen-year-old Em to remember their unpleasant life together, with their parents and then later on their own.

Naylor, P. R. (1986). *The keeper.* New York: Atheneum. ISBN: 0–689–31204–0. 212 pp. MS, HS.

Junior high school student Nick must face the fact that his father is plunging fast into serious mental illness.

Nolan, H. (1997). *Dancing on the edge.* San Diego: Harcourt Brace. ISBN: 0–152–01646–5. 244 pp. HS.

A young girl from a dysfunctional family creates an alternative world for herself which nearly results in her death, but which ultimately leads her to reality.

Rodowsky, C. (1998). *The turnabout shop.* New York: Farrar, Straus and Giroux. ISBN: 0–374–37889–4. 135 pp. MS.

In "conversations" with her dead mother, fifth grader Livvy records her adjustments to living in Baltimore with a woman she had never met, and she comes to see the wisdom of her mother's choice as she gets to know the woman's large, loving family.

Silsbee, P. (1984). *The big way out: A novel.* Scarsdale, NY: Bradbury Press. ISBN: 0–027–82670–8. 180 pp. MS, HS.

Fourteen-year-old Paul tries to save his family after it is split apart over his father's inevitable return to a mental hospital.

Sinykin, S. C. (1991). *Next thing to strangers.* New York: Lothrop, Lee and Shepard. ISBN: 0–688–10694–3. 147 pp. MS, HS.

While visiting their grandparents at a trailer park in Arizona, a diabetic boy and an overweight girl become friends and learn a lesson about self-acceptance.

Sirof, H. (1996). *Bring back yesterday.* New York: Atheneum. ISBN: 0–689–80638–8. 167 pp. MS, HS.

When her parents die in a plane crash, thirteen-year-old Lisa escapes from her grief and her new life with her aunt through returning to the past and an imaginary playmate.

Westall, R. (1996). *Gulf.* New York: Scholastic. ISBN: 0–590–22218–X. 101 pp. MS, HS.

Tom Higgins, a British schoolboy during the Persian Gulf War, narrates his younger brother's struggle with an apparent mental illness or mystery of nature which drives the child to assume the role of an Iraqi.

Mental Health: Nonfiction

Barden, R. (1989). *Fears and phobias.* New York: Crestwood House. ISBN: 0–896–86441–3. 47 pp. MS, HS.

Explains the differences between fears, phobias, and anxieties, and includes some of the most frequent ones.

Gopaul-McNicol, S. (1993). *Working with West Indian families.* New York: Guilford Press. ISBN: 0–898–62229–8. 212 pp. HS, Adult.

Presents a comprehensive assessment of West Indian families living in North America and considerations counselors should employ when treating West Indian families.

Jamiolkowski, R. (1993). *Coping in a dysfunctional family.* New York: Rosen. ISBN: 0–823–91660–X. 130 pp. MS, HS.

Discusses different causes of family problems, including physical and emotional abuse, overprotection, depression or mental illness, and perfectionism and suggests ways of dealing with each situation.

McCoy, K, and C. Wibbelsman (1996). *Life happens.* New York: Berkley. ISBN: 0–399–51987–4. 213 pp. MS, HS.

A teenager's guide to friends, failure, sexuality, love, rejection, addiction, peer pressure, families, loss, depression, change, and other challenges of living.

Ponterotto, J., M. Casas, L. Suzuki, and C. Alexander, eds. (1995). *Handbook of multicultural counseling.* Thousand Oaks, CA: Sage. ISBN: 0–803–95506–5.

Presents a comprehensive review of the literature on the history of multicultural counseling, theoretical approaches to working with clients from diverse backgrounds, and recommendations for treatment.

INTERNET RESOURCES

American Academy of Child and Adolescent Psychiatry. *http://www.aacap.org*

A comprehensive site for information about childhood and adolescent mental health and illness.

Mental Health Net—Child Resources. *http://www.cmhc.com/guide/children.htm*

A twenty-page list of resources related to childhood and adolescent mental health development. This is an excellent list for any individual working with children and adolescents.

REFERENCES

Eisen, A. R., C. E. Schaefer, C. A. Kearney. (1995). *Clinical handbook of anxiety disorders in children and adolescents.* New York: Aronson. ISBN: 1–568–21294–1.

March, J. (1999). *Anxiety disorders in children and adolescents.* New York: Guilford Press. ISBN: 0–898–62834–2.

Rutter, M. (1995). *Psychosocial disturbances in young people: Challenges for prevention.* Cambridge: Cambridge University Press. ISBN: 0–521–46187–1.

CHAPTER 8

The Craziness Within and the Craziness Without: Depression and Anger in *Ironman*

John Noell Moore and David William Hartman

> Kids' isolation in adolescence can be broken with good stories. Their behavior doesn't look like they're scared, but it looks like anger. When we give students stories that talk about what they're going through, we give them a witness.
>
> Chris Crutcher

Students are fascinated by Chris Crutcher's fiction. Why do adolescents like these books so much? The answer is simple: they often see themselves in his characters; Crutcher's novels "give them a witness" to their struggles for identity and selfhood. Crutcher invites us to look deeply into the worlds he creates, and *Ironman*, published in 1995, transports us into the world of Bo Brewster, a depressed and angry young man who is one of the isolated kids to whom Crutcher refers in the epigraph. He is also one of the narrators of the novel, telling us part of the story in the epistolary format in which Crutcher has cast his story. As Bo writes letters to Larry King, the popular talk show host, he writes them to himself and to us as well. As we move with him through the troubling days of *Ironman*, we see how he breaks his own isolation through the power of story.

SCENE ONE

It's 8:30 on a mid-November morning in the local high school. Miss Wahlberg's senior English class is engaged in a lively discussion of *The*

Taming of the Shrew. They've recently seen one of Miss Wahlberg's favorite film versions, a live performance by the San Francisco Repertory Company in commedia de l'arte style. Right away they recognized handsome star Marc Singer in his role as the outrageously macho Petruchio. This morning's escalating debate centers on this question: Is Katherine tamed in the play? Gender issues bounce off the walls; the conversation heats up. Miss Wahlberg smiles and moves toward the back of the room to observe and enjoy the moment.

On her way she notices that Henry Hudson, normally attentive and conversational, is unusually silent this morning, looking beyond the glass that separates him from the graying late autumn world outdoors. He seems oblivious to the buzz around him, and Miss Wahlberg is puzzled. He has been arriving for class just before the bell, sitting in what looks like a daze, and leaving without comment the minute the bell rings.

In an effort to encourage him, she moves near him, asking, "What do you think about all this gender business, Henry?"

"Dunno. Nothing, I guess." He avoids looking at her, his shock of auburn hair masking his eyes.

Miss Wahlberg makes a mental note to chat about this with Anne Alger, her Guidance Department colleague. She suspects that Henry's lethargy, his failure to complete his work on time, and his disinterest in what's going on around him are signs of depression, and she thinks he might use some help from the counselor.

SCENE TWO

As Miss Wahlberg moves to the back of the room, she stops near Matt Higgins' desk. Lately she's noticed that Matt has been irritable, anxious, and extremely critical of the class and the work she asks them to do with her.

"What do you think about this gender business, Matt?"

"Think of *what?*" Matt snarls. "I don't give a damn about gender or about Shakespeare. It's just a *#@# play!" He angrily faces the class.

"Here's what I think of this stupid conversation. Men are men and women are women. This gender crap—forget it. This class, Shakespeare, and you, Miss Wahlberg, always telling us, 'Our language constructs us'—that's all crap, too." His face reddens, and he gesticulates wildly.

"Man, I am outta here." With that, he swirls out of his desk, yanks his red backpack from the floor, and bolts out of the room, slamming the door on his astonished classmates.

Miss Wahlberg attempts damage control, letting her students talk freely about what has just happened, then bringing the discussion back to the play. She thinks, "It's just a few minutes to the bell, and I'd better get right on this when class is over." She decides to ask Sandy Hapgood, the disciplinary principal, to look into the matter. She fears that Matt is potentially dangerous and should probably not attend classes for the rest of the day. Does she think that Matt, like Henry, is depressed? Probably not. She associates depression with withdrawal, but she sees Matt's behavior as a disciplinary issue, and she fears for the safety of the people at her school.

Anger leading to violence in public schools has been front page news in this country. In the 1998–1999 school year, it erupted in October in Pearl, Mississippi; in December in Paducah, Kentucky; in March in Jonesboro, Arkansas; and in April in Littleton, Colorado. "How could this happen?" people everywhere asked.

The kind of violence erupting in schools across America does not take place in Chris Crutcher's *Ironman*, in which Bo Brewster, Crutcher's angry young man, receives therapy and learns to recognize his depression and then to deal with the anger that comes from it. Bo's depression results from a broken relationship with his angry, domineering father, a relationship borne of family guilt and grief. Learning to recognize and deal with his anger, Bo also learns to cope with his depression.

Crutcher sets the story in the context of a triathlon that tests Bo's physical, emotional, mental, and spiritual abilities. As Bo trains for the triathlon, he gets help from a number of sources. As we read and draw out his character, we see how depression leads to anger, and we also see how personal writing, physical training, and group therapy can heal the mind and the heart and renew the spirit.

DEPRESSION

Depression as illness serves as a symbol of the wear and tear of living in our stressed-out world. Cures for depression are everywhere. Television ads proffer the healing powers of herbal medicine in St.-John's-wort. Men and women with calm voices beckon us to check into stately homes turned into mental health care centers so we can work through our despair and overcome our sense of hopelessness. Literature abounds, from scholarly journal articles to media for the masses. Recently someone who knew that I was writing on this subject handed me the pamphlet *Climbing Up from Depression*. It offers plain advice for coping with depression in a sequence of actions: "know what you're dealing with; reach out for help; tend to your feelings; take small definite steps toward hope; be gentle and generous with yourself; and take heart" (Bradshaw & Weber 1996, 3–7). Written for a large general audience, it identifies these symptoms of depression:

- Feeling sad, pessimistic, dissatisfied, guilty, worthless, helpless, hopeless
- Loss of interest in things that used to give pleasure
- Sleep difficulties or the desire to sleep all the time
- Problems with concentration, memory, and decision-making
- Lack of energy, fatigue
- Nervousness, anxiety, irritability
- Loss of appetite or weight gain
- Heart palpitations, dizziness, or recurrent and unexplained aches
- Suicidal thoughts (2–3).

These signs of depression match Ava Siegler's "warning signs of adolescent depression" (1997, 194) and are well documented elsewhere in recent scientific literature: Bell et al. (1998, 173); Steinberg and Levine (1997, 172); Pipher (1994, 149–150); Oster and Montgomery (1995, 5–7); Laufer (1995, 3–20); and Williams (1995, 14–16, 143). Bo Brewster exhibits many of the typical signs of depression, and when I first talked to David Hartman about collaborating with him on this chapter, we discussed the sources of depression in adolescents.

DEPRESSION IN ADOLESCENTS

David Hartman is a distinguished Virginia psychiatrist who is the first blind person in the United States to earn an M.D. He also earned a degree in psychiatry and recently completed studies in therapy for adolescents.

"What brings on depression in adolescence?" I ask.

"I connect it to the moves from childhood to adolescence and adulthood," Hartman tells me. "Kids aged nine to ten, eleven, and twelve are wrapped up in their parents; they're connected and happy. But at ages thirteen and fourteen they want to branch out, to connect to their peer groups, and a consequent struggle begins between parent and child because the child wants to spend more time with friends than with family. This conflict is played out in numerous scenarios. Parents may worry about the kinds of friends their adolescents are developing; as a result, parents exercise more control, which leads the adolescent to pull away, to rebel. This early rebellion may then lead to more complete rebellion against parents as authority figures."

"Rebellion like this can escalate into a battle between the parents' efforts to restrict the behavior and the adolescent's increased efforts toward greater personal freedom. For example, an adolescent girl and her friends may want to do things that the parents consider bizarre, such as dressing all in black, maybe reading about and talking about satanic rituals. Parents fear the outcomes of such behaviors, restrict the adolescent girl's contact with friends even more, and the girl, feeling more and more isolated, falls into a severe depression."

"Why," I want to know, "do parents struggle against their children's efforts to be unique, different?"

"Sometimes," Hartman responds, "parents resist the process of individuation because it separates them from their children. If conflicts continue, adolescents can feel totally abandoned by the parents on whom they have formerly relied completely. Here's another example. A girl and a guy fall deeply in love, and for some reason, one leaves the other. This sense of abandonment can lead to depression, too. Or in the struggle of adolescents to explore their identity, the parents are unclear as to when they should push or pull back, and from the adolescent's viewpoint, the parents make the wrong move at the wrong time."

"Depression in adolescents can also result from a mismatch in the genetic system of child and parent," Hartman continues. "An obsessive compulsive military type of parent is trying to raise a child who is artistic and romantic, who prefers to spend his time daydreaming and doing things that are not valued by the parent. The child is never able to fulfill his parent's wishes and to develop into the kind of adolescent that the parent envisions as a source of pride and as a reflection of the parent's concept of good parenting."

Hartman explains that schools sometimes fail to focus clearly on the problem of a student with attention deficit hyperactivity disorder (ADHD). The child is "wired" and gets marked as a bad child. The result is that the student feels different from all his or her friends or has real trouble making friends. In the absence of friends, adolescents rebel against parents and fall into loneliness, despair, and, finally, depression. Sometimes this leads to the extreme, to feeling that the only way out is to kill oneself.

"Adolescence is so turbulent; everything seems exaggerated; the smallest things can become overwhelming. When a boyfriend and a girl-friend break up or when there's a bad report card which angers parents, some teens cannot cope," Hartman tells me as we continue our conversation. "They decide that life is too tough, not worth living, and they try suicide. Girls tend to overdose on drugs, but this is usually ineffectual, and they become hysterical. Boys turn to firearms, and the results are often fatal. Occasionally boys overdose. In many cases, alcohol is involved with the suicide or the suicide attempt. Sometimes drug abuse precipitates depression, such as in the case where kids get involved with drinking and clique dynamics. Then abuses of alcohol and marijuana can also lead to depression."

"The struggle of adolescence is to try to make sense of all the life-changing information that's coming into the psyche. In my research I've focused recently on these major issues we've been discussing—the separation from parents, individuation, the need to have mastery and competence in one's own life."

"Do teens understand that many factors make them who they are becoming? That they are not solely responsible for their maturation? To use fancy terminology, do they understand that they are really socially constructed, actually made by all the forces that intersect in their lives?" I inquire.

"No, they don't. I'll use my fifteen-year-old son as an example. He is staunchly determined about what he can do; he is quick to say, 'I did that *on my own.*' " Hartman slows down and deliberately emphasizes these last words in the way that his son might say them.

ADOLESCENT DEPRESSION AND ADOLESCENT LITERATURE

In our second meeting Hartman and I talk about the book we want to write about. He suggests that we look for a book in which a young person struggles with the separation from parents in the pursuit of a unique identity. He gives an example of a story in which a boy in Canada, trying to cope with the death of his father, falls into depression. He can't begin to recover until he puts together a team of dogs and enters a race; his commitment to the team and to the victory pulls him out of depression.

"Lots of depression in teenagers stems from loss," Hartman notes. "I've always been fascinated with John Knowles' *A Separate Peace* and the process Gene Forrester goes through in order to come to grips with his identity after the death of his classmate, Phineas."

We talk about several books appropriate for our study of adolescent depression and its manifestation in anger. We decide on Chris Crutcher's *Ironman*, not just because the book is a young adult novel version of the father-son problems in *The Great Santini*, but because Bo Brewster is an athlete, a competitive swimmer, and so is Hartman. We agree quickly.

Hartman speaks very casually about his reading, which surprised me at first since he has been blind since he was eight. I have known David Hartman for about a decade; I first met him when he came to my high school to speak at a career exploration day. I admired his unique combination of intellectual brilliance and the human touch, but I had been somewhat self-conscious about his blindness. I learned how the sighted can sometimes be awkward in dealing with the blind when I invited Hartman to speak to a group at a nearby college. It was getting dark when we arrived at the meeting room.

"Wait a second," I told him as I opened the door, "and I'll turn on the light for you." His laugh startled me.

"Now I know that you're comfortable with my blindness," he said, "because you've started treating me normally."

When Hartman talks about his reading, he means that he listens to books on tape and that his wife reads to him. His computer can also read to him, and his printer prints in Braille.

Hartman uses fiction as part of his treatment for patients of all ages: "Often literature is a much more powerful teacher than a self-help book. I really like giving a novel to someone rather than giving them a book that focuses directly on a psychological issue they're dealing with." Hartman's use of books to help people deal with their psychological lives is a version of bibliotherapy, a term coined in 1916. A more recent definition of the term is "the guided reading of written materials in gaining understanding or solving problems relevant to a person's therapeutic needs" (Riordan & Wilson 1989, 506). Modern bibliotherapy does not suggest that a child or adolescent with problems "can be 'fixed' by the proper application of the right book" (Myracle 1995, 40). Instead, bibliotherapy is effective because it allows the reader to identify with a character and realize that he or she is not the only person with a particular problem. Experiencing a character's process of working through a problem, "the reader is emotionally involved in the struggle and ultimately achieves insight about his or her situation" (Shrodes 1955, 24). Helping students find powerful books and encouraging conversation about their characters helps to draw them out in all directions. In drawing out a character such as Bo Brewster, young readers make a personal connection that helps them draw out themselves. When they make this link, they may open themselves up to new possibilities, and, perhaps, move toward healing.

IRONMAN

Ironman is an unusual book from a therapist's perspective because Bo Brewster receives therapy through his own personal writing and through the school's anger management group. David Hartman will discuss the nature of Bo's therapies, and as a way of introducing his reading of the novel, I will explain how Bo's story is told to us. From my perspective as an English teacher, one of the most fascinating characteristics of *Ironman* is its format. It weaves together two storytellers whose accounts alternate throughout the novel. Bo Brewster writes letters to talk show host Larry King that tell us what Bo is thinking and doing. An omniscient second narrator tells us what is going on in other locales in the story, places where Bo is not. In this way, Crutcher allows readers to construct the story from multiple angles; we're able to draw out many of the characters in the novel and to contextualize Bo's experiences from a much broader angle of vision than if we had to rely only on Bo for the story.

Bo Brewster is a high school senior and a talented athlete, but he is also an angry young man. He is suspended from school because he cannot control his anger; in order to return to classes, he's required to attend an anger management class run by a Japanese man, Mr. Nakatani. The group meets before school, and through his interactions with group members, including his girlfriend Shelly, he learns the sources of his anger and how to control it. Throughout this process he writes letters to Larry King, explaining that he wants to write his memoirs and that he'll give King exclusive rights to a television interview. He doesn't mail the letters, but they are Bo's personal therapy, helping him understand his relationships with Coach Redmond, Lionel Serbousek, his parents, and his peers. Within this large-scale architectural design Crutcher builds his story in many small, complementary sections. Each chapter follows a multisection plan, and some chapters are structurally complicated as Crutcher provides the details of Bo's story.

The story of Bo's girlfriend Shelly demonstrates that adolescent depression and anger are not just a macho thing, a maturing boy's defensive reaction to a perceived offense to his masculinity. Shelly reveals that her history has included treatment in a residential center during junior high and being thrown out of three high schools. She reached a point, she tells Bo, where she was always worn down, depressed, tired of perpetually being in trouble, of having people hate or fear her, and worst, sick of being alone. Her inner turmoil expressed itself physically as her weight yo-yoed from as much as 160 pounds to as little as 103.

When she arrived at Clark Fork High School, Shelly acted out her anger, and Coach Redmond threw her off the basketball team. Bo wonders how Shelly could be the person that she has become after living through such nightmares. He thinks about the power that men like Redmond have over others: "Where does it come from and how do you fight it?" (118). He gets some insight into this power in a conversation with Lionel Serbousek. His struggles are part of being an adolescent, Lion tells him, and although Bo has to fight some battles, he encourages him to look "past the current war" to "separate from your dad to establish who you are" (123).

Bo's problems emerge in response to the common experience that all the anger management group members share: "We all lost something," Shelly tells them. "We lost the truth" (169). Later, Bo explains to Larry what truths he is discovering about himself; anger covers his fear, he realizes, and he will not control his anger until he admits his fear. Anger is natural, Shelly says. Through therapy Bo feels that he is "being handed a secret of the universe" (180), learning to destroy the "monster that lived inside me" (182). Symbolically, he signs his letter "Tower of Power" (183).

At the beginning of the triathlon Bo talks with Lonnie Gerback, an opponent who gives him insight into father-son relationships. Bo's father has given Gerback an expensive ($500) bicycle so that he can outrace Bo. The plan backfires, though, when Gerback gives the bike to Bo. "Why?" Bo asks. Gerback offers two reasons. First, in giving Wyrack, Bo's archrival and a favorite to win, such fierce competition, Bo has been a good model of endurance for Gerback. Second, Gerback's father has cautioned him against getting involved in the "war" (206) between Bo and his father, Lucas Brewster, asking him to consider how he'd feel if he were in Bo's shoes. Gerback's wise father tells his son that if he ever wants "to see how something works, look at it broken" (207). The father's advice highlights the brokenness of Bo's relationship with his father, which is the primary source of Bo's depression. Bo doesn't win the triathlon, but he finishes ahead of Wyrack, and that is what matters to him.

As the novel ends, we see how Mr. Nakatani is a father figure for Bo. Nak tells the story of his own personal tragedy. Years ago, driving drunk cost him the lives of his three small children, two daughters and a son. Nak is tortured, but he has learned that in order to heal, "you beg the universe to teach you the quality of mercy" (199). Bo credits Nak's influence; he tells Larry King that Nakatani has pulled everything together for him.

What is the transforming power of mercy? In his final meeting with the anger management group, Mr. Nakatani explains that mercy "excuses nothing, but it allows for all things" (226). He uses the lives of the people in the group as examples—his story and Bo's. Nak's last words to the group serve as a metaphor for the witness that books can give to adolescents struggling with depression and the traumas of the psyche: "I been payin' attention to other folks' lives—an' learnin' some while I was at it—but now it's time to start payin' attention to my own" (227). He will return to Texas, where his life fell apart, he says, to pick up the pieces and move on.

In his final letter to Larry King, Bo chooses a stance similar to Nakatani's. Armed with new knowledge, he will go forward. His father is seeing a therapist, but Bo will not count on the outcome of that. He can count, however, on his own ability to cope. After eight months in anger management he knows that he has "the power to let the world be every bit as goddamn crazy as it is" (228). In learning to understand the craziness within, Bo Brewster feels confident that he can face the craziness without.

DR. HARTMAN READS *IRONMAN*

Ironman vividly depicts the life of a high school senior who falls into a deep depression characterized by anger and rebellion. His anger stems from a childhood with many intense conflicts with a very critical and overly punitive father. As the novel opens Bo has quit the football team because Coach Redmond has severely humiliated him in front of his teammates. Redmond is also Bo's English teacher, and he confronts Bo in class, again humiliating him publicly. In a fit of temper, Bo lashes out, calling the coach an asshole, which results in his suspension from school. There are other manifestations of Bo's depression—he has been skipping school, has had trouble turning in his assignments on time, and has been having trouble sleeping. Bo may return to Redmond's class only if he attends the school's anger management class.

As the novel unfolds we learn that Bo's parents are divorced, that his father has been a very demanding and inflexible parent, and that Bo's mother has not been strong enough to confront the father. Lucas Brewster's attitude is revealed when Bo awakens his father by shutting a door too loudly. His father makes him close the door ten times to learn how to close it quietly. Humiliated and belittled, Bo gets frustrated and slams the door violently. His father demands that he repeat the entire process, but Bo refuses and is consequently banished to his room for three months. He cannot join in the normal family routines, and his father insists that he stay in his room throughout the Christmas holidays. Neither Bo nor Mr. Brewster will give in on occasions such as this, and anger becomes part of Bo's emerging self-concept. In the incident with Redmond, Bo relives the struggle with his father, and he reacts in the same way, by lashing out in anger. As we learn more about Bo, he tells us how his anger has become a motivating force in this life. He has been able to turn his rage into powerful positive energies, and he has set a major goal for himself, completing the Ironman triathlon. Placing these physical demands on his body is therapeutic for him—exercise generates endorphins that help relieve the intensity of his depression. By using his anger to drive his exercise, Bo inadvertently treats his own depression. After his suspension from high school, he goes to the college gym to work out, and recurring images of Coach Redmond motivate him to push himself to the maximum. He finds that the process of training enables him to focus his thoughts, and he gains self-confidence in the success of his workouts.

Early in his story Bo reveals his fear of looking deeply into himself and confronting his anger. He sees Mr. Nakatani as a man with an uncanny ability to look inside others, and he tells us about his fears of what Mr. Nak will tell him about himself. We may also see another fear of group therapy here, the fear that if he is forced to give up his anger he will discover that there is nothing left inside him. Bo is a proud young man, and he is worried about being humiliated in front of others in the anger management group. After his first meeting with the group, he writes a letter to Larry King and describes his emotional reaction to the group. At the end of the letter he says that he is going for a run. Again, exercise helps Bo cope with situations that make him anxious. Mr. Nakatani helps group members become aware of the disjuncture that occurs when other people's words have told them they were okay but their abusive actions have sent the opposite message. He shares his hatred of the disparity between word and deed, his hatred of other people telling him how he feels or is supposed to feel, and recalls how his adolescent depression led to anger. Nakatani's explanation vividly describes how teenagers feel as they struggle with what adults tell them about how they ought to feel or behave. Adult intervention usually causes teenagers to feel worse and, consequently, to direct their anger inward. When they do so, their bad feelings intensify and spiral downward into depression that can precipitate both emotional and physical conflicts, as we see in the stories of the adolescents in Nakatani's group.

At the heart of Bo's depression is his relationship with his father, who, Bo says, has left bruises on the inside. His main critique of his dad is that Mr. Brewster will never take the time to listen to his side of the story. Whenever Bo gets in trouble at school, his dad automatically assumes that Bo is wrong, and he takes the teacher's side. Bo feels abandoned, disregarded. While his father makes a reasonable argument that Bo should learn to get along with authority figures even though he might not agree with them, Bo effectively counters that he has been working two jobs for several years without being fired. With bosses who have been less than ideal, Bo feels that his success demonstrates that he has been a good worker and that he deserves credit which his father refuses to give him. His father is nearly impossible to please. In Bo's story, Crutcher stresses the traumatic effects of humiliation on the adolescent psyche. Too often teachers and coaches use humiliation as a tool to punish, and, they think, to instruct students. Unfortunately these adults fail to realize that humiliation is never a good way to teach students in either sports or the classroom. Teenagers are vulnerable; they need support, not humiliation. When Bo tries to explain this to his father, Mr. Brewster hears the words, but he does not hear the message. Mr. Brewster's failure to respect Bo's point of view further widens the gap between father and son. At group meetings Mr. Nakatani discusses the power that fathers have over teenagers. He explores the relationship between another group member, Elvis, and his father. When Elvis says that his father intimidates him, Nak understands why. Elvis' father is physically much larger than the boy. In Nakatani's exploration of this relationship, Crutcher suggests that the physical size of Elvis' father may serve as a metaphor—fathers in general have a larger-than-life impact on their sons. They should approach all dealings with their sons with respect for the difficulty of growing into manhood.

In Bo's Christmas Eve visit to his father, Crutcher gives us a glimpse of how Mr. Brewster feels about the father-son issues. He can tell Bo that he wants to be close and that he wants to love him, but his actions negate his words in his compulsion to maintain a critical attitude that he believes is required if he is to raise Bo properly. He sacrifices the warmth of a personal connection to the life lessons he thinks Bo needs to learn. Mr. Brewster is caught in his own struggle—on the one hand, he'd like to love Bo as he is, but, on the other hand, he feels he must enforce at all costs the rules he has established. He creates his own disjuncture between compassion and control. As Bo talks, his father softens, and a breakthrough seems possible, but it does not arrive. Struggling against his sadness, Mr. Brewster drops the topic, and the subsequent conversation leads to more conflict. For example, when Bo talks about his girlfriend Shelly, his father is critical; he is critical, too, of the anger management group. Originally he was a strong advocate for Bo's participation in the group because he considered it a form of punishment that could bring Bo back in line. Now, however, realizing that group therapy is helping Bo address critical issues related to his own anger, Mr. Brewster denigrates Mr. Nak's group. As he tries to turn Bo against Nak we realize the issue—both Mr. Brewster and Coach Redmond, who is also encouraging Bo to leave the group, feel that their power over the boy is being threatened. Perhaps they fear that their own inadequacies will be uncovered if Bo remains in group therapy any longer. In addition to feeling threatened by Bo's relationship with Mr. Nakatani as a surrogate father figure, Lucas Brewster fears the consequences of Bo's closeness to Lionel Serbousek, a supportive teacher whom he fears may be a better father to his son than he has been. Lionel Serbousek plays a key role in Bo's life as he helps him cope with his father's power. Consequently, Mr. Brewster disparages Serbousek by telling Bo that his teacher friend is gay, a revelation that further increases the distance between Bo and his father. Nakatani also acts as a father in helping Bo realize that Lionel Serbousek's homosexuality should not be a reason to stop being his friend.

Bo's sense of his masculinity becomes an issue at this point in the novel. He often says with good humor that Shelly is stronger than he is and very supportive. When his college arch rival Wyrack calls him a weakling and attacks him, Shelly defends Bo. All boys struggle with their emerging masculinity during adolescence, so many of Bo's feelings are very natural. Caught between his father's harsh and constant disapproval and his gay teacher's support, Bo's masculine identity becomes a big issue for him. His poor self-concept, arising from this conflicted identity, exacerbates his depression. Mr. Nak helps Bo realize that he is frightened, that his fear is driving his anger. Larry King functions as a father figure, too. In his many unmailed letters to the talk show superstar, Bo writes freely, discovers what he thinks, and gains insight into how his mind and body work. The letters become a therapeutic journal, a tool that has the power to help young people confronting difficulties in the passage from childhood to adulthood.

Issues of love, hate, anger, and fear are often sources of adolescent depression. The group members bond and rally to support each other. As the novel moves forward, Bo copes with the consequences of his depression. Beating the opposition in the triathlon becomes a metaphor for winning out over his illness, for controlling anger, for achieving understanding. When Mr. Redmond, for example, requests that Bo leave Nakatani's group, Bo refuses politely, explaining that he is learning to deal with his fears and that he needs the group. Another interpretation is that Bo is handling himself better because he is feeling that the void left in his life by his father's abandonment is being filled by Mr. Nakatani and the group and Lionel Serbousek. He feels less isolated, a major cause of his depression. He belongs somewhere, and he is confident in his adolescent supporters. So, here is the dilemma—the struggle between the craziness within and the craziness without. The moment situates Bo in two worlds, the psychical and the physical. If they collide, catastrophe results. If they complement one another, they can create a powerful tension that leads to mental and spiritual harmony.

From this moment the novel speeds forward, its pace paralleling the upcoming triathlon. A crucial event in this momentum occurs in an explosive scene in which father figure and father meet. Nakatani goes to Brewster's Sporting Goods store to talk. Brewster's first response is predictable; he asks if Bo is dropping out of anger management as he dropped out of football. When Nakatani suggests that Bo's problems might be solved if he could resolve the anger issue with his father, Brewster responds defensively. Like many parents, Brewster cannot see that he can help reduce the power struggle through compassion and compromise.

Ironman dramatizes the fact that being a parent is one of the most challenging roles adults can assume in life. Parents often feel that they are inadequate, too, and as children become adolescents, it is easier to respond with the quickness of anger than it is to confront issues of disagreement head on and try to settle these differences. Such differences are normal in the adolescent individuation process. A parent's anger all too often spreads to the child, becoming a malignant tumor that eats away at the parent-child relationship. That relationship is the most critical element of parents' ability to influence their children in positive and nurturing ways.

On the night before the Ironman competition, Bo wants to be alone and to reflect on the next day's test. He camps at a spot where he and his father used to fish, and during the night he tries to recapture the sense of the love they shared when he was a little boy. He remembers how his father taught him to fish and his patience as he allowed the boy to bring in a little fish by himself. When the fishing line gets caught in twigs and rocks, his father patiently untangled it and let Bo bring in the fish alone. This memory serves as a metaphor for how a father can nurture a son's discovery. Now, however, in contrast to that idyllic moment, Mr. Brewster feels obligated to manipulate and control his son's life. Instead of untangling the lifelines that crisscross Bo's world, Mr. Brewster complicates issues, entangling the metaphoric fishing line to ensure his son's defeat. As Bo emerges into manhood, Mr. Brewster seems threatened by his loss of control in his son's life; he panics and exerts too much control, an abuse of power that could destroy a young man lacking Bo's mettle.

Bo does not win the Ironman triathlon, but he defeats Wyrack thanks to Lonnie Gerback's gift of the fast bike and the help of the therapy group who support him on the running, swimming, and biking legs of the race. At the starting block Bo comes face to face with his father. Symbolically the moment represents that Bo's real battle is not with Wyrack or the other competitors but with his father. The moment also symbolizes the brokenness of the father-son relationship. Most fathers would be present to cheer on their sons, but Bo's father is there to challenge him, to watch him lose, to teach him a lesson. Mr. Brewster is present as the biological parent, but he is absent as the loving father. Subsequently, Bo writes the final chapter of his story in a letter to Larry King. After the race, he reveals, Mr. Brewster disappeared and had little contact with Bo before his high school graduation. One interpretation of Brewster's absence is that his father assumed Bo was a quitter, that he would not complete the race just as he had not completed the football season. When Bo proves him wrong, Mr. Brewster's belief in his parenting approach is shattered. At graduation when he asks Bo what he wants for a present, Bo requests that his dad go to counseling with him. They give it a try, but Mr. Brewster cannot endure the psychological stress. In a therapy session Bo discovers that his father was also harshly disciplined as a child. In fact, in a parallel to Bo's trauma in the door-closing episode, his father reveals that he endured a similar experience as a child. Once he left a corral gate open, the cattle roamed free, and a bull worth several thousand dollars was killed on the highway. This scene at the counselor's office is too much for Mr. Brewster, and as the novel ends, Bo tells us that he has not seen his father since that day, although he has noticed his father's car parked at the therapist's office on occasion. The novel ends with Mr. Nakatani's lesson on the quality of mercy, his plans to return to Texas, and Bo's affirmation that he has to "let the world be every bit as goddamn crazy as it is" (228).

Bo's depression and its consequent anger seem to have responded to a number of therapeutic approaches. First, in the anger management group he develops friends he can trust and who support him when he feels abandoned by his father. Second, the insight he gains from the group members allows him to forgive and go forward with his life despite the way he has been mishandled by the significant others in his life, including his parents and Coach Redmond. Third, from the Ironman race he learns how the body can heal the mind through vigorous physical exertion, how the release of powerful endorphins arms his psyche in the battle with anger. Fourth, his girlfriend helps him accept who he is and who he does not have to be. From her love he learns that he does not have to be macho man, a rough and tough guy without sensitivity. Fifth, Nakatani and Serbousek help him see that fear drives his anger, and that confronting fear head on leads to victory in the race of life.

When we think of what a psychiatrist does, listening is probably at the top of the list of healing modalities. Bo offers Larry King an indirect compliment by telling him that he should become a shrink because he has listened—although King has been unaware, since Bo did not mail the letters. King does, however, learn Bo's story, and he responds to him once in the novel. Shelly has sent the celebrity some of Bo's letters, and the therapy group asks King to tape a pep talk to Bo that is played to him on the last leg of the triathlon. Crutcher's novel demonstrates his belief in the power of listening as therapeutic modality. Frequently during the novel he portrays Bo's father as a nonlistener who misses the goodness and beauty of his son. Even without his father's support Bo achieves a number of victories. Through the love of surrogate fathers and good friends, Bo confronts the craziness within—in his mind and heart—and the craziness without—what the world throws at him. He learns that to achieve a measure of happiness a person needs to understand the power of compassion and to stay in touch with his feelings. At the end of the novel, we realize that the Ironman is a metaphor for both physical and emotional endurance, that the powerful body complements the healthy mind, and that, in the end, we cannot run the race alone.

RECOMMENDED READINGS

Depression: Recommended Reading for Young Adults

Armstrong, J. (1996). *The dreams of Maihre Mehan.* New York: Knopf. ISBN: 0–679–88557–9. 199 pp. HS.

Civil War losses lead to depression in Maihre Mehan, an Irish immigrant, whose dreams of a bright future in America seem futile: "when you have nothing at all, a dream will only lead you into dreaming forever" (70). At first she resists the fall into depression, into "shards and fragments" (65), because of the encouragement of Walt Whitman, whom she meets while nursing the wounded in Washington, D.C. By the end of the novel, though, her spirit is broken, and she hopes that, like the wounded soldiers, she will be "put together and be whole again" (119). Poems by Whitman introduce each section of the novel.

Bennett, J. (1990). *I can hear the mourning dove.* New York: Scholastic. ISBN: 0–590–16309–4. 197 pp. HS.

Sixteen-year-old Grace suffers from a curable form of schizophrenia that has grown out of her depression following her father's death. Her mother, also depressed over the death, doesn't know how to help her. They move to a different city where Grace attends a new school and her mother begins a new teaching job. All this change is too much for Grace, but she makes new friends in Dee Dee and Luke, who are able to help her deal with her sense of hopelessness and helplessness.

Bridgers, S. E. (1981). *Notes for another life.* New York: Knopf. ISBN: 0–394–94889–0. 250 pp. HS.

In small-town America, Wren and Kevin Jackson's nuclear family disintegrates when their father Tom is committed to a mental hospital and their mother moves to the city to pursue a career. Left in the care of their grandparents, both teenagers must deal with their loss. Wren, a talented pianist, dreams of a musical career (these are the "notes" for another life). A broken wrist cuts short Kevin's season as the senior star tennis player, and their mother returns to begin divorce proceedings. Kevin falls into a depression and contemplates suicide. A strong family faith keeps him from shattering.

Creech, S. (1994). *Walk two moons*. New York: HarperTrophy. ISBN: 0–06–440517–6. 280 pp. MS, HS.

When thirteen-year-old Salamanca Tree Hiddle's mother dies, Sal will not admit her loss. A weeklong journey of 2,000 miles with her grandparents to Lewiston, Idaho, is the frame within which Sal learns to deal with "piles and piles of unsaid things" (5), a metaphor for her devastating loss. On the journey she tells her grandparents the story of Phoebe Winterbottom, through which she is able to recognize her own loss, accepting that there are "truly awful things in the world," things that "we can't explain" and "we can't fix." We learn to deal with our fears and loss by looking "at the frightening things that are closer to us" and by magnifying "them until they burst open." "Inside," she articulates, "is something we can manage, something that isn't as awful as it had at first seemed" (277).

Crutcher, C. (1996). *Ironman*. New York: Dell. ISBN: 0–440–21971–X. 228 pp. HS.

This novel is discussed in this chapter.

Flipovic, Z. (1994). *Zlata's diary: A child's life in Sarajevo*. Trans. C. Pribichevich-Zoric. ISBN: 0–670–85724–6. 200 pp. MS, HS.

This beautiful book affirms the power of the human spirit. Adolescents who feel overwhelmed by their lives might find courage to face their traumas as they read how thirteen-year-old Zlata copes with the disintegration of her physical world. Though she thinks of suicide, she will not despair, and she looks beyond the destruction of the outer world with inner hope.

Guest, J. (1976). *Ordinary people*. New York: Ballantine. ISBN: 0–345–25755–3. 245 pp. HS.

Conrad Jarrett's depression over the death of his brother in a boating accident is made metaphor in a dream of a metal tunnel where darkness obliterates everything. He is trapped both in the dream tunnel and in his own fragmented language; he is "convulsed with panic, begins to work himself backward and his feet strike the wall of the tunnel, he shifts his position. . . . Oh God he is sealed in this metal tomb . . . he cannot breathe" (71). During his junior year in high school Conrad receives the therapy he needs to begin his recovery. He learns to deal with his grief, his distant mother, and his overprotective father, and, most important, he learns that he is not to blame for his brother's death.

Hinton, S. E. (1997). *The outsiders.* (reissue ed.). New York: Viking Penguin. ISBN: 0–140–38572–X. 180 pp. MS.

Johnny's story reveals the devastating effects of abuse and neglect on adolescent self-esteem; throughout the novel, Johnny is depressed, isolated, and alone. He is a study in the dark despair of the hopeless.

Holland, I. (1972). *The man without a face.* New York: HarperKeyPoint. ISBN: 0–06–447028–8. 157 pp. HS.

During summer vacation fourteen-year-old Charles Norstadt meets Justin McLeod, a mysterious father figure who tutors him for the entrance test for a prestigious private school. In the process, he begins to find a male identity that has eluded him in the loss of his father and a series of stepfathers who have meant little to him. His family is fragmented into a vindictive older sister and a neglectful mother.

Krisher, T. (1994). *Spite fences.* New York: Bantam Doubleday Dell. ISBN: 0–440–22016–5. 238 pp. HS.

Maggie Pugh can see the world clearly, and in this complex novel of the early sixties in Kinship, Georgia, Krisher uses Maggie's camera as a metaphor for a vision of the world torn apart by racism. Maggie's camera ultimately reveals the truth of a town's racial hatred, and seething beneath it is Maggie's mother's violent anger about who she is and the place that she and her family occupy in the socioeconomic strata of Kinship. How Maggie deals with her mother's depression and rage is at the heart of this courageous young girl's story.

LeMieux, A. C. (1995). *Do angels sing the blues?* New York: Avon. ISBN: 0–380–72399–9. 215 pp. HS.

A trio of high school seniors share a passion for music. Theodore Haley Stone falls in love with Carey, an off-the-wall girl who suffers from depression as the result of family problems. When she can't face her family life anymore, she runs away. Theo and his best friend Boog try to stop her, but a freak accident causes Theo's death. Carey falls hopelessly into a deeper depression, but Boog focuses his attention on the future; he finds comfort when he can accept Theo's death and experience peace through the memory of their strong friendship.

Marsden, J. (1993). *Checkers.* New York: Houghton Mifflin. ISBN: 0–395–85754–6. 122 pp. MS, HS.

"Life seems so fragile," Marsden's adolescent female narrator writes, unfolding the story of her guilt and depression at "how I caused the death of my darling dog, Checkers" (122). She writes a metaphor for how life destroys people as they walk down the center of a highway where big trucks rush past them, hitting them, spinning them into oblivion. "It's a miracle anyone survives to be a teenager," she says. "It's a miracle any teenager survives to be an adult" (3). With that she begins this gut-wrenching novel of her life in a mental hospital where trying to write her story is one way to survive a devastating depression. Marsden is Australia's most celebrated author for young adults.

Marsden, J. (1994). *Letters from the inside*. New York: Houghton Mifflin. ISBN: 0–395–68985–6. 146 pp. MS, HS.

In this epistolary novel tenth graders Tracey and Mandy create a friendship that takes surprising twists and turns. Tracey describes an ideal life with a nearly perfect family while Mandy writes of her struggles to survive a dysfunctional family with a violent brother. As they exchange letters, however, we learn that Tracey is being held in a maximum security detention center and that she comes to rely on Mandy's letters for comfort and stability. She resolves to change her ways just as the letters from Mandy stop. From December 26 until February 11 there are no letters, and Tracey's letters are returned. In failing health, Tracey is placed in a medical unit where, it seems, she will spiral downward in helplessness and hopelessness. We can only imagine the worst for Mandy—that her brother has murdered her. The realistic language will shock some readers, but the novel is a gripping tale of the struggles of two young women for whom there is no way out of the depths of depression and loneliness.

Mori, K. (1995). *One bird*. New York: Fawcett. ISBN: 0–449–70453–X. 247 pp. HS.

It's 1975, and fifteen-year-old Megumi Shimuzi's mother tells her that she will not live long enough to see Megumi grow up unless she leaves her husband. In this moment of despair, Megumi learns that she cannot see her mother for seven years (until she finishes college). When she finds the injured bird from which the title is taken, a series of events occur that help her recover from her loss and the cultural shame of being motherless.

Mori, K. (1993). *Shizuko's daughter*. New York: Fawcett Juniper. ISBN: 0–449–70433–5. 214 pp. HS.

In the action to which the entire novel is a reaction, Shizuko Okuda commits suicide, her death a haunting legacy for her daughter Yuki. When Yuki's father marries a distant and difficult woman, the girl grows angry and rebellious, both manifestations of her depression over her mother's death. Eventually, through her understanding of her family's past as she interprets it in her artistic mother's sketchbook, she comes to see her father differently.

Neufeld, J. (1969). *Lisa, bright and dark*. New York: New American Library. ISBN: 0–451–16684–1. 143 pp. HS.

In this well-known novel, sixteen-year-old Lisa Shilling is falling from depression into schizophrenia, but her parents do not realize that she needs professional help. Betsy Goodman tells Lisa's story of how her friends attempt to help her through a form of group therapy. Lisa's suicide attempt, a desperate cry for help, leads to the hospitalization she needs, and in the process, Betsy discovers that she has a gift for helping others heal.

Oneal, Z. (1982). *A formal feeling*. New York: Viking. ISBN: 0–670–32488–4. 162 pp. HS.

The title is taken from Emily Dickinson's poem "After great pain a formal feeling comes." The poem's suggested sequence of recovery from mental disturbances ("First—Chill—then stupor—then the letting go") outlines Anne's story in the novel. Anne is sixteen and just home from boarding school for Christmas; she has to adjust to a stepmother in a house filled with memories of her deceased mother. She goes through many stages of depression: self-blame, isolation, the inability to cope with new situations, reluctance to express her emotions, and even questioning her own identity. She learns to deal with her depression and to handle her new life by opening up to friends, finding solace in her reflective writing, and allowing herself to enjoy the pleasures of ice skating and playing the piano.

Peck, R. (1978). *Father figure*. New York: Viking ISBN: 0–670–30930–3. 192 pp. HS.

Jim Atwater and his brother Byron have lived with their mother and grandmother for nine years since their parents' divorce. When their mother commits suicide, Jim confronts his loss and the attendant anger at his father for being absent from his life. His grandmother sends the brothers to live with their father in Florida, where constant conflict fuels the father-son anger. Jim hates his dad for dating a much younger woman, but in time he discovers more about this man whom he has never really had a chance to know, and he begins to let go of his hatred.

Pfeffer, S. B. (1987). *The year without Michael*. New York: Bantam. ISBN: 0–553–27373–6. 164 pp. MS, HS.

A marriage beset by problems defines the complicated family life of this story in which Jody Chapman's fourteen-year-old brother Michael disappears and never returns. In a world of awful tensions, family members, unable to depend on one another, are forced to deal with the pain of their loss alone. When Jody leaves in a desperate move to find Michael, the family nearly falls apart, but on her safe return both parents acknowledge that they need professional help.

Rylant, C. (1992). *Missing May.* New York: Orchard. ISBN: 0–531–08596–1. 89 pp. MS.

In this extraordinary Appalachian novel set in Deep Water, Fayette County, West Virginia, Summer deals with the depression that her Uncle Ob falls into after the death of her Aunt May. The journey that leads to his recovery has all the magic of a trip to Oz as Summer, Ob, and their friend Cletis set off for the golden-domed state capitol in Charleston. The story of how she and Cletis help Ob recover from his depression is a paean of praise to a love that endures.

Thomas, J. C., ed. (1990). *A gathering of flowers: Stories about being young in America.* New York: HarperKeyPoint. ISBN: 0–06–447082–2. 236 pp. HS.

In this superb collection of modern American short stories, Lois Lowry's "The Harringtons' Daughter" tells the story of a depression turned to insanity, borne of the insurmountable grief of the accidental death of a child. It also reveals the unspoken social stigma surrounding mental illness in the posh East Coast neighborhood in which the story is set.

Wilson, B. (1990). *The leaving and other stories.* New York: Philomel. ISBN: 0–399–21878–5. 206 pp. MS, HS.

In this superb short story collection by the award-winning Nova Scotian writer, we see adolescent depression and its consequences from several different angles. In "The Metaphor" a vivacious and creative seventh grade teacher who is ridiculed by her students when she is transferred to a high school loses touch with her self-worth and dies tragically. In "The Leaving" a mother who is little more than a servant to her husband and sons finds hope and overcomes her depression through a journey that signals a new life for her and her daughter.

Wolff, V. E. (1988). *Probably still Nick Swanson.* New York: Scholastic. ISBN: 0–590–43146–3. 175 pp. MS, HS.

What makes this book extraordinary is that Wolff takes us inside the mind of Nick Swanson, whose uncertainty about his identity is signaled by his repeated use of the word *probably*. Nick suffers from minimal brain dysfunction, and Wolff shows us that he encounters the same identity issues that sometimes depress all adolescents. Finally Nick understands himself more and begins to move forward in his life by sharing the personal nightmare of his sister's death by drowning. Facing what he fears frees him. At novel's end, he affirms his identity in a moment of peace.

Woodson, J. (1994). *I hadn't meant to tell you this*. New York: Bantam Doubleday Dell. ISBN: 0–440–21960–4. 115 pp. MS.

Marie, a popular black adolescent in Chauncey, Ohio, befriends Lena Bright, a transient girl branded by schoolmates and Marie's father as "white trash." Marie describes the depressed Lena as walking "like someone broken" (33). In the course of the time that they know each other, Marie learns that Lena has been broken by her father's abuse. In the end, Lena's agony is more than she can bear, and she and her sister Dion run away, leaving Marie to tell her story.

Other Resources on Adolescent Depression

Bell, R., et al. (1998). *Changing bodies, changing lives*. 3rd ed. New York: Times Books. ISBN: 0–8129–2990–X. 411 pp.

Chapters deal with emotional health (including a section on depression), eating disorders, substance abuse, physical health care, sexually transmitted diseases, birth control, and teen pregnancy. The final chapter, "Changing Things," offers many suggestions on how teenagers can take charge of their lives and work through difficulties with positive attitudes and positive actions.

Holmes, G. H. (1995). *Helping teenagers into adulthood: A guide for the next generation*. Westport, CT: Praeger. ISBN: 0–275–95341–6. 169 pp.

Successive chapters on the history of adolescence and the early, middle, and late stages of teen development serve as prelude to insightful chapters on family, peer groups, separation, love, and work.

Siegler, A. L. (1997). *The essential guide to the new adolescence: How to raise an emotionally healthy teenager*. New York: Dutton. ISBN: 0–525–93970–9. 271 pp.

The chapter titled "A Depressive Response to Adolescence" in this recent and readable book details the symptoms of adolescent depression and offers a case study: "Jennifer: Beating the Blues." Other chapters explore other faces of adolescence: anxiety, rebellion, withdrawal, and overattachment.

Steinberg, L., and A. Levine (1997). *You and your adolescent: A parent's guide for ages 10–20*. New York: HarperPerennial. ISBN: 0–06–273461–X. 431 pp.

This useful text handles depression as well as eating disorders and other emotional disturbances in adolescents. It offers advice on how to get professional help, discusses the risks of depression-related suicide as well as medications for depression, and offers other resources for dealing with the problem.

Stringer, S. A. (1997). *Conflict and connection: The psychology of young adult literature*. Portsmouth, NH: Heinemann Boynton/Cook. ISBN: 0–867–09415–X. 98 pp.

Stringer, a psychologist, discusses young adult fiction and its portrayal of the themes of adolescents as they mature psychologically. Two chapters address adolescent emotional problems: "There's a War Going on Inside My Head" and "I Must Be Going Crazy." In each of these chapters she offers reads of young adult novels and recommends other titles that provide insights into the emotional dilemmas facing today's teens.

REFERENCES

Bradshaw, C., and H. Weber (1996). *Climbing up from depression*. St. Meinard, IN: Abbey Press.

Davis, T. (1997). *Presenting Chris Crutcher*. New York: Twayne. ISBN: 0–805–78223–0.

Laufer, M., ed. (1995). *The suicidal adolescent*. Madison, CT: International Universities Press. ISBN: 0–823–66697–2.

Myracle, L. (1995). "Molding the minds of the young: The history of bibliotherapy as applied to children and adolescents." *ALAN Review* 22, no. 2: 36–40.

Oster, G. D., and S. S. Montgomery (1995). *Helping your depressed teenager: A guide for parents and caregivers*. New York: John Wiley and Sons. ISBN: 0–471–62184–6.

Pipher, M. (1994). *Reviving Ophelia: Saving the selves of adolescent girls*. New York: Putnam. ISBN: 0–399–13944–3.

Riordan, R. J., and L. S. Wilson. (1989). "Bibliotherapy: Does it work?" *Journal of Counseling and Development* 67: 506–507.

Shrodes, C. (1955). "Bibliotherapy." *The Reading Teacher* 9:24–30.

Williams, K. (1995). *A parent's guide for suicidal and depressed teens*. Center City, MN: Hazelden. ISBN: 1–568–38040–2.

CHAPTER 9

Dying to Be Thin: Eating Disorders in Young Adult Literature

Patricia P. Kelly and Marshall D. Tessnear

Billboards and magazines display models who weigh 23 percent less than the average female. Weight reduction programs are heavily marketed. Dancers and gymnasts are encouraged to stay excessively thin, in most cases fighting the natural development of their bodies. Ads for junk food bombard television viewers. These cultural influences are among the reasons that eating disorders, specifically anorexia nervosa and bulimia nervosa, have become a serious health issue for young people. Although there are historical references to starvation, or anorexia, in writings as early as medieval times, generally the concept of eating disorders is a modern phenomenon.

Statistics on the number of people in the United States who suffer from eating disorders vary because many cases go undiagnosed; therefore, many reports are based on estimates. Some estimates from various eating disorders centers are that 720,000 women and 80,000 men in the United States are anorexic, that 7,600,000 women and 380,000 men are bulimic, that 50 percent of girls diet during adolescence, and that up to 3 percent of women are anorexic or bulimic at some time. Marshall Tessnear suggests that one in five college women have an eating disorder. He says that research supports a more conservative estimate of one in twenty-five college women who fit all the diagnostic criteria for anorexia and bulimia. That means, however, that, on average, every floor of every residence hall on college campuses has one young woman with a severe eating disorder. Because eating disorders can begin as early as ten or eleven years of age and because the incidence of bulimia seems to be increasing in recent years, many medical and psychological experts are concerned about what they see as an eating disorders epidemic among middle school, high school, and college age students, often continuing into the early years of work.

We chose two novels for our discussion so that we could reflect on both anorexia and bulimia as they are portrayed in young adult literature. The first, Steven Levenkron's *The Best Little Girl in the World*, originally published in 1978, became a classic among the young adult novels dealing with anorexia. Levenkron, who is a therapist and an authority on eating disorders, bases Kessa, the main character in this novel, on real-life patients. In this way, he helps readers understand the behaviors and thinking associated with anorexia nervosa from the perspective of a girl suffering from the disorder, her family, and her therapist. The novel also deals with both types of anorexia: the restrictive type and the binge/purge type. Though an older novel, Levenkron's depiction is excellent, and was one of the first to break the silence about anorexia nervosa.

Although anorexia is more noticeable and perhaps more deadly than bulimia, more adolescents struggle with bulimia, both purging and non-purging types, than any other eating disorder. Therefore, we chose a second, more recent novel, Lesléa Newman's *Fat Chance* (1996), which shows two bulimics, one who becomes anorexic and the other who uses purging as a way of losing some weight. Through Judi Liebowitz's diary, readers see her progression from dieting to purging to her recognition that she must stop even though she cannot relinquish her desire to be thin. Newman's emphasis on self-image as an important factor in eating disorders is realistically portrayed.

We then met to discuss eating disorders as they are depicted in these two books. Following each summary, Tessnear, the therapist, responds to questions posed by Kelly, the young adult literature specialist.

THE BEST LITTLE GIRL IN THE WORLD

Ostensibly, fifteen-year-old Francesca Dietrich's view of herself as fat begins when her ballet teacher tells her, "Now stay slim—perhaps even a pound less here" as she touches Francesca's rear lightly (11). "Slim, firm" becomes a mantra that sounds in her head as she exercises, trying to eliminate the fat from her body, trying to eliminate Fat Francesca, who weighs ninety-eight pounds. From the mantra and exercise, someone she names Kessa emerges in her mind, the person who will beat everyone at being slim and in control.

Francesca (Kessa) combs through fashion magazines, cutting out pictures and ranking them in order of slimness. She then rates her own progress by these models, tearing up each picture as she surpasses the model in thinness; "the thinner is the winner" (24).

The youngest of three children, Kessa is "too good to be true" (14) and a relief to her mother and father because she doesn't disrupt their lives. Her grades are high, she's compulsively neat, and she never demands attention. She tries to be the "best little girl in the world." But despite exterior calmness, Kessa feels she has "no control over anything" (15). She lives in the shadow of her brother Gregg, who is at Harvard and whose grades and awards are a source of pride for the parents; but he has isolated himself emotionally from the family. In contrast, her sister Susanna, argumentative and indomitable, has quit college and moves from one commune to another. After years of family arguments over Susanna's behavior, she gets attention and dominates the family even in her absence.

Kessa develops rituals to manage her desire for food. Her fingers tap a magic formula on the table, on her thigh, or in her head, "Kes-sa, Kes-sa"; she drinks water to fill her stomach and stop the hunger pangs; she cuts her food into pieces, moving them around into geometric patterns on her plate. When her father forces her to eat, she does so, carefully removing the food from the fork with her teeth so that none touches her lips. Then she goes to the bathroom and forces herself to vomit. She can appear to be the obedient Francesca and still win. She exercises, walking long distances or dancing her ballet exercises for hours, to rid her body of its hated fat.

Kessa's losing weight soon becomes a battle of wills. Her mother, Grace, who has done everything for her family, believes the situation is her fault. Her father, Hal, a self-made successful businessman, demands obedience, especially when he is drinking. When Kessa loses ten pounds and her period stops, her family physician, Evelyn Gordon, starts monitoring Kessa's weight, only to have it slip further, to eighty-one pounds. Dr. Gordon prescribes medication to increase her appetite, which terrifies Kessa. Even with purging, Kessa fears that the "medicine would remain in her stomach, churning it up with an insatiable hunger, forcing her to eat against her will, forcing Kessa to give in to Francesca, forcing thin, self-controlled Kessa to become fat, fearful Francesca" (67). Dr. Gordon also puts a name to what Kessa is suffering from, anorexia nervosa, and recommends a psychiatrist.

When Kessa begins seeing Alexander Smith, a Park Avenue psychiatrist, she feels only fear and vows to "lie as much as necessary, but the doctor must not find out about Kessa and all the important habits and practices that kept her alive" (82). Kessa's father grumbles about the cost; her mother feels guilty and responsible, and Kessa quits going after six appointments. She is now seventy-eight pounds, cold all the time, and developing downy hair on her body. She is tired and cannot concentrate on schoolwork. Yet with her grades slipping and her health failing, Kessa feels in control and very powerful. Kessa continues to throw up when she is forced to eat. She keeps herself in control by organizing very carefully when she will exercise, what she will eat, how many pieces she will divide her food into, how many bites she will eat. "Kessa's body was starving for food, but her mind was drowning in it" (106). She thinks of food all the time but is terrified of it.

In desperation, Mr. Dietrich takes Kessa to an old family friend, a physician who though well intentioned has no idea what to do other than to tell the girl to eat. But Kessa continues losing weight, throwing up when necessary. When she reaches seventy-three pounds, "a picture of the models she'd cut out of the magazine flashed through Kessa's mind. And the winner is . . . seventy-three!" (115).

Dr. Gordon then suggests that Kessa see a psychologist, Sandy Sherman, who is currently treating two anorexic patients. Dr. Gordon is surprised that Sandy has two of them, explaining that most psychiatrists hesitate to take them on. Anorexics can be uncooperative and sneaky and aren't always very likeable (117). Sandy Sherman begins the process of counseling Kessa, but in two weeks she drops another pound and her vital signs have slipped dangerously. Hospitalization is the only answer at this point. Kessa is angry and sulks. The staff see her as a "sullen, difficult girl" (142) whose chart reads "depressive—hostile" (143) and one of "the skinnies" (149). Although her parents cannot see her for a month, Kessa harasses them by calling so frequently that they take the phone off the hook to get sleep. Kessa complains to her mother that the nurses ignore her and that the food isn't good, although she never eats it. Sandy tries to explain to Mrs. Dietrich:

Kessa is not only not logical now, she isn't even competent. . . . Try to remember that next time Kessa begins to manipulate you . . . I'm not suggesting her problem is as simple as a [power struggle], but I am suggesting her need to manipulate you is part of the problem, a part we're all going to have to work on . . . We can't let Kessa continue to manipulate, and we have to be especially wary of letting her pit you against me or against any of the doctors. I suspect that's one of the things that keep girls like Kessa from getting well. And we can't allow her to keep herself from getting well. (155–156)

It is ironic that Kessa sees Myrna, another anorexic, as horribly thin but cannot see herself that way. Myrna has been in and out of hospitals for three years; she considers herself a "pro." Myrna is also a binger, who vomits to purge. In the hospital, she walks incessantly to rid herself of calories.

Kessa now is in constant pain, falling from weakness, walking on feet stripped of padding, and sitting on hard chairs with uncushioned bones. She does not eat and drops to sixty-nine and a half pounds when she collapses and almost dies from shock. As they insert the intravenous tube to supply her body with nutrients in liquid form, Kessa is only worried about whether it will make her fat. Because of her condition, they decide to start hyperalimentation, which involves a catheter being inserted below the collarbone and intercepting the jugular vein approximately two inches above the heart (171). This painful procedure provides more nutrition than intravenous feeding.

Myrna feels threatened by the attention Kessa receives because Myrna always wants to be the worst. She is gleeful when she tells Kessa that she'll now gain weight. Ironically, Kessa is caught with hoarded food that has spoiled; she doesn't eat the food, but the hoarding is part of a ritual.

Sandy tells her that her obsession "with weight is not the real problem," that the "fear is coming from someplace else in your head," that "when we find out what it is, you'll be free from this terrible trap" (176–177). During therapy sessions Kessa talks of never feeling that she belonged, even in her family; and Sandy suggests that she rejects people first before they can reject her, as well as sending out messages that say "you don't want to belong" (198). Then he tells her that he would probably do just what Kessa is doing, making up games and magic tricks to protect himself from others' feelings (199). Kessa admits that her "life *is* magic tricks" (200). Sandy says that talking about them is the beginning of getting rid of them. He tells her it won't be easy; it will take a long time, but that he won't stop pushing her. He holds a family conference at which emotions erupt: Susanna and her father in angry confrontation and her mother wishing for peace and quiet. Finally Kessa explodes with years of pent-up anger: "I've asked for nothing, and that's what I got. Gregg got admiration and Susanna got attention and I got nothing. Nothing from you and nothing from Mommy. She doesn't even like me" (231). This confrontation is the breakthrough that begins Kessa's healing.

In the end, when Kessa is eating some food and has gained enough weight to leave the hospital, her father takes the day off so that the family can bring her home. His understanding that this is an important part of bringing the family together shows hope that the family can support Kessa's recovery. Sandy will continue as Kessa's therapist, but he also agrees to take on Myrna, who will represent a different challenge.

■

A THERAPIST RESPONDS

Kelly: When Dr. Gordon, the family physician, tries to explain anorexia nervosa to Kessa's mother, she provides information (68) that was known in 1978, when this book was originally published. What are some current theories about "causes" of anorexia nervosa?

Tessnear: The theories described by Kessa's doctors are rather old theories. Although in some instances there can be a mother/daughter struggle, most writers and therapists in the field look at reasons for both anorexia and bulimia in terms of three things. Of course, as with any broad generalizations, individual cases may differ. First are the societal or cultural causes with all the attention to and emphasis on thinness and appearance in advertising, magazines, and television. But we're all part of this culture, and not everyone responds to those stimuli by developing an eating disorder.

Second, there are some descriptors of family relationships that seem to correlate in a lot of instances with the development of eating disorders. However, for many of my clients this is not descriptive of their families. On the other hand, many of the women or girls come from families that place a premium on appearance, and that is not only physical appearance but other kinds of appearances, such as what would people think about our family if they knew something or the other? So there is often a heavy emphasis on how the family is perceived by the outside world. The patient's mother is often described as being overinvolved, often almost enmeshed in the daughter's life. And the fathers are described as being somewhat absent, if not physically at least emotionally, not available. Those are two of the more local family kinds of things that are often associated with eating disorders.

Third, given the societal pressures and family environment associated with eating disorders, there are personal characteristics of girls or young women that might make them more susceptible to developing an eating disorder. Here again, I've seen many who don't fit the description, but in general they are sometimes described as perfectionists and pleasers. For these young women it is very important to make a good impression, to please people, to avoid conflict, to basically live up to real or perceived expectations. Although I have seen a number of cases where these generalizations were not necessarily descriptive of the family nor of the individual, I do think the pleaser part is fairly common. In my experience it is rare that a woman who has developed bulimia or anorexia might not be described as a pleaser in some sense.

Those are the three general causes. There are, however, more immediate causes. Most eating disorders do begin with a diet. In that sense, you could say some sort of initially successful diet would be the cause, a trigger of sorts. On the other hand, a high percentage of teenage girls go on diets and not all of them develop eating disorders; but again, it seems that a diet, usually somewhere in early adolescence, may be instrumental in initiating an eating disorder. Beyond that, we can't really nail down specific causes.

Practically no one subscribes to the old psychodynamic notion of a young woman who is trying to repress her emerging sexuality or the mother/daughter conflict that is alluded to in Steven Levenkron's book. Often there is a child/parent conflict going on, but most of the time the conflict has emerged as a result of the family trying to cope with the eating disorder. I typically don't see family conflict as necessarily the root of an eating disorder. Often families have not developed the skills for dealing with conflict; so an eating disorder may be ignored for awhile. Once the eating disorder is confronted and the conflict begins, the problem is exacerbated because the family does not have good strategies for resolving conflict.

Kelly: At one point Kessa's physician in the hospital notes that he doesn't think anorexia can be cured, that it can be managed but never actually conquered (167). From your experience how would you characterize this statement?

Tessnear: With anorexia particularly, that is true. Below a certain critical body weight, all you can do is manage them medically. It is usually ineffective to try to convince a severely anorexic patient that she is too thin, that her health is being jeopardized, or even that people care about her: the distortions are fairly fixed and immutable at that point. Levenkron's book more or less suggests the same thing. It seemed they made very little progress with Kessa until they forced her weight up through IV or hyperalimentation. It was only after she began to gain some weight that psychotherapy was effective. In my experience early intervention with a good therapist in a good therapeutic program offers a reasonable chance for success. This fall I began treating a young woman who was five feet, two inches and came in at about 85 or 86 pounds. That is a low body weight, but she was not overtly resistant at first; she was in therapy because that's what her parents and her doctors wanted. I was fairly persistent, and when she missed appointments, I called her. I also told her that, if we didn't make progress, she would need something more intensive. I don't know if that scared her, but she did continue to come in, and we focused not only on her weight and health but on other things that were going on in her life. Prior to the holidays, she weighed 96 pounds. I'm hopeful, but we'll see how she is after the holidays. If she had been much less than 85 pounds when we started therapy, I'm not sure that it would have been effective. Frankly, I'm still not sure what exactly made the difference.

As for "cures," people do have relapses; particularly, those who have been at a much lower weight and regain that weight are much more likely to have a relapse. Recently at a conference one of the speakers was talking about how much worse the prognosis is for someone who has gotten to a dangerously low weight even though they were able to regain the weight, perhaps in a hospital, perhaps through IV, or whatever. It is important to intervene early. A major difference today is that the current definition of anorexia is 15 percent rather than 25 percent loss of normal body weight. This allows for earlier intervention than when Levenkron wrote his book.

Kelly: Steven Levenkron developed what he called a nurturing-authoritative therapy, an approach he has his fictional psychologist, Sandy Sherman, use. How do you feel about this approach? What are other treatments for anorexia?

Tessnear: That's a much better approach for anorexics than a reflective, client-centered approach. We also use a multimodal or two-track approach to therapy. Two-track means that there is a physical aspect and a psychological aspect of eating disorders. The multimodal approach involves a combination of medical, nutritional, cognitive therapy, and attending to the patient's feelings and emotions as well. It also involves the family if possible.

In the mid-seventies, when I first saw some women with eating disorders, the predominant thought at that point, and you still hear it echoed today, was that this doesn't have anything to do with eating; it's a psychological thing. In one respect I guess that's true, but in another respect it does have to do with eating, in the sense that if an anorexic person is not eating, you can do all of the best psychotherapy in the world and it won't be effective. Likewise, if a woman is in a binge/purge cycle, the purging is a setup for the bingeing; you can't ignore the fact that they have starved themselves all day. It's not just a psychological thing of having no willpower or losing control or being unable to deal with feelings. If you haven't eaten for twenty-four hours, the likelihood is that when you do eat, you will eat more than usual. The notion that it doesn't have anything to do with eating paints too broad a stroke; it does have to do with eating but, ironically, it doesn't have to do with just eating. With the two-track approach we attend to the physiological component of the eating disorder and at the same time deal with the emotional/cognitive component. We don't deal with just one or the other.

Kelly: Myrna is both anorexic and bulimic. Are the two disorders frequently found in one person like this?

Tessnear: They go together fairly often. One pattern we see is an anorexic who loses a lot of weight through restriction of eating and then regains the weight either through some treatment intervention or for some other reason, and then develops the bulimic cycle. There are two forms of anorexia: there is the restricting form and then there is the more bulimic form, which is the bingeing/purging. It's not at all unusual to see both illnesses in the same person.

FAT CHANCE

Judi Liebowitz, almost fourteen, begins keeping a diary as a requirement of her eighth grade English teacher. Because the diary is personal, Judi can write her secret thoughts and desires, and one of those desires is to be the thinnest girl in the eighth grade. The diary covers almost a semester, and each entry is dated, beginning with "Dear Diary." The first-person diary format allows Lesléa Newman to show Judi's thinking as she becomes more and more obsessive about her weight. One of her favorite expressions throughout the diary is "fat chance," which means no way, or it won't happen. But the expression is also a plaintive cry: Why me? Why am I fat? Why can't I be like everyone else? As Judi eventually figures out, "a fat chance and a slim chance are really the very same thing" (214).

At five feet, four inches and 127 pounds, Judi is not fat, but she calls herself "full-figured" and wears baggy, dark-colored clothes. She constantly calculates calories, both for what she eats and what others eat. She also has the emotionally destructive habit of classifying herself as "good" on days she's able to diet, but once she has been "bad" by not sticking to her diet, she pigs out on the theory that the day is ruined anyway and that she'll start over tomorrow. She hates her clothes because they're size 11/12, and she hates her body. She's an avid reader of *Seventeen* and judges herself and others by its standards.

Throughout her diary, Judi uses language that negates her self-image: "I look like an elephant"; "I pigged out last night"; "I have absolutely no willpower"; "I feel too fat to even leave the house"; "I'm such a blimp" (16–42). She thinks everything in her life would be wonderful if she could just lose weight. She skips breakfast when she can, eats little lunch, and then wonders why she can't control her eating at night. She wishes she could have her stomach stapled or her jaws wired shut or be locked up away from food.

Judi longs to get control of her eating, but anything can trigger an eating episode. Once, while babysitting, she sees an "ad for frozen yogurt and as soon as I saw it, I knew I was a goner . . . voices were coming from the kitchen" (46). As she's pigging out, the family comes home. Not wanting to get caught eating, she shoves a bowl of ice cream under the sofa and tells them she cannot babysit for them anymore. Another way she tries to get control is to make bargains with herself: if she loses weight, she'll go to the party or she'll audition for a play or she'll buy herself something new. She decides that fasting is the best way to get control; so she fasts for a week before her mother finds out and makes her eat. Judi longs to talk to her mother about her obsession with food, but she knows her mother wouldn't understand: "She would just tell me I have a nice figure or I'll grow out of it, or something else that just isn't true" (77). Later, her mother tells her that "food is something to be enjoyed, not something to torture yourself with" (86). But the harassment of a boy at school making fun of her bouncing breasts when she runs and making oinking noises at her has much more impact on Judi's view of herself than her mother's words.

Two girls at school serve as counterpoint for Judi: Nancy Pratt, who is thin and beautiful in Judi's eyes but doesn't know that Judi exists; and Monica Pellegro, a thin, not yet developed musician, who is Judi's best friend. Monica doesn't understand Judi's obsession with weight. "She's thin, so she has no idea what it's like," writes Judi (80). But when Judi finds Nancy throwing up in the bathroom at school, Judi is initiated into purging. Nancy tells her that models and actresses and dancers do it, that she can eat and then get rid of it. And "it's not as disgusting as being fat" (84). Judi asks her how it's done, and Nancy tells her but warns her to be careful if she's using anything but her fingers.

After Judi eats a big meal at her mother's insistence, she tries what Nancy has taught her. She writes in her diary: "It wasn't bad, Dear Diary. I hope you don't think I'm too disgusting. I mean, Nancy Pratt does it, and she says lots of other girls do, too . . . I'm really relieved because now I know I can eat whatever I want, as long as I have my new 'secret weapon' " (99).

So Judi begins a regimen of exercise and eating one meal a day, which she throws up. She doesn't want anyone to know because it's disgusting, but it's also "too good to be true. I can eat and lose weight at the same time!" (102). She begins standing guard for Nancy at the school bathroom while she vomits. An up and down movement with two fingers becomes their signal. They figure they'll have to do it every day for the rest of their lives. Judi continues to lose weight but keeps setting her goal lower as she measures herself against Nancy and a picture of a five foot, ten inch model who weighs 115 pounds.

As Judi loses weight, she thinks she has gotten control, which is ironic because she has lost control. However, in some ways vomiting makes a bulimic feel she has gained control of how to lose weight. When Nancy Pratt collapses in the school bathroom, her hair covered with her vomit, and is taken to the hospital, Judi is frightened, but not enough to stop. In fact, she gets progressively worse. Judi tries to stop but, when she starts gaining weight, she begins vomiting again. She thinks people will be disappointed in her if it looks as though she's lost her willpower, and she knows they would be disgusted if they knew what she does to lose weight. She continues to binge, sometimes vomiting, sometimes not. When Nancy asks her to smuggle laxatives into the hospital, Judi begins trying laxatives too. Now she's bingeing, vomiting, and taking laxatives. Judi sees that Nancy is truly emaciated yet terrified of gaining weight. When Nancy is placed in a residential center, where she can be better monitored, Judi tells first Monica and then her English teacher about her problem. Eventually she lets her mother read her diary.

In the end she is seeing a counselor, Miss Fiorino, who talked with the student body about eating disorders after Nancy collapsed. In the school assembly the counselor explains the dangers of bulimia: "You can rip the lining of your throat or rot the enamel off your teeth or get ulcers or even stomach cancer . . . Once the lining of your stomach disintegrates, that's it. You don't get a second chance" (172). She goes on to talk about societal pressures on females to be thin, and the impact of models on women's images: Twiggy in the sixties and Kate Moss with the "waif look" in the nineties. She tells the students that dieting leads to frustration and frustration leads to bingeing and bingeing leads to frustration. It's a vicious circle. Miss Fiorino also tells them that people do not get better by themselves, that, if they know of a friend who is bulimic, they should tell. "Girls who are bulimic can be very sneaky and clever, and lots of times even the people they live with don't know what's going on. Sometimes a girl is actually very relieved to know that someone is on to her, and she doesn't have to deal with this all alone"(177).

A THERAPIST RESPONDS

Kelly: How important is self-image in developing eating disorders, especially bulimia?

Tessnear: Obviously, body image is important in both of the disorders. However, self-image is more important although patients end up focusing a lot on body image, which is often an inaccurate view of their bodies. For example, in the book, Nancy's boyfriend was saying she was too skinny, and asked why she was still losing weight. Self-image, to me, includes more than just body image. It involves how effective you are as a person and qualities you have as a person. Judi, the main character, is preoccupied with her weight and her appearance, but she also cannot come up with an occupation that she thinks she can do. She also uses negative words about herself all the time, which only adds to her poor self-image.

Kelly: What is the prognosis for recovering adolescent bulimics as adult women?

Tessnear: The prognosis for the character, Judi, looks hopeful, partly because I think she has a supportive mother and a supportive friend; she even has this guy who says he's not going to tease her about her weight anymore. She is connected with a counselor, whom she apparently has some confidence in; so this book ends with some optimism, I think, especially since she has had early intervention. However, one of the problems with identifying bulimics early on is that their weight may not fluctuate drastically; you can't look at them and tell they have an eating disorder.

Many, many women who begin dealing with bulimia as teenagers continue to deal with it in their twenties, thirties, and forties. I've had cases of girls who report that their mothers have eating disorders. But to have an eating disorder in one's twenties and not have it still be a problem at all ten years later, probably is very much an exception rather than the rule. It may be very much like Judi saying, "I'm a recovering bulimic; I threw up for my last time yesterday." It sounds as though she has it under control, but she really doesn't. Patients with eating disorders are very difficult for therapists to deal with, but I wouldn't dread seeing a person like Judi; I would dread seeing a person like Nancy Pratt, at least the way she is portrayed.

Kelly: Are the physical problems associated with bulimia accurately described by the counselor in this book? Are there others?

Tessnear: Some were mentioned in the book: the chance of tearing your esophagus from throwing up, dental damage, swollen neck glands, and so forth. With more severe cases of bulimia where the patient has been purging for quite a while, at least once a day, one of the biggest risks is heart damage, which is not mentioned. The purging will often create an electrolyte imbalance that causes irregular heart rhythms and can create permanent heart damage. We had at least one case this year, where we had to hospitalize a woman because her potassium was messed up and she was starting to develop EKG patterns that were irregular, and the risk of a heart attack was imminent. So heart damage is one of the more serious medical risks from bulimia. The laxative abuse, also, has some very serious consequences; the person may actually become dependent on the laxative. I would say that anyone who is a serious laxative abuser and decides not to do that anymore should actually withdraw from laxatives under medical supervision because abrupt withdrawal from laxatives can actually be fairly dangerous. Serious laxative abuse can result in the lining of the intestines becoming paper thin and tearing. Aside from the ones mentioned in the book, I would say the risk of heart disease and serious gastrointestinal problems are major health consequences of bulimia.

Kelly: How do you work with patients to stop the binge/purge cycle?

Tessnear: A few patients engage in purging after eating very little; however, usually purging is associated with bingeing. In therapy groups, I actually draw the cycle and talk about it. Let's start with someone who decides not to eat for a day; so they restrict themselves. That obviously leads to hunger, which may lead to a binge, which is usually followed by physical and psychological discomfort and a lot of anxieties and anger with yourself. So then what you might do is purge, get rid of it in some fashion, which leads to immediate physical relief but also some sort of guilt. This might be followed with what Judi did a lot of times, which is called a purification promise: "I'll never do that again, I'm going to be good, I'm not going to binge anymore." So that you won't binge again, you avoid food situations, which starts the restricting again—it just goes in a circle. When women with bulimia come in, they want to stop bingeing, but what I try to get them to understand is that this is a cycle and that you really have to address everything along the cycle. When you throw up everything and then don't eat for awhile, you're setting yourself up for a binge. It's not a lack of self-control; it's hunger.

So the first step is not to purge; however, then we have to deal with the fear of getting fat. But it is a cycle, and I think to simply look at it as avoiding bingeing often makes the mistake of not seeing how purging and restriction leads irrevocably to the binge. That sounds like simple stuff; but believe me, to try to have someone see it that way who is in a binge/purge cycle, their fear of gaining weight is so intense that stopping that purge really requires self-control and willpower. But stopping purging gives better control over the binge, and most of the time the weight gain isn't that much, if any. The problem is they don't want to stay the way they are; they want less.

RECOMMENDED READINGS

Eating Disorders: Fiction

Bauer, J. (1992). *Squashed*. New York: Delacorte. ISBN: 0–385–30793–4. 208 pp. MS, HS.

Sixteen-year-old Ellie Morgan is consumed by two goals: to raise the largest pumpkin (a squash) for the state festival and to lose twenty pounds. As Max, the pumpkin, grows to record proportions, Ellie ironically fluctuates between weight gain and weight loss. Filled with humor and some suspense, the novel also shows that, no matter how accomplished a young woman is, she always thinks that losing a few pounds would make her happier and more successful.

(A *School Library Journal* Best Book and winner of the Ninth Annual Delacorte Press Prize for an Outstanding First Young Adult Novel)

Bennett, C. (1998). *Life in the fat lane.* New York: Delacorte. ISBN: 0–385–32274–1. 260 pp. MS, HS.

A beauty pageant winner, Lara Ardeche has a perfect life, but a rare metabolic disorder called Axell-Crowne syndrome with no known cure changes all that. Although she eats little and exercises excessively, she goes from 118 pounds to 218 and finds herself an outsider and a target of cruelty, some of it well-meaning advice that she herself had given to others when she was thin. Lara experiences the social costs of being fat and the destruction of her self-image. Although Lara is fortunate to begin losing weight at the end, she may never be truly thin again; however, she has changed forever the things she values in life.

Blume, J. (1976). *Blubber.* New York: Bantam Doubleday Dell. ISBN: 0–440–40707–9. 160 pp. ES, MS.

This classic story of the cruel tormenting of an overweight kid remains ageless, because every year in every school across the nation, the same story is acted out again and again. Jill Brenner, a fifth grader, relates how Wendy leads the abuse against Linda, an overweight girl she calls Blubber after Linda gives a report on whales. Eventually, Wendy manipulates almost everyone in the class to become involved in ostracizing first one, then another member of the class until it's Jill's turn. (A *New York Times* Outstanding Book of the Year and a Child's Study Children's Book Committee Children's Book of the Year)

Cruise, B. (1995). *Picture perfect.* New York: Simon and Schuster. ISBN: 0–689–80093–2. 125 pp. ES, MS.

Zack, Kelly, and Screech chaperone a camping trip for a group of ten-year-olds, only to discover that one of the girls, Lisa, is taking her dieting too far. They do some research on anorexia and develop a plan to convince Lisa she is perfect the way she is.

Crutcher, C. (1993). *Staying fat for Sarah Byrnes.* New York: Green-willow. ISBN: 0–688–11552–7. 224 pp. HS.

Although much more than the story of an overweight boy, this novel does deal with the ostracism of obese people. As Eric loses weight because of swimming, his friendship with Sarah, a victim of psychological and physical abuse, is jeopardized. To save their friendship and help Sarah, Eric eats gluttonously to regain weight, for Sarah will not accept him if he becomes "normal." (An American Library Association Best Book for Young Adults)

Frank, L. (1995). *I am an artichoke.* New York: Holiday House. ISBN: 0–823–41150–8. 187 pp. MS, HS.

Fifteen-year-old Sarah takes a summer job as a mother's helper in New York City, only to find that she's been hired to be a role model for Emily, a twelve-year-old anorexic, whose divorced parents fight over how to deal with her. Emily fears being fat like her mother, and her father threatens to have Emily hospitalized. When Emily runs away, Sarah finds her and takes her to Sarah's parents. It is there that Sarah sees the power that Emily holds over her parents by not eating. Through a doctor's care and continued friendship with Sarah, Emily's prognosis for recovery appears good.

Hall, L. F. (1997). *Perk! The story of a teenager with bulimia.* Carlsbad, CA: Gurze Books. ISBN: 0–936–07727–1. 128 pp. MS, HS.

Priscilla, better known as Perk, is a high school student with problems that push her into bulimia: self-doubt and insecurity, concern about her weight, and a first love.

Hamilton, V. (1985). *A little love.* New York: Berkley Books. ISBN: 0–425–08424–8. 207 pp. HS.

Sheema, deserted by her father, longs for some security and a little love. Food is comforting, and so are the boys she used to get into cars with. She just needs to be held and get a little love. Forrest accepts her as she is—her overweight body, her longing to find her father—and sets out with Sheema to find him. Rejected again, she will survive, but there will always be a hunger inside. (A Coretta Scott King Honor Book)

Hanauer, C. (1997). *My sister's bones: A novel.* New York: Dell. ISBN: 0–385–31704–2. 272 pp. HS.

Because Billie Weinstein finally sees the destructive patterns of her family, there is hope that she can escape serious consequences. Her father, a dominating surgeon who demands perfection, and her mother, meek and subservient, have eroded the well-being of Cassie, Billie's older sister. When Cassie returns from college emaciated and refusing to eat, she is eventually hospitalized. However, she and her parents remain locked in a deadly battle of wills.

Lemieux, A. C. (1997). *Dare to be, M.E.!* New York: Avon. ISBN: 0–380–97496–7. 240 pp. MS.

Justine returns from Paris obsessed with food and dieting and how she looks. In seventh grade with her friend, Mary Ellen, Justine also has problems with her parents' separation and her own lack of self-esteem. Soon Mary Ellen realizes that Justine has a serious eating disorder, bulimia, and she decides to tell in order to get help for Justine. In the end Justine is seeing a therapist.

Levenkron, S. (1986). *Kessa.* New York: Warner Books. ISBN: 0–445–20175–4. 256 pp. MS, HS.

In the phenomenal sequel to *The Best Little Girl in the World,* readers get a chance to see Kessa's continued battle with anorexia. Recovery does not happen overnight and there are no quick fixes; therefore, this book adds a useful dimension for readers. Currently out of print, this novel is well worth the search in public libraries.

Levenkron, S. (1989). *The best little girl in the world.* New York: Warner Books. ISBN: 0–446–35865–7. 256 pp. MS, HS.

This book is discussed in depth in this chapter.

Medoff, J. (1997). *Hunger point: A novel.* New York: HarperCollins. ISBN: 0–060–39189–8. 288 pp. HS.

Frannie Hunter, though a college graduate, works as a waitress and lives at home with her mother, who pops Valium and diets compulsively; her father, who spends his time preparing gourmet meals; and her sister, who appears perfect but is anorexic and eventually commits suicide. Frannie is also obsessed with food and her fluctuating weight. Medoff, who reveals that she had suffered from a long-term eating disorder, deals with the symptoms of anorexia and its effects on a family while exploring the politics of food, women, and self-image. The novel is funny, graphic, and painful.

Newman, L. (1996). *Fat chance.* New York: Putnam. ISBN: 0–698–11306–X. 214 pp. MS, HS.

This novel is also highlighted in this chapter.

Shute, J. (1997). *Life-size.* New York: Avon. ISBN: 0–380–73021–9. 308 pp. HS.

Josie, a twenty-five-year-old graduate student, weighs sixty-seven pounds when she is forcibly hospitalized for anorexia. She sees food as disgusting and obscene and longs to live on air like a plant. She revels in her willpower and begins each day with a ritualistic fingering of her bones. Although Josie begins dieting because she hates her plump body, the problem soon goes beyond body image to a psychological one. Once forced to eat, she begins a slow recovery and understanding of herself.

Snyder, A. (1988). *Goodbye, paper doll*. New York: New American Library. ISBN: 0–451–15943–8. 155 pp. HS.

Rosemary Norton is a young woman who sets goals for herself and accomplishes them, but when she sets out to make herself look like a thin billboard model, she slips into compulsive and ritualistic behaviors about food. She either doesn't eat or she binges and vomits; she is destroying herself emotionally and physically. Rosemary is a classic example of how an anorexic's deceitfulness inhibits recovery because both family and therapists are frequently deceived.

Woodson, J. (1995). *Between Madison and Palmetto*. New York: Dell. ISBN: 0–440–41062–2. 112 pp. MS.

In this final volume of the trilogy about Margaret and Maizon (*Last Summer with Maizon*, 1991; *Maizon at Blue Hill*, 1993) changes are occurring rapidly for both of them. Maizon's father, who deserted her as a baby, comes back; Margaret's body begins developing in ways she doesn't like; and a white girl, Caroline, moves into the neighborhood and wants to be friends. Fearful of becoming fat, Margaret begins dieting and vomiting. Maizon is angry with her and says she can't be friends as long as Margaret does that. When Margaret's mother finds out, she strongly intervenes, taking Margaret to a doctor, monitoring her, and suggesting she start running to gain control of her body. Although Margaret says she still thinks about vomiting, in the end she seems to be on her way to recovery.

Eating Disorders: Memoirs and Diaries

Apostolides, M. (1998). *Inner hunger: A young woman's struggle through anorexia and bulimia*. New York: W. W. Norton. ISBN: 0–393–04590–0. 192 pp. HS.

Apostolides chronicles a decade-long battle with eating disorders from junior high through college and into work, with her weight ranging from 80 at times to 160 at other times. She finally learns how to deal with her disorders. This journal is straightforward, painful, and powerful.

Bitter, C. N. (1998). *Good enough*. Penfield, NY: HopeLines. ISBN: 0–965–77556–9. 285 pp. HS.

This memoir describes a twenty-five-year near-fatal struggle with anorexia and bulimia that includes not only the eating disorder symptoms but also the obsessive thinking that only someone who has been there can describe.

Hornbacher, M. (1997). *Wasted: A memoir of anorexia and bulimia.* New York: HarperCollins. ISBN: 0–060–18739–5. 304 pp. HS.

At twenty-three, Hornbacher has dieted nearly all her life, beginning, she says, at four. In this memoir she discusses complex causes: some cultural, some familial, and some personal. She tells her story candidly with no self-pity. She has not triumphed over her eating disorders and is convinced she will die young because when she steps on a scale, she's still overjoyed if she's lost weight. (A *Health and Fitness* Editor's Recommended Book)

Krasnow, M. (1996). *My life as a male anorexic.* Binghamton, NY: Harrington Park Press. ISBN: 1–560–23883–6. 152 pp. HS.

Published before his death in 1997, Krasnow's memoir describes his horrible experience with anorexia from age fourteen to just before his death at age twenty-eight. Michael had difficulty getting help because anorexia is frequently considered a female eating disorder and some treatment centers will not accept males. He lived his last five years at a grotesquely dangerous weight. This account shows the devastating human suffering and utter helplessness wrought by anorexia.

Miller, C. A. (1991). *My name is Caroline.* Carlsbad, CA: Gurze Books. ISBN: 0–936–07707–7. 288 pp. HS.

Miller writes of her obsession with food, overeating, bulimia, and her eventual recovery. Her story provides hope for other victims and their families.

Phillips. K. A. (1995). *Diary of an anorexic.* West Palm Beach, FL: Palm Bay Publications. ISBN: 0–964–45270–7. 139 pp. MS, HS.

This diary takes readers into the mind of a young woman as she struggles with an obsession that distorts reality and can kill. It shows her obsessive thought processes and the emotional devastation of anorexia, but it also reveals how she breaks through the self-destruction to recovery.

Smith, C., and B. Runyon (1998). *Diary of an eating disorder: A mother and daughter share their healing journey.* ISBN: 0–878–33971–X. Dallas: Taylor Publishing. 232 pp. HS.

This diary covers Smith's two-year bout with anorexia and bulimia, caused by her self-hatred of her body, and her eventual recovery. Interspersed throughout the diary are her mother's insights and messages to those who love someone with an eating disorder.

Eating Disorders: Nonfiction

Boskind-White, M., and W. C. White (Forthcoming). *Bulimarexia*. New York: W. W. Norton. ISBN: 0–393–31923–7. HS.

This revised third edition of a comprehensive, practical, and helpful resource on bulimia discusses the dynamics of the binge/purge cycle, adolescent danger signals, and bulimia in the college years and early years of work. The authors use a decidedly behavioral approach with a feminist perspective, the first step being encouraging the binger/purger to take responsibility.

Claude-Pierre, P. (1997). *The secret language of eating disorders*. New York: Times Books. ISBN: 0–812–92842–3. 288 pp. HS.

Founder of a Canadian eating disorder clinic and a parent of two anorexic daughters, the author discusses her theories about eating disorders and the treatment strategies she prefers. Case studies provide examples of her theory, confirmed negativity condition (CNC), a term she coined for feelings of worthlessness and self-loathing. However, there is not agreement among professionals regarding her approach.

Costin, C. (1996). *The eating disorder sourcebook*. Los Angeles: Lowell House. ISBN: 1–565–65463–3. 304 pp. HS.

A recovered anorexic and eating disorder specialist, the author is in a unique position to discuss eating disorders from both a personal and professional perspective. She examines individual and family dynamics and helps readers assess symptoms.

Kinoy, B. P., ed. (1994). *Eating disorders: New directions in treatment and recovery*. New York: Columbia University Press. ISBN: 0–231–09695–X. 166 pp. HS.

Ten professionals from medical, psychological, and nutritional fields, writing for a general audience, discuss their views and experiences with patients who have eating disorders.

Kolodny, N. J. (1998). *When food is foe: How you can confront and conquer your eating disorder*. Boston: Little, Brown. ISBN: 0–316–55843–5. 224 pp. MS, HS.

This newly revised paperback edition examines the causes and effects of bulimia and anorexia and discusses ways to treat and prevent these disorders. Specifically for a young adult audience, this book is an excellent resource.

Maloney, M., R. Kranz, and L. de Bernieres (1991). *Straight talk about eating disorders*. New York: Facts on File. ISBN: 0–816–02414–6. 128 pp. MS, HS.

Written specifically for the young adult female, this book examines the psychological causes and symptoms of anorexia, bulimia, and compulsive eating. It also looks at society's mixed messages about eating, weight, diet, and appearance, and how these messages can be destructive to young women.

Pipher, M. (1997). *Hunger pains: The modern woman's tragic quest for thinness*. New York: Ballantine. ISBN: 0–345–41393–8. 120 pp. HS.

Our appearance-obsessed culture has idealized a body type that most women cannot achieve. In this newly reissued edition, Pipher offers advice about understanding ways to live with our bodies and appetites.

Sherman, R. T., and R. A. Thompson (1996). *Bulimia: A guide for family and friends*. San Francisco: Jossey-Bass. ISBN: 0–787–90361–2. 155 pp. HS.

This book by two leading experts on eating disorders, written in question and answer format, focuses on bulimia: an overview, possible causes, and psychological dynamics of the disorder. The authors' message is that bulimia is a complicated disorder that can be successfully treated.

Siegel, M., J. Brisman, and M. Weinshel (1997). *Surviving an eating disorder: New perspectives and strategies for family and friends*. New York: HarperCollins. ISBN: 0–060–95233–4. 256 pp. HS.

Newly updated to include the latest advances in family therapy, psychopharmacology, hospitalization policies, insurance coverage, and support services, this guide provides a wealth of information and strategies for dealing with anorexia, bulimia, and binge eating. Updated readings and support organizations are also included.

INTERNET RESOURCES

The American Anorexia/Bulimia Association: *http://members.aol.com/amanbu*

The web site for the American Anorexia/Bulimia Association, a nonprofit organization, offers information for those suffering from eating disorders, their friends and family, and professionals, as well as general information.

The Center for Eating Disorders: *http://www.eatingdisorder.org*

This web site is operated by the Center for Eating Disorders of the St. Joseph Medical Center, the University of Maryland. A comprehensive, user-friendly site that offers excellent information and links to other sites.

The Something Fishy Website on Eating Disorders: *http://www.something-fishy.org*

This premier web site provides comprehensive resources.

CHAPTER 10

Reading Anorexia in *Nell's Quilt*

Nancy Mellin McCracken and Jan Carli

Nell's Quilt by Susan Terris, published in 1981, is choice reading for young adults and the older adults in their lives. It provides insights into the range of possible causes of anorexia nervosa, rather than placing the entire blame on contemporary fashion or peer pressure to be thin. Viewing models in magazine ads and TV, it might be easy to forget that causes other than current fashion underlie eating disorders. Joan Jacobs Brumberg's *Fasting Girls* (1988) is the best history of anorexia nervosa. She concludes that "today's anorectic is one of a long line of women and girls throughout history who have used control of appetite, food, and the body as a focus of their symbolic language" (2). Scholars have pointed out that fasting, even to death, is a practice with a long history. Catherine of Siena was sainted in recognition of her fasting. John the Baptist's decision to live on honey and locusts was not viewed as an illness. Brumberg views the disease as it has manifested itself since the latter nineteenth century as "a secular addiction to a new kind of perfectionism, one that links personal salvation to the achievement of an external body configuration rather than an internal spiritual state" (7).

Since the 1970s more and more girls, and some boys, have been identified as having anorexia nervosa. The disorder has been reclassified by the American Psychiatric Association (Zerbe 1995), and it continues to be studied from a variety of perspectives. Because anorexia is life-threatening, it is absolutely essential that those who work with young adults understand this disorder, or complex of disorders. The challenge is to understand how even Princess Diana, one of the most beautiful women in the world, could risk her life as a bulimic, how today's liberated young women, who have more power than their mothers or grandmothers could have imagined, use that power and money to distort and weaken their bodies.

The psychological and counseling perspective reminds us that eating disorders serve a purpose. It is not only the desire to look like the rail-thin models they see in the media that drives some young people to restrict their eating to the point of starvation. Some who suffer from anorexia are seeking a means to gain control over some small part of a life that seems otherwise to be completely controlled by others. Others starve themselves to death trying to stave off the sexual demands and sex roles scripted by society for adults by retaining the shape of a child's body. Carolyn Costin, an author and the director of the Eating Disorder Center of California, for example, includes her anorexia in the list of acknowledgments for her book, *Your Dieting Daughter: Is She Dying for Attention?* (1997): "And finally, last but not least, I am indebted to my own suffering, battle, and victory over an old enemy *and* friend, anorexia nervosa, without whom I would not be the person I am today" (ix). A number of young adult books on the shelves today appear to deal with eating disorders, but those novels that fail to recognize the complexity of the disorders and the positive functions they serve in the lives of the young people who suffer them are not helpful. *Nell's Quilt* is one novel that is sufficiently complex and insightful to be useful for both young people in danger of developing anorexia nervosa and those adults and peers who know them.

Anorexia was first described in medical literature three centuries ago. The case was a female whose eating changed at age eighteen; she was dead by twenty (Bode 1997, 12). While not a new disease, anorexia continues to be lethal for an estimated 10 to 20 percent of its victims. Those who work with adolescents should know how to recognize the signs that a student may be suffering from an eating disorder and should refer such students for professional clinical assessment and therapy. While there is no substitute for professional clinical referral, the fact remains that even once they have been referred, and certainly before referral, all but the most severely ill students with eating disorders continue going to school. Teachers and guidance counselors, who see endangered adolescents daily both before and after referral, are in a position to educate all students about their risk from eating disorders, and they are in a position to support diagnosed students as they continue in school.

In this chapter, Nancy McCracken, English education professor, discusses *Nell's Quilt* by Susan Terris as an outstanding work of young adult fiction that illuminates anorexia nervosa, a sometimes lethal and still puzzling eating disorder. We believe that by reading and discussing *Nell's Quilt*, young adults and their teachers and counselors will gain valuable insights into this disease. Following the discussion of the novel and some suggestions for teaching it as a literary work, we move from historical fiction to the present, and high school guidance counselor Jan Carli sketches two cases based on students she has worked with. Carli offers suggestions framed around Jacquelyn Small's *Becoming Naturally Therapeutic* for teachers and others who work with adolescents who may be troubled by eating disorders. The chapter concludes with a selected annotated bibliography of fiction and nonfiction works recommended for young adults and those who work with them.

When I first started thinking about writing this chapter, my sense of eating disorders was that they are caused by sexism, in a culture that denies its girls and women the pleasures and health of eating—seemingly in direct proportion to their potential for economic and political equality. The liberated flappers of the twenties were held as firmly to the ideal of the childlike body as the aspiring supermoms of the seventies were held to the ideal of the model Twiggy. In the nineties, a decade that has been called postfeminist because it is often perceived that women have achieved freedom, high fashion celebrates the woman in the style that has been called "heroin chic," with models portrayed as starved addicts, dark circles under lifeless eyes, arms wasted, body prone.

Reading Joan Brumberg's *Fasting Girls* and Mary Pipher's *Hunger Pains* and *Reviving Ophelia*, we learn of the social forces that appear to be the leading cause of eating disorders in adolescent girls. Surely, the opening scene in Steven Levenkron's *The Best Little Girl in the World* has been replayed in some variation in the lives of girls who spend some portion of their adolescence in the high risk behavior of eating disorders. Levenkron's best-selling novel is the classic fictional work about anorexia. Like many of the young girls in young adult literature and in life who suffer from anorexia nervosa, Levenkron's fifteen-year-old Francesca/Kessa experiences an event that initiates her focus on food. *Nell's Quilt* shows a different sort of trigger for the protagonist, one that represents some of the underlying functions of the disorder.

NELL'S QUILT

The quilt in the novel serves as a motif and a metaphor for anorexia nervosa: a "crazy quilt" made from daily work, a kind of creativity, an effort to create a new body and a new self—to work away at the small scraps and gradually build a beautiful cover to warm the isolated heart within. Nell begins her quilt the day her parents announce their intention to marry her off to a young widower. She has been thinking that she would like to go to Boston to work, as her Grandmother Shaw had, to further the cause of women's rights. Nell's mother has been encouraging her to make a quilt from the basket of fabric scraps Grandmother Shaw had been saving, but was too busy to get to. As Nell tells it, her grandmother had been planning to make them into a crazy quilt, "but she'd been so busy marching and campaigning for women's rights that she hadn't taken time to do it" (3). Faced with the abrupt loss of the possibility for her to get an education and live an independent life, Nell turns to the scraps, the only remaining legacy of her grandmother.

Ironically, we learn that the quilt scraps are fake. They were purchased from a department store as a kit. And we learn that Grandmother Shaw's good works for women's rights did not extend to her daughters: "And as for the Shaw money, Harvard had inherited it when there was no male to carry on the family name" (5). Indeed, the achievements of the first wave of feminism in the United States were modest. Nell is horrified to discover that she can be given away in marriage. She muses: "Was this truly 1899, only ten months shy of the beginning of the twentieth century? Or had I been catapulted back into the Middle Ages?" (5). The trigger for Nell's anorexia is not a desire to lose weight.

INSIGHTS INTO THE FUNCTIONS OF ANOREXIA

Early in the novel, Nell looks into the chicken coop and considers the chicken's lot: "Eat, lay, and then, soon, die. Not what I wanted for myself" (7). She flings a chicken egg away and, at the same time, begins her anorexic struggle against what appears an inevitable future as wife and mother. That night, for the first time, Nell loses her appetite and notes that "they watched me push food around my plate. I was glad to see they were alarmed. I wanted them to suffer" (8). This motive for not eating is one of the reported reasons for the onset of anorexia: a kind of rebellion in the one area of life where a good girl may safely rebel against her parents and assert her displeasure. But to the credit of Susan Terris and this novel, no such simple single cause is offered for Nell's anorexia.

In fact, the roots of all the causes that have been proposed in the medical and psychological literature on anorexia nervosa are illustrated in the novel. When Terris' Nell loses her appetite, she enters the psychological "golden cage of anorexia" described by Hilde Bruch in her classic medical work on the subject, *The Golden Cage: The Enigma of Anorexia Nervosa* (1978). After studying over seventy anorexics, Bruch concluded that often the causes of anorexia include fear of adult responsibilities and sexuality, and she discovered that many of the effects of anorexia were identical to those exhibited by people suffering from famine. "What has been called 'anorexic behavior,' as if it were specific to anorexia nervosa, such as obsessive, ruminative preoccupation with food, narcissistic self-absorption, infantile regression, is identical with what occurs during externally induced starvation" (9).

Nell's consciousness is deeply influenced by fear of the sexual role that has been scripted for her. In addition, there is a strong suggestion in the novel of prior or potential sexual abuse by the neighbor's hired hand, Tobias. Throughout the novel, Nell says, Tobias "made my flesh creep" (6). He appears to lurk around all the time, ogling both Nell and her younger sister and making them uncomfortable. Nell's parents ignore this danger even when Tobias is found lurking in places where he should not be. In several scenes in the novel, merely seeing Tobias makes Nell literally sick to her stomach. At one point when she is knocked unconscious by a fall, Nell awakens to find to her horror that Tobias has carried her to the stable and lain with her while she was unconscious. Zerbe cites a number of recent studies showing that "50%–60% of all eating disorder patients report a history of physical or sexual assault" (200). Another factor underlying anorexia—rebellion against always having to be "the best girl in the world"—is evident throughout *Nell's Quilt*. Her family needs money, so Nell reasons she will marry Anson Tanner, but when she does her sister will have to fill in to help her mother. Since her sister has been the weak one, Nell decides to change places with her, growing smaller and weaker.

Besides showing the range of functions anorexia can serve for its victims, *Nell's Quilt* clearly illustrates the effects of gradual starvation on the victims of anorexia as reported in the current medical literature. In this regard the quilt serves as a metaphor. In the beginning, the quilt is merely a basket of scraps, aptly called the makings of a crazy quilt, which Nell explains is useful only as an ornament. It will not keep anyone warm. As the novel progresses, the quilt mirrors changes in Nell's condition. At first the quilt is simply a way to fill the time until her arranged marriage. Nell announces that she won't marry Anson Tanner until she finishes the quilt, so it is a way to buy herself time. Before long, as Nell's anorexia progresses, the quilt becomes an obsession, gorgeously embroidered, one square for each important person in her life. At the height of Nell's disease and the beginning of her most intense work on the quilt, Terris shifts the narrator's focus, as Nell begins speaking of herself in the third person, as if she were someone else. Nell represents the ego-splitting that accompanies starvation in anorexics studied by Bruch and others.

This shift in the narrator's perspective happens just after Nell's childhood friend Rob leaves without kissing her goodbye, because, he explains, "you're not the same person. Not the old Nell—not my Nell. You're different now" (90). Nell looks in the mirror and discovers that she does indeed look like a boy. She cuts off her long braid and looks back into the mirror, and from this point until the end of the story, Nell speaks of herself only in the third person: "I saw someone I liked. It was Nell Edmonds. She was lean and smooth. Her belly was flat" (91). The starvation of anorexia has bought Nell the apparent safety of a pre-adolescent's body, but it has cost her her health, and it threatens her very life.

The crazy quilt, like Nell's illness, grows as her body shrinks. She embroiders ever more colorful patterns on each square of the quilt, even as she begins to hallucinate and grows steadily weaker and less able to think straight. Finally, when the quilt has taken over her entire life, Nell decides to dye it black, to cover all the bright color and beauty that was her life before the illness. The scene of the dyeing and Terris' language are evocative of a failed suicide:

> The crazy quilt on which she'd spent nearly a year of her life was dark now. . . . The quilt should have been uniform in color—a solid, coal black. It was, instead, a quirky melange of blacks, bronzes, buffs, mahogany browns, and other charred, soot tones. Different fabrics had absorbed the dye in different ways. . . . "That was the best, the very best I could do."
> (158)

Nell carries the quilt up to her bed and lays it over her shrunken body and prepares to die. But she doesn't. Like 80 to 95 percent of her contemporary nonfiction counterparts, Nell survives her anorexia. Like the quilt, whose persistent underlying colors and patterns resist absorbing the black dye, Nell's spirit resists death. As a survivor of a severe eating disorder, her life will be different, but beautiful in its own way and with its earlier color showing through.

At the end of the novel Nell speaks again directly of herself in the first-person narrative voice: "I, Eleanor Sara Edmonds, was trapped there, unable to move, unable to change anything. Death was going to stalk in at *my* door and take *me*. . . . I sat up and took hold of the dark, heavy quilt. 'No, no, no . . . ' " (162).

The novel ends as it began, "No, no, no."

TEACHING IDEAS

Nell's Quilt may be studied for its literary qualities as well as for its health insights, and there are many extension activities that all students might do to enrich their reading of the novel. A few are suggested here.

Literary Allusions

Terris makes good use of literary allusions throughout the novel. Poets Emily Dickinson (13) and Robert Frost are alluded to (" 'What a day,' Rob kept repeating. 'First fire and then ice. Fire and ice, fire and ice' " ([15]). George Bernard Shaw is suggested in Grandmother Shaw, and Ralph Waldo Emerson's statement "The only gift is a portion of thyself" (55) is the text for a sermon Nell finds herself resisting. The name Nell recalls Charles Dickens' Nell of *The Old Curiosity Shop*. When Terris' Nell lies dying, we think of Kit's tender lines at the end of the novel, "Why dost thou lie so idle there, dear Nell . . . when there are bright red berries out of doors waiting for thee to pluck them?" Nell's description of herself early in the novel—"Nell the Good. Dependable Nell. Our Nell—is one in a million"—echoes the description of Dickens' Nell: "She was dead. Dear, gentle, patient, noble Nell was dead." It is interesting to compare and contrast the nineteenth-century notions of the good girl as presented in both novels. Terris' character Tobias is also reminiscent of Dickens' minor villains, preying on innocent girls, abusive toward his poor wife.

Point of View

First-person point of view, particularly stream-of-consciousness techniques employed in *Nell's Quilt*, might be studied alongside Katherine Porter's "The Jilting of Granny Wetherall" with older readers. Students might be encouraged to keep a journal as they respond to Nell's. Certainly the students can be asked to consider the shift in point of view discussed earlier. They might try writing about themselves in the third person to see how doing so offers a different perspective.

Symbolism

Symbolism, as the discussion at the beginning of this chapter demonstrates, is well exemplified in Terris' use of the quilt itself for Nell's illness. Another fruitful exploration for students would be the use of color symbolism. Each square of the quilt is done in different colors to represent relationships and people in Nell's life. Artistic students in a literature circle would find it profitable to trace the use of color imagery, and even to draw the quilt squares as they are described in the novel. Students might design quilt squares for the characters in this novel or others.

Students could also write on the use of color throughout the novel, paralleling the way the scraps grow from a colorless basket of "silk and velvet scraps" and "the basket full of patches" (4) into the lushly colored quilt near the end of the story. They could follow the way Susan Terris abruptly inserts a colorful image into Nell's landscape, for example, the "bluish shadows" on the cheeks of Anson Tanner (4).

Historical Research

Nell's Quilt is historical fiction. It may seem odd to some readers to recommend a historical novel as a way of understanding a contemporary disease such as anorexia, and yet that is one of the most interesting aspects of the novel. Older students could profitably read some of Shaw's plays, especially *Major Barbara*. Some might choose to research early U.S. feminists such as Lucy Stone, who is named in the novel. The hunger-striking British feminists, and their punishment by force-feeding in prisons, would be interesting collateral reading for *Nell's Quilt*. Students might also enjoy reading some of Shaw's Fabian tracts and the discussion of Victorian feminism in Barbara B. Watson's *A Shavian Guide to the Intelligent Woman*.

Relationships and Characterization

The novel shows, through Nell's eyes, the anguish and helplessness of the family and friends of a person suffering with anorexia. Terris does a good job depicting the relationships between Nell and the secondary characters in the novel, especially Rob, her best friend. Readers can easily see the ineffectiveness of the scolding offered by Nell's father and the cajoling of her mother. In contrast, the slow development of the relationship between Nell and Tobias' abused wife Ludie shows the role that nonjudgmental caring can play in the recovery from anorexia. In addition to opportunities to study techniques of characterization, the novel provides important lessons in relationships for readers who have friends or relatives who appear to be suffering from anorexia. By exploring the responses of the secondary characters to Nell's illness, readers will gain insights into ways to respond to eating-disordered individuals. As Janet Bode writes in *Food Fight*, "There is no mandatory accreditation for those who treat eating disorders. There is no universal treatment for adolescents let alone preteens, eight to twelve" (119). The fictional world of *Nell's Quilt* does provide opportunities for young people to explore the very real world of eating disorders, and perhaps by looking inward through Nell's eyes they may be better armed against anorexia's lethal threats.

OUT OF THE NOVEL AND INTO THE CLASSROOM: TODAY'S ANOREXIC YOUNG ADULTS

Jenny's Story

Word floated up to the high school from the middle school that an eighth grade phenom was on the way. Jen started running distance in seventh grade and said she immediately knew what God wanted for her. She would be a witness with her running. She won cross-country and track meets and made a countrywide reputation as a freshman. She returned to school for her sophomore year looking gaunt. Teachers commented on her weight loss. The school nurse reported that Jen had weighed 121 pounds for her freshman athletic physical and now weighed 103 pounds. Jenny's only comment was that she had stepped up her training. Her coach and her parents were not concerned. They knew how hard she worked. At the home opener of the girls' basketball season, Jen's appearance stunned the crowd. Her upper arms jutted from the flapping team jersey like twigs. Most shockingly, her skull appeared to be protruding from her forehead. Her countenance in class and on the court was grim. As she slipped below 95 pounds, the cross-country coach and the school nurse supplemented my calls home with calls of their own. Jen's mother grudgingly took her to the family physician, who asked her to record what she ate. He was satisfied with the menus she produced and suggested that she let up a little on her training.

Jen told me she read everything she could find on Olympic marathon champion Greta Weiss and modeled her training regimen after hers. She had no intention of changing her routine or of seeking therapy.

Her goal to be a witness for God with her running was firm. She was patient, polite, but seemingly unmoved by our continuing efforts to stay in touch with her on this issue for the remainder of tenth grade. And she lost no more weight that year.

That summer, her high school coach introduced her to the local college cross-country coach and team members. Jen's ability allowed her to work out at their level. She made friends and was invited to join in Christian activities at the college. Jen returned to school her junior year to start the season with a running weight that floated between 112 and 115 pounds. She won the State Division I cross-country title. Her face was rounder and softer, and her eyes were open and friendly. She surprised her teachers, displaying a cunning wit and a taste for subtle sarcastic humor never heard from her before. When she won her second state title in her senior year, after rebounding from a serious back injury, she was soaring. Offers from the most prestigious running programs in the country were politely refused. Jen would attend the local college (which, by the way, has a national reputation in distance running), where she is already considered a team member. Jen refuses to call her sophomore episode an eating disorder. She views it as a training error that God and her coaches helped her correct. When I see Jen in easy conversation with friends in the hall these days, she witnesses to me of the gifts of recovery.

Sue's Story

The adopted daughter of professional parents, Sue followed a brother who was a stand-out diver and pole vaulter for our high school. She was painstakingly perfect in her written work. A grade of 97 on a geometry exam brought mortification. Sue's eyes were usually downcast. If a teacher worked at it, she could coax a quick, nervous smile. Dramatic weight loss came between grades nine and ten. She began to tell her parents that she needed to lose even more weight. She told me that the only problem she had was her weight and appetite, and she seemed astonished that so many people were starting to mention it. As she lost weight, she became more defiant and assertive on the topic. When speaking about her body, her head rose, her eyes met mine, and she was in charge. First attempts at therapy seemingly made no difference in her determination to lose more. When her weight approached ninety pounds, her parents had her admitted to the local city children's hospital. Throughout her decline and hospitalization, both of Sue's parents maintained a downright cheerful attitude. Yes, they said, things were a little out of control, but the staff at the hospital had positive encouragement for them, and would I please ask her teachers for more homework to take to the eating disorder unit. They didn't want her to lose her 4.0 grade point average. Sue was hospitalized three times in all. As she improved over the next two years, she talked about feeling more relaxed and confident, and she credited her therapist with helping her see good things in her life other than weight loss. She always maintained her 4.0 and always smiled tightly in her mother's presence. She became a registered dietitian, went on to manage the dietary units for a chain of nursing homes, and is happily married to a chemical dependency counselor.

BECOMING A THERAPEUTIC TEACHER

Literally translated, anorexia nervosa means a "nervous loss of appetite." In fact, sufferers of the disease report extreme hunger pains and obsessive thoughts and dreams of food, but, even so, they severely restrict their eating in pursuit of thinness. The disease has serious psychological as well as physical complications. Young people afflicted with anorexia today often have an extreme fear of becoming obese and express bizarre distortions of their body image. They frequently express feelings of unworthiness and extreme self-loathing. Self-starvation interrupts the body's biochemistry, affecting body temperature, heart rate, hormone balance, and the menstrual cycle.

The onset of this disease is usually in early adolescence. Puberty arrives. Young minds focus on their bodies, and weight concerns take center stage. Today the onset of anorexia nervosa typically occurs during the transition from middle school to high school. Bulimia frequently develops when young women make the transition from high school to college. And compulsive overeating can manifest itself as a coping device anytime from puberty to well into middle age. These three eating disorders have distinct characteristics and require distinctly different treatment approaches. But their common theme is using food, weight, or dieting to solve social and emotional problems. And it is here that the alert and caring classroom teacher can take a therapeutic role.

WHAT MIGHT ANOREXIA NERVOSA LOOK LIKE IN THE CLASSROOM?

- The student loses significant amounts of weight yet persists in dieting behaviors. In extreme cases where the victims are obviously emaciated, they still avow the need to work harder on their diet. Expressions of concern may be interpreted as jealousy at how thin they are becoming.

- Victims claim to feel fat even though they are obviously underweight. They frequently obsess on one particular body part, such as stomach or thighs, which they claim to be grossly fat. Sufferers frequently work conversations, note writing to friends, or writing assignments around to how grotesque their body is. No amount of reality checking from the outside world seems to penetrate their point of view.

- Victims express intense fear and loathing of becoming fat. Their fear and disgust does not diminish as they lose weight. Girls will frequently embark on intense research on the fat content of foods and memorize impressive calorie-count lists. Oddly enough, some girls become fascinated with recipes and cooking or express the desire to become a chef or a dietitian, or pursue some other career related to food!

- Ritualistic behavior may appear. Such behaviors as elaborately arranging and rearranging their lunch food or rigidly intense exercise programs may be seen.

- Withdrawal from friends, preoccupation with perfecting their assignments, and bouts of depression and irritability may be noticed.

RECOMMENDATIONS FOR TEACHERS

While most girls in any given classroom are not actively involved in clinically disordered behavior, a teacher can be sure that today's classes are filled with girls who are obsessing about the size and appearance of their bodies most of the time. Knowledge, grades, and issues of character take a backseat to the study of diet strategy, exercise regimens, and fashion. Students who are suffering from full-blown eating disorders are painful to watch and puzzling to attempt to help. Lay on top of this whatever skewed attitudes and problem histories with weight and eating teachers themselves may bring into the classroom, and the mix is further muddled. What follows are some thoughts on the teacher's role in dealing with eating disorders and cultural attitudes about weight and the body in the classroom:

- Acquire and stay current on basic information about eating disorders. We have already discussed how the three disorders may take shape in students. Alongside the poisonous messages displayed in the mass media today are numerous articles about these diseases. (It is often mind-boggling to see a magazine issue carry a serious article about the perils of eating disorders alongside articles about getting one's body ready for bathing suit season and recipes for chocolate suicide cake!) Newspapers, popular magazines, and web sites offer current thinking from experts in the field. These articles make interesting bulletin board material in the classroom. Displayed alongside questionable photos and headlines from the magazines you see carried around by your students, these articles need no comment from the teacher. You can be sure they will be read.

- Be aware of toxic cultural messages in your classroom and in your students' world. Make note of the points of view presented on the TV channels and shows your students discuss. Notice the popular reading material your students bring to class. Write down harmful comments about weight, fashion, bodies, or eating that you hear in the halls and the cafeteria. Find an appropriate way to lay out these toxic messages in front of your students, and ask them to respond.

- Be aware of the attitudes about your relationship to your students that you carry around unconsciously. One study reports that many anorexics have at least one parent working in the "helping professions." It is a well-intentioned, yet not helpful attitude to present oneself as a healthy, complete, untroubled individual—someone who has all the answers. After all, we're the teachers. Shouldn't we have all the answers? People with eating disorders of any kind experience untold amounts of shame and guilt about their eating behaviors, their weight, and their appearance. They are embarrassed by their imperfect attempts to cope with their perceived world. They fear that if their friends, parents, and teachers saw them as they really are, they would recoil in horror and reject them. It is painful to be who they really are, so eating-disordered people use their behaviors of starvation, bingeing, and purging as ways of coping. It is not healing for them to be around others who carry the attitude that they are perfect people.

In a wonderfully practical book, *Becoming Naturally Therapeutic*, Jacquelyn Small describes how people take on the persona of the Preacher, Judge, or Savior in an effort to be helpful. When teachers become the Preacher, they take on a moralistic tone. "There is a right way and a wrong way to behave. Shame on you. You chose the wrong way. Do it this way and you will be living correctly and everything will be fine."

We have all seen the Judge at work in our school. The Judge often tells students, "Your actions are wrong. There is a penalty to pay for the way you have behaved. I will set down a way for you to pay for what you have done wrong. Do this, this, and this and you will return to good standing in our community." And how hard is it to resist taking on the role of Savior? To swoop in and save the day and see the gratitude in a student's eyes? Leading rescue missions to bring quick solutions to a student's problems is a role teachers frequently take on. Saviors can impart the idea that those they seek to save do not have the innate tools to save themselves. Many teachers need to be needed, but in doing so leave students stuck with the role of being the needy, helpless ones; in the process, such teachers never lead students to learn how to use their own emotional strengths to save themselves. Sometimes teachers do need to intervene in situations of imminent danger to a student. But on a day-to-day basis Preachers, Judges, and Saviors who set themselves up as all-knowing and untroubled individuals leave students feeling inadequate, hopeless, or resentful.

There is nothing evil or malicious behind the need to take on these personalities. It is how human beings protect themselves in situations that are hard to face. It is scary to see students struggling with eating disorders. Teachers are supposed to have all the answers, but, of course, we don't. It is easy to pick up the Preacher, Judge, or Savior as a way of handling situations for which we know we don't have all the answers. We can become mindful of the attitudes we adopt as teachers. We can notice the Preacher, Judge, and Savior when they put in an appearance in our classroom. And we can also learn some easy therapeutic attitudes to practice in the classroom.

There are some basic, healthy ways of relating to your students that make your classroom a safe place for students to explore not only fear-ridden teenage attitudes toward weight and body image, but the myriad of other sensitive issues high school students must face. If teachers want to have an impact on the lives of their students, eating-disordered or not, there are some simple healing attitudes that can really help their cause. These therapeutic attitudes are easy for anyone to learn, and give teachers a practical tool for helping their students grow. In fact, these attitudes are useful as a personal orientation in any relationship with others.

We are all helped to move toward healing in the presence of those who display *respect, empathy*, and *warmth*. When we practice respect, empathy, and warmth, we are asked to clear out a space in our mind and our heart to see our students unclouded by judgment.

Therapeutic teachers make it known in dozens of spoken and unspoken ways that they believe each student has the strength and ability built into them to make it in life. Further, they communicate that every individual has the right to make his or her own decisions and the capacity to make good decisions. Their attitude of *respect* informs students of the teacher's belief that all students are equal and capable. Toxic teachers make it clear that they find the so-called problems of certain students to be small and inconsequential. They indicate that such students should just get over it, or they find ways to inform students that they are not smart enough to make their own decisions and that they always make bad choices. Toxic teachers who are low in respect for their students become narrow-minded and believe that their own way of thinking is the only correct way. Students don't thrive in the presence of a teacher who does not respect them, their right to be their own person, and their natural strengths and abilities. Without respect, eating-disordered students do not feel safe to discard their harmful behaviors and practice other ways of existing in the world. Without a continuous attitude of respect flowing from the therapeutic teacher to a student with eating problems, all attempts to help a student are useless.

Toxic teachers have a really difficult time displaying *empathy*. Their need to be right is so strong that it blocks out their ability to put themselves in their students' place. The therapeutic teacher attempts to join the student and see the world through her eyes. Empathetic teachers make clear their desire to know what the student feels, fears or seeks. To empathize, one does not have to agree with the student's feelings. We might feel that other positions would be wiser or more helpful in solving their problems. An empathetic listener attempts to stand beside the student and see the world through her eyes. It is important to mirror back or restate to the student what you believe you see. At the same time, one must be open for corrections or revisions of those perceptions. One can make simple statements of the image or sense of her experience. For example: "It's as though you are so tired of fighting this battle. I sense that you never feel good enough." Then, by asking if the perception is correct, the teacher indicates further willingness to join the student in comprehending her view of the situation. Practicing empathy demonstrates respect, conveys genuine interest, and shows the desire to understand what the student needs. The sufferer of an eating disorder may not yet know what she fears or what she needs, but continuing demonstrations of empathy are comforting and therapeutic. The therapeutic teacher may be one of the few people in her life making a sincere effort to understand her. The battered self-esteem of an eating-disordered individual is desperately in need of these healing displays of empathy.

Students suffering from eating disorders experience lots of shame about their thoughts and behaviors. They often refuse to seek help, believing they are not worthy of the concern of others and are beyond hope. They desperately need displays of *warmth* from therapeutic teachers to learn that they are deserving of love and care. A spontaneous hand on the shoulder, an affectionate teasing remark, or a simple sincere smile frequently offered is powerfully healing for those with severe self-esteem problems. Asking the student to act as an aide doing useful tasks alongside the teacher demonstrates that the student is seen as more than her disorder, more than a set of symptoms occupying a desk. Toxic teachers find all kinds of ways to avoid genuine displays of emotion in the classroom. Throwing up the need to stay in character as the authority figure, toxic teachers intellectualize feelings rather than experience them. Or they discount and trivialize emotions, suggesting that the student should just cheer up or suck it up or simply get over all these messy feelings. Not everyone is comfortable expressing warmth, and displays should never be forced. Students have an uncanny ability for spotting a fake. It would be better to work on simply being genuine, natural, and friendly than to act out uncomfortable gestures. Warmth, of course, is not sexual, and carries a tone that is easy to differentiate from seductive behavior. Expressions of sincere warmth help eating-disordered students take steps toward self-acceptance and healing.

People who have recovered from eating disorders report that it was important that the people around them kept delivering messages of interest, concern, respect, and love over and over again. In the worst days of dealing with their disorder those messages were heard from a distance. Gradually it became possible to hear messages more clearly. Those in recovery from eating disorders remember that their own internal voices were shouting messages of self-hate and shame so loudly that they could barely respond to others. Therapeutic teachers speaking empathetic words of encouragement with warmth and respect again and again are powerful, healing individuals.

- Know when to refer. Never fail to pass along worrisome concerns for fear of looking foolish or out of line. Concerns about a student who may have an eating disorder are always appropriate to pass along to school staff members. School nurses and guidance counselors have access to information and professional help. They can deal with the problem from other angles of assistance than you can from your classroom. Your report of classroom behavior provides valuable material in convincing parents of the need to seek intervention. School officials are often met with skepticism or outright hostility when attempting to report concerns about eating disorders to parents. It seems to go with the territory that parents are often just as unwilling to seek help as the child is. A great deal of fear surrounds the presence of an eating disorder. Therapeutic teachers can rest in the assurance that their practice of warm, respectful, and empathetic behaviors can help move the student and the family toward healing.

When life presents stressful situations for which an adolescent has developed few coping skills, eating disorders may ensue. Young adult literature like *Nell's Quilt* has the potential to reach student readers, and perhaps the historical distance provided by Terris' novel can be a starting point for discussion or journaling for students who are similarly at risk of retreating under a deadly quilt of anorexia.

RECOMMENDED READINGS

Eating Disorders: Fiction

Hautzig, D. (1999). *Second star to the right*. New York: Puffin Books. ISBN: 0–141–30580–0. 176 pp. MS, HS.

This novel implicates the smothering mother and the Holocaust history as well as the perfect daughter syndrome. *Second Star* is pretty unrelentingly sad as the protagonist gradually starves.

Kerr, M. E. (1989). *Dinky Hocker shoots smack*. New York: Harper Trophy. ISBN: 0–064–47006–7. MS, HS.

A good choice for insights into the functions of compulsive overeating. "To ask someone like Dinky to go into Woerner's Restaurant just to pick up pies for her mother was to ask a wino to drop in at a vineyard just to watch the bottling process" (19).

Lipsyte, R. (1991). *One fat summer*. New York: HarperCollins. ISBN: 0–064–47073–3. 232 pp. MS, HS.

Bobby Marks hates summertime because he can't hide under baggy winter clothing. When he gets a job taking care of the grounds of a doctor's home, he experiences "one fat summer."

Strasser, T. (1996). *How I changed my life*. New York: Simon and Schuster. ISBN: 0–606–10846–7. 256 pp. HS.

Kyle Winthrop suffers a knee injury, and Bolita Vine decides to lose weight and change her image. They both become involved in the school play and develop a close friendship.

Terris, S. (1996). *Nell's Quilt*. New York: Farrar, Straus and Giroux. ISBN: 0–374–45497–3. 176 pp. MS, HS.

This book is the focus of this chapter.

Eating Disorders: Nonfiction

Bode, J. (1997). *Food fight: A guide to eating disorders for pre-teens and their parents*. New York: Simon and Schuster. ISBN: 0–689–80272–2. 153 pp. ES, MS.

Because eating disorders are occurring at ever younger ages, Bode targets this book to preteens. Noting that anorexia, bulimia, and compulsive eating rarely have physiological causes, she discusses the psychological and social pressures that cause eating disorders. Interviews with children who suffer from eating disorders provide an important touchstone for the preteen reader. In the parents' section Bode includes sources for help and further reading as well as discussion of insurance plans, which usually do not cover hospitalization for eating disorders even when medically necessary.

Bordo, S. (1993). *Unbearable weight: Feminism, Western culture, and the body*. Berkeley: University of California Press. ISBN: 0–520–07979–5. 362 pp. HS.

A feminist cultural critique of the idea that girls' preoccupation with the body and fear of fat is always pathological. As Bordo writes, the pathology approach "ignores the fact that for most people in our culture, slenderness is indeed equated with competence, self-control, and intelligence, and feminine curvaceousness (in particular, large breasts) with wide-eyed, giggly vapidity. Virtually every proposed hallmark of 'underlying psychopathology' in eating disorders has been deconstructed to reveal a more widespread cultural disorder. A dramatic example is the case of BIDS, or body image distortion syndrome" (75).

Bruch, H. (1978). *The golden cage: The enigma of anorexia nervosa*. New York: Vintage Random House. ISBN: 0–674–35650–0. 150 pp. HS.

This is the classic medical and psychological study of anorexia.

Brumberg, J. J. (1997). *The body project: An intimate history of American girls.* New York: Random House. ISBN: 0–679–40297–7. 304 pp. HS.

Based on a comparison of diaries written by girls in the late nineteenth and twentieth centuries, Brumberg illustrates the cultural shift from Victorian girls' projects to improve their characters or skills to postmodern girls' projects to improve their appearance by losing weight, body piercing, etc. "At the end of the twentieth century, living in a girl's body is more complicated than it was a century ago. On the one hand, their parents and teachers told them that being female was no bar to accomplishment. Yet girls of their generation learned from a very early age that the power of their gender was tied to what they looked like—and how 'sexy' they were—rather than to character or achievement" (195).

Brumberg, J. J. (1988). *Fasting girls: The emergence of anorexia nervosa as a modern disease.* Cambridge, MA: Harvard University Press. ISBN: 0–452–26327–1. 376 pp. HS.

Traces the phenomenon of fasting from "sainthood to patienthood" and reminds us that food is symbolic, and thus anorexia has had distinctive social and cultural contexts.

Costin, C. (1997). *Your dieting daughter: Is she dying for attention?* New York: Brunner/Mazel. ISBN: 0–876–30836–1. 240 pp.

Costin, a therapist and former eating disorder victim, offers a coping guide for patients and families.

Elisabeth, L. (1989). *Keep coming back: The spiritual journey of recovery in Overeaters Anonymous.* New York: Harper. ISBN: 0–894–86527–7. 128 pp. (Out of print)

Discusses the use of meditation and spiritual awareness as a part of recovery.

Heywood, L. (1996). *Dedication to hunger: The anorexic aesthetic in modern culture.* Berkeley: University of California Press. ISBN: 0–520–20117–5. 243 pp.

Heywood, "a lapsed anorexic," studies the links between anorexia and modernist academic imperatives to use "anorexic logic." She concludes: "Bodies in pieces: I'd like to hold on to each one. Heal the scar between 'theory' and 'living' that often surfaces in practice, the privilege sometimes extended to cynical toughness, unemotional prose, theory without organs, detachable floating minds. Anorexic language, whistling through space, empty as trees. We've been Hegelian 'shadows' long enough. We've been anorexic long enough" (202). A scholarly and readable study of the link between physical anorexia and textual anorexia.

Pipher, M. (1994). *Reviving Ophelia.* New York: Putnam's. ISBN: 0–399–13944–3. 304 pp.

The chapter "Worshipping the Gods of Thinness" is a good overview of the various eating disorders, including compulsive overeating, in the context of contemporary mass culture: "For example, in 1950 the White Rock mineral water girl was 5 feet 4 inches tall and weighed 140 pounds. Today she is 5 feet 10 inches and weighs 110 pounds." Pipher summarizes studies that report that "on any given day in America, half of our teenage girls are dieting and that one in five young women has an eating disorder. Eight million women have eating disorders in America" (184–185).

Small, J. (1990). *Becoming naturally therapeutic: A return to the true essence of helping.* New York: Bantam. 0–553–34800–0. 148 pp.

Discusses the personal characteristics of therapists—how to care, empathize and heal.

Watson, B. B. (1972). *A Shavian guide to the intelligent woman.* New York: Norton.

Zerbe, K. J. (1993/1995). *The body betrayed: A deeper understanding of women, eating disorders, and treatment.* Carlsbad, CA: Gurze Books. ISBN: 0–936–07723–9.

CHAPTER 11

HIV/AIDS: *What You Don't Know Can Kill You*

Nancy Prosenjak, and Laura Sullivan and Diane Hartman

The first young adult case of AIDS in the United States was reported in 1986. In reaction to this event, young adult books about HIV/AIDS quickly began to appear. Within the year, the first young adult novel using AIDS as a plot problem was published, M. E. Kerr's *Night Kites* (1986), as well as an informational book on how one contracts and transmits the human immunodeficiency virus (HIV) and acquired immunodeficiency syndrome (AIDS). More than one hundred informational books have been published for the audience of young adults; however, the topic of HIV/AIDS is nearly nonexistent within the body of young adult contemporary realistic fiction. As of 1999, a total of just nineteen young adult novels about HIV/AIDS have been published, even though according to the Centers for Disease Control there have been 7,902 HIV/AIDS cases of children under age thirteen, 4,602 deaths, and 1,586 newly reported HIV infection cases during 1998–1999 within this age group. There have been 4,805 cases among young adults ages thirteen to nineteen, with about 2,787 deaths. In addition, many children and young adults are living with or know people who are HIV/AIDS patients. The HIV/AIDS epidemic has touched the young adult community with dramatic consequences, yet the realm of contemporary fiction has rarely offered young adult readers a realistic view of the disease.

Many of the novels use a protagonist who is a healthy teenager whose normal life crises are supplanted by the need to deal with the emotions of knowing and/or loving a minor character with HIV/AIDS. Medical treatment the patient receives and names of typical AIDS medications are rarely mentioned, as the protagonist is not old enough to be included in the conversations between the patient and the physicians. In most of the novels, the symptoms of full-blown AIDS are realistically depicted, as the protagonist is often in daily contact with the patient and notices physical changes, including frequent bouts with opportunistic diseases such as pneumocystis carinii pneumonia (PCP), a specialized type of pneumonia that affects only AIDS patients; Kaposi's sarcoma, a specialized type of cancer that appears as purple blotches on the skin; a decreased number of helper T-cells; swollen glands and lymph nodes; thrush, a mouth infection; and diarrhea. None of these related diseases is fatal to people whose immune system is intact. The majority of the characters with AIDS die within the course of the novels, most fairly quickly after diagnosis. In reality, health care professionals state that HIV/AIDS patients who are under the care of an infectious disease specialist are living increasingly long and productive lives that young adult fiction does not represent.

Two of the novels included in the nineteen insert AIDS-related issues in the very briefest of ways (Morris Gleitzman's *Two Weeks with the Queen* [1989] and Ron Koertge's *The Arizona Kid* [1988]. The remaining seventeen novels use illness with AIDS as a major plot problem that affects the life of the main character with varying degrees of drama and trauma through the device of a minor character who contracts HIV/AIDS. The infected characters are related to the narrator/protagonist in a number of ways but are most often an adult family member or a peer. This device of not having the teen narrator contract the disease provides a bit of distance for the young adult reader, perhaps softening the potential impact of the death of a character the reader has come to like. There are not a lot of young adult novels in which a teen dies of disease and, indeed, no teen protagonists die in these nineteen novels on the topic of AIDS.

Of the nineteen novels published to date, six use blood transfusion as a mode of HIV infection, perhaps because the infected person is then an innocent, rather than a person who is gay or an intravenous drug user whose morality the reader may judge. In these novels, the infected characters include one uncle, in Alida E. Young's *I Never Got to Say Goodbye* (1988); one teacher's spouse, in Patricia Hermes' *Be Still My Heart* (1989); one friend, in Lee Bantle's *Diving for the Moon* (1995); and two schoolmates, in Gloria Miklowitz's *Good-bye Tomorrow* (1987) and Miriam Cohen's *Laura Leonora's First Amendment* (1990).

The possibility of becoming infected because of a blood transfusion was virtually eliminated in 1985 by new regulations for testing donated blood. The U.S. Department of Health's Center for Disease Control and Prevention (CDC) reports a fraction of 1 percent of newly reported cases as listing blood transfusion as the mode of transmission. Since HIV can remain dormant within the human body for more than ten years, patients who contracted it through transfusions are still undergoing treatment. However, new cases contracted through transfusion will be extremely rare. This makes the most recently published novel, Lee Bantle's *Diving for the Moon* (1995), which uses the plot problem of a hemophiliac contracting HIV through a transfusion, appear rather irresponsible, as young adults should no longer fear blood donation or transfusion.

In the novels most recently published (there have been no new novels about AIDS for this age group between 1996 and 1999), a change in method of transmission is evidenced, perhaps because of the rising incidence of gay men who have contracted HIV. Of these more recent novels, seven hint at homosexual intercourse as the cause of transmission, since the infected characters are known to be gay. Instead of the infected characters being teenagers they are either gay or bisexual adult males, including two dads, in Paula Fox's *Eagle Kite* (1995) and Theresa Nelson's *Earthshine* (1994); two older adult brothers, in M. E. Kerr's *Night Kites* and Deborah Davis' *My Brother Has AIDS* (1994); one uncle, in Penny Raife Durant's *When Heroes Die* (1994); and two teachers, in Marilyn Levy's *Rumors and Whispers* (1990) and Marilyn Kaye's *Real Heroes* (1993). A third novel, Patricia Hermes' *Be Still My Heart*, uses a teacher's heterosexual spouse who has received a transfusion of tainted blood and becomes HIV-positive. These three novels use the device of a teacher or link to a teacher to portray the fear and stigmatization within the community, as parents and school administrators thoroughly discuss the research on the possibilities of casual transmission in the school setting.

In another novel, the infected aren't developed as characters, but are babies who are HIV-positive because of their mothers' infection, mainly through intravenous drug use. These babies are cared for by the protagonist, a female teen in Lurlene McDaniel's *Baby Alicia is Dying* (1993); through hearing about the care of these infants, the reader understands the depth of the problem of the largest growing population of HIV patients—newborn infants who contract HIV from their mothers, either perinatally, postnatally, or during breast feeding.

The majority of the characters who become infected are male. In only three of the nineteen novels are the characters who contract the disease female: one mother who has been married to an intravenous drug user in Barbara Ann Porte's *Something Terrible Happened* (1994), and two teen female characters who are infected through heterosexual intercourse, one older sister in Fran Arrick's *What You Don't Know Can Kill You* (1992), the focus novel of this chapter; and one teenage friend in Clayton Bess' *The Mayday Rampage* (1993).

The majority of the characters who become infected are adults. In only four of the novels are the infected characters teenagers who contract HIV, but in each of these novels, a healthy friend or sister of the infected teen narrates the story, so the voice of the protagonist who is living with the illness is not always heard in a powerful way. The device of observing infected characters and reporting on their emotions and the progress of their disease does not carry the same impact as hearing from the character who has contracted a fatal disease might. In Bantle's *Diving for the Moon*, the sixth grade narrator learns that her best friend, a hemophiliac, contracted HIV as a child through a blood transfusion. In Miriam Cohen's *Laura Leonora's First Amendment*, a peer's right to attend school is defended by the news columns of a teen who renews a friendship with the infected character. In Clayton Bess' *The Mayday Rampage*, the teen co-narrator discloses her HIV status, but only on the last few pages of the novel. The progress of her illness is related in the epilogue's factual chronology, rather than through the plot. In the most realistically plotted novel, Fran Arrick's *What You Don't Know Can Kill You*, the eighteen-year-old sister of the protagonist becomes HIV-positive after sexual intercourse with an infected boyfriend.

THE FACTS OF HIV/AIDS

Fictional literature written for the reading audience of children and young adults usually reflects the common experiences of the lives they lead and the world in which they live, but in the case of HIV/AIDS, young adult literary characters appear to be falsely protected against the syndrome. In the world of the contemporary realistic fiction novel, teenagers rarely contract HIV, only two contract it through sexual intercourse, none contract it through intravenous drug use, and none die. In reality, young adults *do* contract HIV and face the problem of becoming symptomatic when the virus becomes full-blown AIDS. In reality, the person who contracts HIV/AIDS may be a classmate, friend, or sibling, not just a distant relative, teacher, or person in your town. In reality, approximately 40 percent of the reported AIDS cases of young adults ages thirteen to nineteen contract the disease through sexual intercourse, whether heterosexual or homosexual, and another 9 percent through injected drugs.

- **Children and adults contract HIV and become victims of AIDS**. In fact, AIDS is the sixth most prevalent cause of death in the 0–24 age group. According to statistics compiled by the U.S. Department of Health's Centers for Disease Control and Prevention from 1981 through June 1997, a cumulative total of 612,078 persons with AIDS had been reported. Of these 84 percent were adult and teen males, 15 percent adult and teen females, and 1 percent children under age 13. To date, there have been 6,218 cases of children ages 0–5, 90 percent of these infected perinatally; 2,953 teens age 13–19, and 22,070 young adults ages 20–24. Incidence in the age groups for children and young adults is nearly equally divided between males and females, with the exception of the age 20–24 group, in which 75 percent of the reported cases are males. During this same period of data collection, a total of 230 children ages 0–13 died of AIDS; 374,656 persons age 13 and older have died of AIDS. An additional 86,792 persons have been diagnosed with HIV, but not yet with AIDS. It is hypothesized that because the AIDS virus can remain dormant in the body for more than ten years, many adults may have become infected with HIV in their teenage years, but are not yet symptomatic. AIDS is the leading cause of death for those in the 25–44 age group.

- **Adults and teenagers other than gay males contract AIDS**. Initially AIDS was thought to be a disease most likely to affect the gay male population, but the numbers of heterosexuals and women with the disease has steadily increased. CDC reports that about 15 percent of total cases in all age groups are women; about 40 percent of the reported cases for males ages 13–19 were exposed through sex with men; 41 percent of the women in this age group contracted HIV through heterosexual contact; and approximately 30 percent of the babies born to HIV mothers contract HIV, either perinatally, during birth, or through breast feeding. The majority of new cases reported for children under age 13 is through transmission from mother to child. The incidence of newborns contracting HIV is dramatically lessened (from 25 percent to 7 percent) if the mother takes appropriate medication during pregnancy.

- **Adults and teenagers in all cultures and racial groups contract AIDS**. The CDC reports that in the last data period, July 1996—June 1997, 36 percent of the newly reported cases were white, 43 percent black, and 20 percent Hispanic.

- **Children and young adults attend school with peers who have HIV/ AIDS**. People with AIDS are protected by the Americans with Disabilities Act and are not legally bound to disclose their medical status, so cases of school age students with HIV/AIDS are only known to school administrators or health personnel when students require medication during school hours. Widely publicized cases such as that of Ryan White have challenged and changed procedures schools follow. Every teen and every teacher needs to be aware of, and implement, universal precautions to avoid infection and transmission.

- **Children and young adults will have relatives, friends, neighbors, and acquaintances who are infected with HIV/AIDS**. In the data reporting year July 1996 to June 1997, 62,649 new cases of AIDS were reported, bringing the total number of cases reported since data collection began in 1981 to 612,078. Some of these are people we know and love; every teen needs to be able to react with compassion and caring.

- **There is medical treatment for HIV/AIDS patients**. Medication options continue to advance, and new medications offer AIDS patients the prognosis of a longer life and an improved quality of life, but AIDS is still considered a terminal disease. No method has yet been discovered to remove HIV from the body, so it continues to work to destroy the body's immune system. Diseases and opportunistic infections are able to affect the overall health of the patient, because the immune system is compromised. With the implementation of new drugs and combinations of drugs into triple therapy, there has been a substantial decrease in deaths of persons with AIDS.

- **AIDS is preventable**. All teens need to know more about how HIV/ AIDS is transmitted, what activities put an individual at risk, and what they can do to protect themselves against infection. HIV is spread through bodily fluids: blood, breast milk, semen, and vaginal secretions. The most common ways to contract HIV are through unprotected sex and sharing needles from intravenous drug use. If teens are sexually active, they should insist that their partner use a latex condom. If teens come into contact with blood or other bodily fluids, they should use rubber gloves and disinfect the area of spilled fluids with a solution of diluted bleach water. They should not be afraid to come into casual contact with HIV/AIDS patients, as there is not a single known case of a student accidentally transmitting HIV at school.

WHAT YOU DON'T KNOW CAN KILL YOU

The novel we find most realistic, from the stance of the medical diagnosis of HIV/AIDS as well as the psychosocial and emotional effects of the illness on the patient and the family members, is Fran Arrick's

What You Don't Know Can Kill You (1992). Although this novel is not the most recently published, we find it the best example of a young adult novel with a teenager who contracts HIV and whose entire circle of family and friends must deal with the reality of this event. In addition, the novel responsibly challenges the stereotype that HIV/AIDS only affects a particular group of people, that is, gay men and intravenous drug users, and presents a story in which two middle-class, small-town, teenage characters become infected with HIV.

The narrator of the novel is Debra, just completing seventh grade as her eighteen-year-old sister Ellen gets ready for the senior prom, graduation, and college. Debra expresses her desire to one day emulate Ellen's exciting social life, while showing a bit of jealousy over the family attention lavished on Ellen. The method of disclosure is quickly uncovered; chapter one, a local family is in an auto accident and in need of blood. Debra helps to organize a community blood drive, held at the high school as the students hang prom decorations. Ellen generously donates blood.

The hospital lab calls the family because "something showed up in Ellen's blood" (21) during the routine blood screening conducted on all donated blood (mandatory since 1985). Ellen and a parent are asked to make an appointment with the family physician. Because the Geddes family lives in a small town and the family physician has treated the children all his life, he misinforms Ellen and her mother, stating that he's certain the ELISA test has produced a false positive result. Ellen does not fit the stereotypic candidate Doctor Merlini perceives as at risk of HIV infection, since she has no tattoos or body piercing, is in good health, does not appear to be an IV drug user, and most of all, is from a family known personally to the doctor. Doctor Merlini proposes a second blood test, the Western Blot, which he suggests will surely show the error of the first positive result. The family dismisses the potential danger and waits for the results of further testing, as the doctor advises.

Once the initial test results are confirmed, Ellen and her family fall apart. Ellen stays in her room for days; her mother and father ignore their jobs and refuse to talk to anyone, including each other. Debra is seen as the most normal during this initial period of discovery: she continues to see her friends, attends outings, and confides in her best friend Brenda, although she follows her mother's admonition that no one must know of this disgrace. Instead, Debra tells her friend that Ellen has missed her period and she may be pregnant. In the town of Shelter Rock, being pregnant out of wedlock would be less humiliating than being ill with a deadly disease. Debra, a middle-school student, is well informed about HIV because of a mandatory sex education class. She sprinkles her narrative dialogue with practical advice, reminding readers that AIDS is transmitted only through exchange of bodily fluids.

The reader later discovers that Ellen has also taken this sex education class in which the need for latex condoms was emphasized, but had trusted her boyfriend Jack because their first sexual intercourse was with one another. In fact, Ellen is so certain of Jack's love for her that she mentally assumes the blame for being a carrier of HIV, thinking she must have contracted the virus in some new manner, yet unknown to her doctor. Meanwhile Jack provides a contrasting attitude by taking no responsibility for his actions. He was evidently exposed to the HIV virus during a fraternity party where both alcohol and prostitutes were provided; he had never disclosed this incident to Ellen because to him it wasn't important since he didn't "love" the girls. After Ellen discovers Jack's infidelity, she abandons him, refusing to accept his calls.

Jack's suicide is the true tragedy of this novel. He isolates himself, as he thinks his parents aren't interested in hearing about his troubles. The author emphasizes the apparent distance of Jack from his parents, who play bridge and take vacations, never touching base with Jack. He feels alone. Jack has not asked for support from his family, has no friends in which he feels he can confide, does not seek medical treatment, and makes no effort to disclose his concerns to anyone. He turns to alcohol, but no one recognizes his distress signals; he mistakenly thinks his parents will still be proud of him if he dies before the truth is discovered. Against the portrayal of Jack's dysfunctional family, we see the parallel of the more solid Geddes family, which is temporarily stunned, but who will eventually close their circle and heal themselves and their family relationships.

Although this story cannot have a happy ending, the potential for a successful handling of the plot problem is present. Ellen is referred to an infectious disease specialist in the nearby city and begins to attend a support group for PWA (People with AIDS). She makes the decision to begin college and move to an apartment of her own. It seems she won't be missing out on the college experiences she has dreamed of all her life. Although the novel ends before Ellen goes off on her own, the reader predicts that she will make new friends and be strong enough to disclose her condition to them. Ellen and Debra talk about insisting that their parents join a support group, too, so the parents will have the assistance they need to deal with their own personal issues.

Through the avenue of realistic fiction, this novel allows the reader to take a glimpse into the lives of the characters who are struggling in their individual ways with the emotions and personal interactions within the context of family, friends, and the larger communities of school and town. The reader sees the consequences of choices, both good and poor, as well as a variety of coping skills employed by family members and friends. Chris Crutcher (1992), an author who writes for the young adult audience, stated that "stories can help teenagers look at their feelings, or come to emotional resolution, from a safe distance. If as an author, I can make an emotional connection with my reader, I have already started him or her to heal . . . *I am not alone* is powerful medicine" (39). In *What You Don't Know Can Kill You*, the reader sees that the characters who do not remain alone, but seek the help of supporters (both in their circle of family and friends and within the caregivers of social service) begin the process of healing; those who don't look outside themselves (notably Jack and his mother) may be unable to survive. Readers, one hopes, will understand that making the choice to take one's own life is not an acceptable one, as Jack is characterized as self-centered and dysfunctional.

DESIGNING A TREATMENT PLAN FOR ELLEN AND HER FAMILY

The impact that HIV/AIDS has on individuals, families, and friends is devastating from both a medical and psychosocial perspective. A multitude of stressors accompany the notification of HIV-seropositive status. These stressors include confronting a life-threatening illness, discrimination, stigmatization, isolation, and the disruption of relationships. Stabilizing interventions during this time is vital for those infected or affected by HIV/AIDS in order to assist in reestablishing equilibrium within their lives.

In the novel *What You Don't Know Can Kill You*, the fictional Geddes family is faced with the news that their daughter Ellen is HIV-positive. The emotional responses of the various family members are consistent with the actual reactions of individuals; fear, anxiety, denial, depression, anger, guilt, shame, and powerlessness are all common emotional responses people initially experience (Rapaport 1970). The family expresses these feelings both verbally and behaviorally. Maladaptive coping behaviors, common during such times of crisis, including regression, shutting oneself off from the outside world, withdrawing, and disruption in communication (Rapaport 1970), are all apparent in the Geddes family. Adjusting to being HIV-positive is a process that will occur over a period of time and that can be aided by the interventions of health care professionals.

The standard of care for HIV patients is to have an infectious disease physician manage the case. In fact, Ellen's family doctor might have referred her earlier than he did to the specialist in the larger city near Shelter Rock. His hesitation was based on what he thought he knew about Ellen and her family, not the facts that presented themselves through reputable blood tests. It has been demonstrated that patients who go to physicians who are knowledgeable about HIV live a longer and healthier life, because infectious disease physicians keep up to date on new medications and treatment options (Kitahata et al. 1996).

Another option for referral would have been a pediatric infectious disease clinic that treats patients, prenatal to age twenty-four. Many large cities and regional hospitals have such a clinic that uses a multidisciplinary approach involving specialists in various fields related to the illness. In this way, the physical, emotional, nutritional, and psychosocial needs of the child are met with greater success. If Ellen Geddes had entered the treatment program of a pediatric clinic, she would have encountered a variety of specialists.

A typical pediatric infectious disease clinic offers a multidisciplinary approach to treatment that includes counseling interventions to help deal with psychosocial issues. Crisis intervention is a common strategy that involves providing immediate help to a person or family in order to return the person to a state of homeostasis. These interventions are time-limited, present-oriented, and focus on the presenting problem. Some or all of the following strategies may be involved: providing support, problem solving, goal setting, identifying and accessing resources, education, and altering cognitive processes regarding thoughts and feelings (Poindexter 1997). Both Ellen and Jack were shocked by the knowledge that Ellen tested HIV-seropositive, but they reacted in different manners. These teens, their parents, and their siblings would have benefited from the intervention of professionals.

In expectation of Ellen's arrival, the clinic team would have already met and pooled knowledge about Ellen's case, including all test results, the medical history of the case, potential family psychosocial needs, and the family's insurance status (AIDS medications are expensive, and their cost may not be fully covered under family insurance plans; private funding often underwrites the cost of medication). Decisions about which team members would need to see Ellen during the clinic visit would be made cooperatively. Members of the team might include infectious disease doctors, a nutritionist, a pharmacist, two nurse practitioners, two social workers, a neuro-developmental psychologist, and a nurse coordinator. With children younger than Ellen, issues of physical and cognitive development are also addressed in order to assess potential school-related problems. Team members would each track specific elements of Ellen's care, then meet as a multidisciplinary team to plan continuous, integrated care under the guidance of the assigned case manager.

A multidisciplinary team of this kind would be a great asset, as it could offer Ellen and her family a multitude of resources and support. Team members would provide crisis intervention, emotional support, education about HIV for all family members, counseling, dietary advice, and the opportunity to be part of a clinical trial for new medication, as well as assisting families in making informed decisions and choices. Access to additional supportive services is important during this time of initial crisis. By conducting a brief assessment of Ellen's and her family's needs, including strengths and available resources, a team social worker would have determined the types of needed sustaining services. Wraparound services might include some or all of the following: counseling, support groups, HIV educational opportunities, advocacy, legal services, and case management (Poindexter 1997). For some people, assistance in accessing concrete services such as medical care, housing, medical insurance, and food is necessary.

Interventions that would have been helpful initially to Ellen and her family include active empathic listening, creating a safe environment where the family could begin to verbalize and explore their thoughts and feelings. The counselor, by validating and normalizing their emotional responses, would provide psychic space for the Geddes family to anticipate and plan for future responses. This type of planning allows for the enhancement of coping styles, while exerting a sense of control in some areas of their lives.

If needed, the social worker might have discussed with Ellen and her family the options for enrolling in college and living independently from her family, assisting Ellen with informing her parents of her wishes. The novel depicts Ellen declaring a manifesto for moving out; she later confides in her younger sister Debra that she feels she has abandoned her parents, but must consider her own future. The impact of this new situation involving the temporary loss of Ellen, especially now that her parents are worried about her, also becomes an issue with which the family must struggle.

During this early period of HIV/AIDS diagnosis, families often express concern about issues of disclosure. The decision to tell family and friends about an HIV-seropositive status is difficult. For many people, the opportunity to disclose presents a double-edged sword—disclosing could provide the opportunity for needed social support, but may also cause additional stress due to discrimination and stigmatization (Hays et al. 1993). The characters in *What You Don't Know Can Kill You* experience both of these scenarios. Jack and the members of the Geddes family are each depicted as handling disclosure of Ellen's illness in different manners. Jack seeks a time to tell his parents, but never finds a perfect occasion. Debra, Ellen, and Mrs. Geddes each finally tell their best friend, but the friends are all insulted that they have taken so long and shown so little trust. The reactions the family received from members of the town of Shelter Rock were quite different and, for the most part, less supportive.

The protagonist, Debra, experiences the full range of reactions, from the support of her close friends to an unknown townswoman throwing water on her and verbally abusing her, saying, "You don't belong in a school with decent people! You and your whoring family! Maybe this will clean you up!" (142). Ellen receives abusive phone calls from a woman who thinks "that because I'm [i.e., Ellen] HIV-positive, everyone in town is going to die" (141). Ellen's mother Pam experiences changes in her work relationships severe enough to consider quitting when she notes that a customer refused to let her wrap a gift. Her business partners fear that people will be afraid to shop in their store because "everyone is terrified of getting AIDS" (139). These incidents are very consistent with actual experiences. Irrationality, hysteria, and ignorance are often the impetus for acts lacking compassion and for severe discrimination that can include such atrocities as ostracism, being ejected from neighborhoods and churches, having pets killed, physical and psychological threats, and loss of relationships. Given that all people may not respond in a compassionate manner, one must be judicious in deciding with whom to share this sensitive information (Hays et al. 1993).

Given the nature of HIV/AIDS, it is possible that an individual or family will face various crises throughout the course of the disease. Crisis intervention strategies should be employed when new losses or traumas surface. Flexibility on the part of the case manager to move from the treatment plans to crisis intervention modalities will assist the individual in facilitating emotional and psychological growth, while successfully negotiating stress and regaining some balance and control (Poindexter 1997).

Education about HIV/AIDS is extremely important and beneficial to newly diagnosed individuals, since it can address different aspects of well-being including social, psychological, spiritual, and physical needs. Attention to these areas can help one feel better and stay healthier longer. Understanding how the virus works, treatment options, new medication, better nutrition, and the latest protocols can be empowering to an individual in helping to make important decisions about their care. Information on HIV/AIDS can be obtained through medical care providers, social workers, books, pamphlets, the local state health department, and the Internet.

Ellen and Jack needed to be made aware of their medical options. Jack also needed to be referred to a doctor in order to seek care. The clinic team would have helped him disclose his illness to his parents, and perhaps saved Jack's life by offering him the hope of a productive life with his HIV controlled by medication therapy. One clear choice for Ellen and Jack was to be placed on an immediate regimen of care; another was to reject medication. The current standard of care is to quickly begin medical treatment, as the faster a person gets started on medicine, the more quickly there is an increase in the immune system's effectiveness, as measured with a blood test of the CD4 count, and a decrease in the viral load (the amount of virus replicating in the bloodstream). Currently medication recommendations include multiple doses of antiretroviral medication, with at least three different medications that work on preventing replication and resistance to three different parts of the human immunodeficiency virus.

Group therapy in the form of support groups and psychoeducational groups has been found to be very effective for those living with HIV and for their caretakers. Support groups such as People with AIDS can provide the therapeutic factors of group experiences, instillation of hope, universality, information, socializing techniques, and imitative behavior. Ellen's initial experiences with a support group are depicted as very positive, and she states, "[I]t isn't so much what they tell you. It's that with these people you know that you're not alone" (152). Group therapy decreased Ellen's levels of anxiety, depression, guilt, and stress while assisting her to find acceptance, peer support, strength, and new ways of problem solving (Chung & Magraw 1992; Mayers & Spiegal 1992; Pomeroy, Rubin, & Walker 1996).

Because of her success with a support group, Ellen encourages Debra to help the family seek out a group as well. During the course of the novel, Ellen's parents are initially shown as unreceptive to the idea of sharing family issues with strangers, but the novel ends before this situation can be resolved. The reader is left hoping the family will become more emotionally available and open to this modality, reaching out for the help they need. During this crisis intervention stage of treatment, the team social worker might have offered such services, at the same time being cognizant of the fact that the adjustment period for processing such life-altering news varies for individuals, and some people will be less open to this modality. Group therapy for the Geddes family would have been effective and meaningful if designed to address a wide range of needs. On the final pages of the novel, the reader arrives at resolution of the initial impact of Ellen's disclosure, as we hear Ellen explain her motivations to Debra, saying, "I'm not alone like Jack felt he was. If I felt that way maybe I'd give up too. But I've decided I won't give up. You can't either. All we have is hope" (153).

ANOTHER FACE OF HIV/AIDS

The story of Ellen and the Geddes family is becoming more common as the AIDS epidemic continues to spread; however, as members of a middle-class family from a small town, their experiences are not typical of all families dealing with HIV/AIDS. Not everyone has the same social supports or economic and emotional resources that were available to Ellen. Many individuals, including teens, struggle with additional psychosocial stressors including homelessness, poverty, substance abuse, mental health issues, and lack of support systems. The example of Annie, who is currently a patient at a regional AIDS clinic, presents another face of HIV/AIDS not seen in the novel under study.

At age sixteen and two months pregnant, Annie was referred to the infectious disease clinic after testing positive for HIV at the obstetric clinic where she was receiving prenatal care. As part of her prenatal care, her doctor offered an HIV test. All health care professionals caring for pregnant women should offer the test in conjunction with other prenatal tests, since perinatal transmission can be reduced dramatically when treatment is begun during pregnancy (U.S. Public Health Service 1995). The pregnant woman can help herself by starting antiretroviral medication that can potentially help her immune system by increasing her CD4 count and decreasing the amount of virus in her body (the viral load).

Annie's pregnancy was quite a shock to her, but nothing could have prepared her for the news that she was HIV-positive.

Life has been difficult for Annie. She lives with her older brother and father in a tough inner-city neighborhood. Although family members are close, they struggle with many issues including drug abuse, alcoholism, and finances. When Annie's mother died a few years ago, her father began to drink more and soon lost his job. As the family relationship began to deteriorate, Annie occasionally lived with friends who were older, finally prostituting herself to finance her drug habit.

By entering an infectious disease clinic program, Annie has received the support she needs to create a better life for herself. She attends a support group of teens and young adults who are HIV-positive. Her family has attended a series of counseling sessions as a means of assisting Annie by gaining understanding of the nature of her illness and her physical needs. Annie's social worker has tapped a number of community resources to provide an apartment, daily meals, and medical care for the family. By seeking medical treatment for herself and her baby, Annie, just like the fictional character Ellen, has chosen to tackle her illness head on and to improve her quality of life by adding hope.

RECOMMENDED READINGS

HIV/AIDS: Fiction

Note: Novels in which HIV/AIDS is a part of the main plot and purpose of the novel are marked with an asterisk (*). Others listed use AIDS as a minor plot device, but are useful in building a nonjudgmental attitude in young adult readers. Some treatment patterns were accurate at the time a novel was published, but no longer meet the standard of care implemented by infectious disease health care professionals.

*Arrick, F. (1992). *What you don't know can kill you*. New York: Bantam Books. ISBN: 0–440–21894–2. 154 pp. HS.

This book is discussed in detail in this chapter.

Bantle, L. (1995). *Diving for the moon*. New York: Macmillan. ISBN: 0–689–80004–5. 163 pp. ES, MS.

A sixth grade girl learns that her best friend Josh, a hemophiliac, is HIV-positive because of a transfusion of tainted blood. Through the course of their summer vacation, Carolina learns more about HIV, worrying about Josh when he contracts pneumonia. What she learns is that Josh needs to be independent, and she helps him develop additional inner strength. The reader sees the concerns and supportive behaviors of his family. Josh never becomes symptomatic during this novel, and appears to go on with a normal life except for the necessity of taking medication regularly. One additional plot device involves a gay neighbor couple the teens are friends with. This book provides a very light treatment of AIDS, embedded in a book about friendship.

Bess, C. (1993). *The Mayday rampage*. Sacramento, CA: Lookout Press. ISBN: 1–882405–00–5. 199 pp. HS. (Also on audiocassette, ISBN: 1–882405–02–1.)

The format of this book creates a complex task for the reader. There is no narration; the reader encounters a script of the conversation between two teens, Jess and Molly, who are reporting on recent incidents in their lives. They are a writing team for a high school newspaper and have published a controversial series of articles on AIDS and sex. The reader sees the articles as well as an advice column Molly writes. Both written products provide factual information about the transmission of HIV. When they are suspended from school, the duo has sex. At the very end of the dialogue, Molly confesses that she had unprotected sex a year ago with another partner; because of their research, they know they need a blood test. Molly tests HIV-positive. The epilogue presents a chronology of her illness and death.

Cohen, M. (1990). *Laura Leonora's first amendment*. New York: Lodestar/Dutton. ISBN: 0–525–67317–2. 134 pp. MS.

A thirteen-year-old girl makes an initial attempt at friendship with a boy new to the school, whose diagnosis with AIDS has been widely publicized. The main content of this storyline is learning about yourself and forms of courage, while interacting with friends in the schoolroom. The character with AIDS is rarely mentioned until Chapter 13, when he enrolls in school. Laura does all the talking, and we don't hear his voice.

*Davis, D. (1994). *My brother has AIDS*. New York: Atheneum. ISBN: 0–689–31922–3. 186 pp. MS.

Lacy is thirteen years old when her twenty-five-year-old brother, who has been infected with HIV/AIDS by his gay lover, comes home to die. Because she is closed out of the family's discussions about Jack and his disease, Lacy interviews the family physician and researches AIDS to learn more about the progression of her brother's illness. She goes public through an oral report in her health class, bringing attention to her family's problems. Through the concerns of her parents that Jack's condition remain secret, the reader gains an understanding of the potential for stigmatization by friends and townspeople, whose lack of knowledge about the syndrome causes fear and overreaction. Through Lacy's journal, the reader gains an understanding of the emotional strain on family members and the individual ways she and her parents deal with Jack being gay.

*Durant, P. R. (1992). *When heroes die.* New York: Atheneum. ISBN: 0–689–31764–6. 136 pp. MS.

Gary's favorite uncle Rob, who has been his role model and pseudo-parent in the absence of a father, becomes symptomatic with AIDS-related pneumonia, confesses he's gay, and quickly dies. Meanwhile, Gary must defend himself from an insensitive friend who labels all non-macho actions "fagot," but is supported by a neighbor girl who provides him with factual information about AIDS as well as unquestioning friendship. Gary is only twelve, and many of his reactions seem immature. The facts about contracting AIDS and treatment efforts are realistically presented.

Fox, P. (1995). *Eagle kite.* New York: Orchard Books. ISBN: 0–531–06892–7. 127 pp. MS.

Liam's dad leaves home to live in an isolated cabin two hours away, after his mother explains that his father is ill from a transfusion of tainted blood received during surgery. But Liam has seen his father with another man on the beach, so he suspects that her story is untruthful and that his father is bisexual. For months Liam ignores his father, but finally goes to visit when he is ill and dying of AIDS. The mother's attitude is clear to the reader as selfish, wishing only to protect herself from rumor within her community. The boy's attitude depicts personal struggle with the issue, and an aunt's attitude depicts rejection and unwillingness to forgive. Thus three typical reactions are shown by the characters of the novel.

Hermes, P. (1989). *Be still my heart.* New York: Putnam. ISBN: 0–399–21917–X; paperback, ISBN: 0–671–70645. 144 pp. MS, HS.

This book is mainly a romance. Allison, a fifteen-year-old, confides her attraction to a classmate. The title is a phrase interspersed after her casual encounters with this boy. As a subplot, Allison leads a team of yearbook writers to protect the job of their advisor, whose husband has just been diagnosed with AIDS as the result of a blood transfusion. These teens do provide a positive example of taking action against adults (the PTO) by gathering facts, rather than being swayed by emotion and fear.

Humphries, M. (1991). *Until whatever.* New York: Clarion. ISBN: 0–395–58022–6. 150 pp. HS.

This novel is unique in that the high school protagonist, Karen renews a friendship with a childhood friend, Connie, who discloses that she contracted AIDS through heterosexual sex. Both must deal with the disapproval of family and friends, evidencing social stigma clearly. Karen stands up for Connie and becomes involved with every aspect of her life, as well as preparing for her eventual death.

*Kaye, M. (1993). *Real heroes.* San Diego, CA: Harcourt. ISBN: 0–15–200563–3. 139 pp. MS.

The community discovers that the sixth grade gym teacher, Mr. Logan, has tested HIV-positive. Kevin, his friends, and their parents exemplify the various attitudes toward AIDS and gays that are prevalent in our society. One of the boys has a brother who is gay, and he provides good information about contracting the disease. One of the boys is very vocal in mocking his friends for their support of the teacher and calls gays all the typical rude names. The teacher's health class lessons serve as a venue for providing readers with clear information on sexual transmission. Kevin's father, a police hero, is the leader of a parent group that demands the teacher's dismissal. Although Kevin likes Mr. Logan, he is unable to stand up to his father or most vocal friends to present a defense, but he does begin to see his father's actions in a more realistic light and is able to judge his actions more accurately.

*Kerr, M. E. (1986). *Night kites.* New York: Harper. ISBN: 0–06–023253–6; paper, ISBN: 0–06–447035–0. 216 pp. HS.

Told by seventeen-year-old Erick, whose twenty-seven-year-old brother Pete, a homosexual who is a writer and teacher, contracts AIDS and returns home. Pete does not die during the course of the novel and begins to know some success as a writer, although he is too ill to continue teaching. Erick's girlfriend abandons him, and the reader sees his emotional ups and downs as he tries to maintain a normal life while caring for his brother. "Night kites" are individualists, unafraid to be different.

Koertge, R. (1988). *The Arizona kid.* Boston: Little, Brown. ISBN: 0–380–77–0776–4. 228 pp. HS.

Billy, age sixteen, spends a summer with a gay uncle, so he has social encounters with a number of gay men, some of whom have AIDS. The plot of this novel is about first love and racehorses, not AIDS, but the uncle's advice on safe sex before Billy's first heterosexual sexual experience includes the possibility of contracting AIDS if a condom is not used.

Levy, M. (1990). *Rumors and whispers*. New York: Fawcett. ISBN: 0–449–70327–4. 144 pp. HS.

Sarah, a high school senior, discovers that her brother and her art teacher are gay. When the teacher develops AIDS, Sarah's parents try to insist that she drop the class. The novel discusses safer sex as a sign of a caring relationship. Because Sarah's boyfriend is an AIDS researcher, the facts of HIV/AIDS are well presented.

*McDaniel, L. (1993). *Baby Alicia is dying*. New York: Bantam Books. ISBN: 0–553–29605–1. 185 pp. MS, HS.

This book provides a heart-rending look at the institutional care of HIV/AIDS infants. The featured baby, Alicia, is placed at the center while the teenage mother undergoes drug rehabilitation. One of her volunteer caretakers is Desi, a fourteen-year-old ninth grader who takes Alicia's case to heart. Within the course of the novel, Alicia becomes symptomatic and dies, while Desi provides round-the-clock care at the hospital, skipping school to do so. The novel's premise that young teens are permitted to take such a leadership role in providing infant care is potentially misleading, but the increased incidence of infants contracting HIV from their mothers in utero, placing a burden on the traditional foster care system, is accurately portrayed.

*Miklowitz, G. (1987). *Good-bye tomorrow*. New York: Delacorte Press. ISBN: 0–385–29562–6. 150 pp. HS.

A seventeen-year-old boy contracts AIDS because of a blood transfusion. As Alex is diagnosed and becomes symptomatic, the reader sees the reactions of his friends and family as they become afraid of casual contact with him. He is removed from school and the swim team as officials and friends lack factual information about the illness. Alex's HIV infection is represented realistically, but the progression of HIV to AIDS is misrepresented. His doctor reassures him he will not likely get AIDS. It is now believed that most HIV-positive people will develop full-blown AIDS, although this may take more than ten years.

*Nelson, T. (1994). *Earthshine*. New York: Orchard Books. ISBN: 0–531–06867–6. 182 pp. MS.

Slim, who is twelve years old, lives with her gay father and his partner during the time of her dad's treatment for AIDS and his eventual death. In a PWA (People with AIDS) support group, Slim makes a friend whose mother is expecting a baby that may be HIV-positive because the father died of AIDS. This plot device helps readers to see that others beyond the gay population contract AIDS and to understand the value of family support groups. Other valuable understandings that are touched on include a realistic look at the physical progress of the disease, the lack of government funding for AIDS research, the value of telephone hotlines and PWA support groups, and the strain placed on families of AIDS patients, both emotionally and financially.

*Porte, B. A. (1994). *Something terrible happened.* New York: Orchard Books. ISBN: 0–531–06869–2. 210 pp. MS.

Gillian's mother has contracted AIDS from her husband, an intravenous drug user who died of a drug overdose when Gillian was only four. When she becomes symptomatic, she first takes Gillian with her from New York City to Florida to search for cures, staying until they are penniless. At age ten, Gillian is sent to her father's relatives in Tennessee. The reader sees her emotions and the events of her life through letters written to a family friend, the book's narrator.

Young, A. E. (1988). *I never got to say goodbye.* Columbus, OH: Willowisp Press. ISBN: 0–87406–359–0. MS.

A fourteen-year-old girl has a twenty-year-old uncle who contracts HIV through a blood transfusion. She must deal with friends who avoid her for fear of catching the virus from her. While visiting her uncle in the hospital, Traci meets a boy her age who later dies from AIDS, which he contracted from intravenous drug use. The reactions of the characters demonstrate the need for compassion for patients as well as irrational fears of friends.

HIV/AIDS: Informational

Blake, J.(1990). *Risky times: How to be AIDS-smart and stay healthy.* New York: Workman Publishing. ISBN: 0–89480–656–4. 151 pp. MS, HS.

A great, easy-to-read resource offering factual definitions, answers to specific questions, personal narratives of HIV/AIDS teenagers and young adults, and parallel narratives of friends, relatives, and sexual partners of the HIV/AIDS speakers. The narratives are truthful in describing the various ways the speakers contracted the disease. Photos and quotes of the featured speakers, as well as famous people teen readers will recognize, are interspersed within the text.

Ford, M. T. (1992). *100 questions and answers about AIDS: A guide for young people.* New Discovery. ISBN: 0–02–735424–5. 202 pp. MS, HS.

Presents clear, factual responses to questions about HIV/AIDS. Provides historical background on the progress of AIDS in the United States. Interspersed with the text are interviews with two males and two females from different walks of life, including one male runaway/prostitute and one who contracted the disease through intravenous drug use and was diagnosed during a pregnancy.

Johnson, E. "Magic" (1992). *What you can do to avoid AIDS.* New York: Times Books. ISBN: 0–8129–2063–5. 192 pp. MS, HS.

Question and answer format plus interviews. This book provides in-depth, honest responses to questions related to sexually transmitted diseases. Each answer is based on current medical knowledge. When Magic Johnson, a public figure with high recognition value, disclosed his HIV infection on November 7, 1991, more governmental funding was applied to AIDS research, and laws on discrimination related to athletes in contact sports were reviewed. (A *Booklist* Editors' Choice and YALSA [Young Adult Library Services Association] Best Book for Young Adults)

Jussim, D. (1997). *AIDS and HIV: Risky business.* Springfield, NJ: Enslow. ISBN: 0–89490–917–7. 112 pp. HS.

Scattered throughout this book are the stories of young adults with AIDS, with an example for each of the types of transmission. National facts and statistics are presented clearly, in a readable fashion, including how the body reacts to the syndrome and a variety of common medical treatments. Especially valuable are the real school stories of AIDS patients in Chapter 3, including that of Ryan White, and a concise double-page list of "How to Practice Safer Sex" embedded in the great advice in Chapter 5. Chapter 6 provides solid advice for readers who consider themselves at risk of infection.

Klein, M., ed. (1989). *Poets for life: Seventy-six poets respond to AIDS.* New York: Crown. ISBN: 0–892–55170–4. 220 pp. HS.

A collection of poetry written in response to AIDS. These poems create a powerful way to experience the emotional impact of the disease on patients as well as friends and family members.

Kuklin, S. (1989). *Fighting back: What some people are doing about AIDS.* New York: Putnam. ISBN: 9–992–15935–9. 110 pp.

Photos of volunteers working with AIDS patients. (An ALA Best Book for Young Adults)

Walter, V. A., and M. Gross (1996). *HIV and AIDS information for children: A guide to issues and resources*. New York: H. W. Wilson. ISBN: 0–824–20902–8. 261 pp. HS.

This book provides resources mainly for adults working with children and young adults. Includes suggestions for working with social issues, annotations of books, and lists of books and resources in a broad range of categories beyond AIDS.

HIV/AIDS: Autobiographies/Biographies

Ford, M. T. (1995). *The voices of AIDS: Twelve unforgettable people talk about how AIDS has changed their lives*. New York: Morrow Junior Books. ISBN: 0–688–05322–X. 221 pp. HS.

Interviews with young adults with AIDS and friends and family members are presented with Ford's original question and the response. "Fast Facts" are mixed in with interviews as a means of presenting condensed informational material just as a reader might be open to absorbing such facts. The purpose of this book seems to be expressed in Gabriel Morales' response to Ford's question, "What do young people need to know most?" Morales states, "By putting a face on HIV, we are showing young people that it can and will happen to some of them" (19).

Gonzales, D. (1996). *AIDS: Ten stories of courage*. Springfield, NJ: Enslow, ISBN: 0–89490–766–2. 112 pp. MS.

Collective biographies and photos of ten famous people with AIDS, making the point that the disease affects people in all walks of life, all cultural groups, and with all sexual orientations. The author states that AIDS has robbed the world of some great talents. Entries include athletes Magic Johnson (the only one still living) and Arthur Ashe, actor Anthony Perkins, author/journalist Randy Shilts, artists Alison Gertz and Keith Haring, dancer Rudolf Nureyev, Elizabeth Glaser, and musician Freddie Mercury.

Landau, E. (1990). *We have AIDS*. New York: Franklin Watts. ISBN: 0–531–15152–2. 126 pp. HS.

A mixed format including excerpts from personal interviews with nine teenagers with HIV/AIDS, known only by first name. Informational pieces present facts relevant to each case in a question/answer format. The emotional reactions of the teens are clear, as are their personal and physical problems. The resource list in this book is too old to be helpful, but the personal nature of the stories makes a powerful read.

Reese, L. K. (1997). *A young man's journey with AIDS: The story of Nick Trevor*. New York: Franklin Watts. ISBN: 0–531–11366–3. 159 pp. HS.

Published after Nick's death, this book provides a powerful first-person narrative based on journal entries written by Nick, diagnosed at age twenty-one, and his mother, the author. Her purpose is to make the daily experiences of living with AIDS tangible to teens, especially because teens tend to take an "it can't happen to me" attitude. The narrative provides an accurate description of medical treatment and common opportunistic illnesses. Nick's story evidences the stigma society places on people with AIDS and their families.

Sparks, B., ed. (1994). *It happened to Nancy*. New York: Avon. ISBN: 0–380–77315–5. 236 pp. MS, HS.

The story of this anonymous fourteen-year-old is told through diary entries, as edited by her professional counselor after her death of AIDS. Nancy was date raped, a scene which is described in one short paragraph. The book shows her emotions and struggle to not love the man, who had posed as an eighteen-year-old college student. Nancy's dialogue demonstrates the need to resolve her dilemma with her upbringing and religious training. The book ends with answers to the questions Nancy had about AIDS. The editor also wrote *Go Ask Alice*, the story of a teen drug abuser.

White, R., and A. M. Cunningham (1991). *Ryan White: My own story*. New York: Dial. ISBN: 0–803–70977–3. 227 pp. MS. (Also available as an audiocassette from Dove Audio.)

Ryan was a hemophiliac and perhaps the most publicized case of AIDS because of the media treatment of public stigma in his town and school. This autobiography, published after his death, describes Ryan's diagnosis with AIDS, his legal battles to remain in school, and his efforts to publicize his dilemma. Includes photos and answers to frequently asked questions on AIDS, as well as his testimony to the President's Commission on AIDS.

AUDIOVISUAL RESOURCES

Johnson, Magic, and Arsenio Hall, hosts (1992). *Time out: The truth about HIV and AIDS*. Paramount Pictures. [Video.] (Free rental at many video stores.)

This video is professionally produced, set to music, and very engaging. A number of professionals—actors, athletes, and musicians—make appearances to share the facts about HIV/AIDS. A study guide for teachers is included in the package.

Koop, C. E. (host). *AIDS: Everything you and your family need to know but were afraid to ask*. Video.

Shilts, R. (1988). *And the band played on*. Audiotape. Read by Willem DaFoe. New York: Simon and Schuster Audio Works.

Presents a chronology of the AIDS virus' increasing hold on America. Statistics are effectively integrated to demonstrate the rapid spread of the disease and the ratio of those infected to those who died in the early stages of the epidemic. Points out that government research funding was minimal when the disease was considered one that only affected gay men. When women began to test positive and movie actor Rock Hudson died of ARC (AIDS Related Complex), more attention and more research money followed. Also a book (St. Martin's Press, 630 pp., ISBN: 0–312–00994–1), but the tape is more accessible to teens.

INTERNET SITES AND OTHER RESOURCES

American Institute for Teen AIDS Prevention: (817) 237–0230

CDC (Centers for Disease Control) National AIDS Hotline: 1–800–342–2437: *http://www.cdc.gov*

Children's Hospital Immunodeficiency Program (CHIP), Denver, Colorado: (303) 861–6981:*http://www.chipteam.com*

Names Project Foundation: *http://www.aidsquilt.org*

National AIDS Hotline: 1–800–342–2437

National STD Hotline: 1–800–227–8922

People with AIDS Health Group: (212) 255–0520

Teen HIV Hotline: 1–800–440–TEEN (8336)

REFERENCES

Chung, J. Y., and M. M. Magraw (1992). "A group approach to psychosocial issues faced by HIV-positive women." *Hospital and Community Psychiatry* 43, 891–894.

Crutcher, C. (1992). "Healing through literature." In D. Gallo, ed., *Authors' insights*. Portsmouth, NH: Boynton Cook.

Hays, R. B., et al. (1993). "Disclosing HIV seropositivity to significant others." *AIDS* 7, 425–431.

Kitahata, M. M., et al. (1996). "Physicians' experience with AIDS as a factor in patients' survival." *New England Journal of Medicine* 334, 701–706.

Mayers, A., and L. Spiegel (1992). "A parental support group in a pediatric AIDS clinic: Its usefulness and limitations." *Health and Social Work* 17, 183–191.

Poindexter, C. C. (1997). "In the aftermath: Serial crisis intervention for people with HIV." *Health and Social Work* 22, 125–132.

Pomeroy, E. C., A. Rubin, and R. J. Walker (1996). "A psychoeducational group intervention for family members of persons with HIV/AIDS." *Family Process* 35, 299–312.

Rapaport, L. (1970). "Crisis intervention as a mode of brief treatment." In R. Roberts and R. Nee, eds., *Theories of social casework*. Chicago: University of Chicago Press.

Rodriquez, E. M., L. M. Mofenson, and B. H. Chang (1996). "Association of maternal drug use during pregnancy with maternal HIV culture positivity and perinatal HIV transmission." *AIDS* 10, 273–282.

"U.S. Public Health Service recommendations for human immunodeficiency virus counseling and voluntary testing for pregnant women" (1995). *MMWR (Morbidity and Mortality Weekly Report)* 44: 1–14.

CHAPTER 12

Conquering Alcoholism in *Imitate the Tiger*

Margaret Ford and Danna Bozick

First, when you're using drugs, and booze is a drug, there is often a huge gulf separating one's expectations of oneself and one's behavior. One presumes that at some time in the future somehow things will just work out. Even for those young people who strike the cynical and existential pose that "I'll be dead by the time I'm twenty-five anyway, so what the hell," there still is a presumption that even if dead I will survive. This is a most ingenious self-deception that many of us engage in: We ignore the inevitable. The reality is that Chris Serbo's behavior is growing more and more out of control. He's on the edge of doing something very destructive to himself and others. Is Chris an addict?

Those kids who say strongly that Chris is addicted have had some exposure to addiction, usually because a parent or another close relative is drinking or using drugs. Those who vehemently deny Chris's addiction are usually drinking and taking drugs themselves.

Jan Cheripko

According to the National Institute on Drug Abuse (1999), approximately 9.5 million Americans between the ages of twelve and twenty have had at least one drink this month; 4.4 million have consumed five or more drinks in a row; and 1.9 million have been heavy drinkers for five consecutive days. During the last month, 8 percent of our nation's eighth graders, 22 percent of our tenth graders, and 34 percent of our twelfth graders have been drunk. Among teenagers who abuse alcohol, 39 percent drink alone, 58 percent drink when they are upset, 30 percent drink when they are bored, and 37 percent drink to feel high. Adolescents typically begin using alcohol around age thirteen. The earlier adolescents begin drinking, the more likely they will develop a problem with alcohol or other drugs later in life and the more likely they are to be involved in traffic accidents, sexual assaults, vandalism, and other crimes.

Drivers under age twenty-five had the highest intoxication rates for fatal crashes (National Highway Traffic Safety Administration 1999). According to the U.S. Department of Justice (1999), 32 percent of adolescents in juvenile institutions were under the influence of alcohol at the time of their arrest and 22 percent of the clients admitted to drug treatment programs were under age twenty. Alcohol use is implicated in two-thirds of sexual assault cases among teens, and among sexually active teens, those who drink daily are three times less likely to use condoms, placing them at a higher risk of HIV infection.

If we care about the health of our children, we must understand alcohol and substance abuse and become proactive in counseling teens who turn to alcohol. Alcoholism is a disease with genetic, psychosocial, and environmental roots.

We began our collaboration at the local Barnes and Noble café, close to the two staples that would see us through this project—books and caffeine. Our task was to examine alcoholism through literature as a health issue affecting adolescents. We, Danna Bozick, an adolescent chemical dependency counselor, and Marge Ford, a school library/media specialist, became acquainted nearly twenty years ago over a mutual love of young adult literature as we prepared to participate in the Youngstown State University English Festival.

IMITATE THE TIGER

Imitate the Tiger by Jan Cheripko was the winner of the 1997 Joan Fassler Memorial Award, presented by the Association for the Care of Children's Health (ACCH) for a book for children or young people that deals with medical and health-related issues. Recognizing that genetic predisposition toward alcoholism is debated as an additional mitigating factor, the family struggles portrayed make this novel especially appropriate.

The guiding spirit of *Imitate the Tiger* is born in the mind of the main character. Chris Serbo imagines himself a brave warrior serving under King Henry V of England who, when the odds are overwhelming, rallies his troops with the battle cry "Imitate the action of the tiger." The reader is left to discover the many battles Chris must wage in his fight to become a man. He battles his own alcoholism and that of his father. He skirmishes on the football field with opposing teams and even with the friends and coaches who would help him if he could admit he has a problem. He engages in real battles in the bars and streets of his town and rolls over friends and family whose spirits he wounds even as they try to help him.

Imitate the Tiger is a complex novel both in structure and theme. Chris Serbo, the seventeen-year-old protagonist, tells the story from two different platforms. Each chapter begins with a diary entry that comments on his progress or lack of progress at Opportunity School, a resident facility for youths with alcohol and drug problems. Following each diary entry, Chris leads the reader back to Valley View High and into the football locker room, the cafeteria, or home to Aunt Catherine's, where his father has left him after the death of his mother. Each story then links back to Chris' diary and creates a mesh of first-and third-person narratives that gradually reveal his character and his life story.

Aunt Catherine has cared for Chris since he was five years old. His father, whose alcohol abuse led to the destruction of a promising army career, visits Chris infrequently. His father's distance, both physically and emotionally, leaves Chris unable to relate to those around him. He pushes his girlfriend Marissa away because of his drinking and possessiveness; takes advantage of Aunt Catherine and does nothing to help her around the house; uses his friend Polly to deliver messages and steal homework; patronizes Jesse, his African American teammate; and betrays Billy, his best friend. He does as little as possible in school and resents Mrs. Whittaker, the teacher he admires most, when she challenges him to grow up. This litany of behavior flaws can be traced, in part, to the growing abuse of alcohol that he cannot admit.

The power of this novel lies in the realism with which the characters and situations are portrayed. Chris Serbo, as the son of an absentee alcoholic father, clearly lacks parental guidance. After the death of their mother, responsibility for Chris and his sister falls to Aunt Catherine, who is older and not up to the rigors of raising an adolescent boy. It seems that throughout the novel Chris is actually searching for what it means to be a man. When Mrs. Whittaker challenges him to do better in advanced placement history, he says, "Something inside of me knows she's telling the truth. I want very much to take responsibility for my life, like she says, but I don't know how. I don't have any strength to do that" (52). Hanging around with the older guys he met through football and drinking provides the blueprint for his twisted view of manhood. After he is beaten and made to grovel drunkenly at the feet of Tony Salerio, he observes, "For a moment I am actually proud of what I look like. As strange as that may seem, I really think this is what it means to be a man. To drink, to get sick, to have a fight" (124).

As he searches for the manhood rulebook, he looks to football to give him structure and discipline. The football scenes are many and detailed, often reading like a playbook. While he snaps back at Aunt Catherine, he takes any verbal abuse from John "Pappy" Papano, his coach. He drives himself to his physical limits doing wind sprints, gets hit mercilessly by Panda Bear Johnson, and takes on the team for bull-in-the-ring. He even admits in his diary sequence, "And always I come back to this football team. It's like some mystery is hidden there, and if I just talk enough I'll figure out what it is" (86).

His search for structure keeps the football image as a primary focus, but he also admits enjoying the structure of grammar. Even though he hates those times when Coach Jones takes over practice, he loves his emphasis on the strategy of each play, allowing him "to see all of the intricate parts of the offense start to move and in only a couple of seconds while someone is rushing at me to knock me on my ass, figure out who's playing what part, where they're going and then smash their plans to pieces with a jarring tackle or, even better, an interception" (152). It's this ability to predict that early in the novel convinces the team that Pappy is their man as he predicts the plays called by the opposite team when Valley View scores their first massive victory of the year. As Chris goes back and forth between his life and the football field, the reader can see the order of one and the complete chaos of the other.

Chris conceals a brutal anger in his alcoholism. In his Opportunity School diary, he admits that he is always angry. In one of the early scenes at Connie's Bar and Grill, his friends have to restrain him when he discovers that Marissa is dating his friend, Bill Schumacher. He calls her a whore and then goes out and gets drunk. Later in the novel, he admits to having slapped her when she called him a drunk. His anger flares when he tries to rake the leaves in the yard and the rake breaks. His solution is to throw the rake head into the woods and smash the handle against a tree. Then he drives off with his friends to drink some moonshine they have brought along. When Aunt Catherine finally confronts him about his drinking, he punches his fist through the glass in the door and storms out of the house. He is constantly whirling in this chaos of anger, for which drinking appears to be a solution.

The effects of his drinking are always portrayed in a brutally realistic light. When he's drinking, his homework goes undone despite his best intentions, and he takes advantage of his friend Polly to copy assignments. His schoolwork suffers, showing a gradual decline from his sophomore to senior years. He is content to do just enough to get by with a barely passing grade. Even though he criticizes his father for making Aunt Catherine hound him for support checks which he should be sending regularly, Chris does the same thing when he shirks all responsibility, even for household chores. Cheripko really paints a dismal picture of Chris' feeling of powerlessness when he describes the effects of shirking such a simple job as taking out the garbage. When he finally takes the trash bag to the burner in the yard, the rancid contents have attracted an army of ants. "I light the trash bag and watch the ants scurry around trying to get away from the fire. Faster and faster they run, but they can't escape. The flames race after them and they fall into the red and yellow heat. I feel magnificently strong that I can burn them out of existence, these little creatures that I hate so much" (30–31). The reader is left to wonder: Who are the ants in Chris' life?

The physical effects of Chris' drinking are also very realistic. When he wakes up in the morning after the near-fight at Connie's, Chris discovers that he is still in his clothes. On other occasions in the novel, he rummages through dirty clothing to find something that doesn't look or smell too bad. When he waters down the gin in Aunt Catherine's liquor cabinet, the only container he can find in which to pour the stolen gin is a shampoo bottle. The combination of shampoo and gin makes him deathly sick, and he stumbles out of the school dance, refuses a ride with Johnny because Bill and Marissa are in the car, and finds himself in the gutter. He graphically describes plunging into blackberry bushes that tear chunks out of his face. It becomes apparent that he is describing a scene that has clearly happened before. "I've had plenty of practice, so I stick my fingers down my throat and up come the gin-soaked, soapy potato chips. Then come those horrible, wrenching convulsions in your gut— dry heaves" (109). At that point, he passes out. Add to this dismal physical description the blood gushing from his nose and gouged face after an encounter with Tony Salerio and friends, and getting drunk at the school dance loses all its allure.

In fact, that is the strength of this novel—there is absolutely no attempt to make alcoholism pretty. There is no romantic interest who stands by her man and rescues him from his affliction. There is no kind and gentle counselor who manages to turn around this life in the final chapter. In fact, there is no final resolution, much like the reality of the recovery process. This honest fictional portrayal of the consequences of adolescent alcoholism provides many launching points for classroom exploration.

TEACHING STRATEGIES

The point of view and the use of diary entries to open and link each chapter make this novel an effective introduction to the power of journal writing and memoir. For that reason, the list of recommended works at the end of this chapter includes several other first-person narratives of adolescents dealing with adverse conditions, even if not linked to substance abuse. A classic such as *Anne Frank: The Diary of a Young Girl*, when linked with more contemporary journals such as *Red Scarf Girl: A Memoir of the Cultural Revolution, Zlata's Diary: A Child's Life in Sarajevo*, or *The Diary of LaToya Harper* can provide a solid discussion of the importance of the journal in exploring emotions and recording events. Students could be encouraged to keep a journal of their own using *Imitate the Tiger* or these diaries as models. They might even choose to keep an electronic journal using word processing software or a dedicated program like Diarymaker using three of the works mentioned above. A moderated chat might also expand the personal sharing, perhaps even linking to students in other classrooms or schools.

As students give some thought to sharing with each other, they might also explore some cross-age sharing. Several works on the list are picture books that could be used in several ways. Teachers might use picture books to introduce the serious concept of alcoholism to older students or even adults. The simplicity of the text and illustrations often opens up more complex discussions that could be further explored through the fiction and nonfiction selections in the bibliography. Older students might read to younger students under the supervision of a teacher or school health care professional and record the reactions of their young audiences. Students might even try to write their own picture book based on some of the other books to which they have access. Students with greater accessibility to technology might also create a hypermedia presentation based either on the fictional portrayal of alcoholism or the factual issues raised in many of the books cited. After checking such products for accuracy, they might be posted on the school web site to be shared with the school and local communities—a truly global audience.

Danna has speculated that Chris' story might have evolved differently if someone had intervened earlier in his addiction. Teachers might have students suggest different scenarios for such interventions and have students complete the story. For example, what if Chris' father had been enrolled in a successful recovery program and had not been absent from home? What if Chris had then joined Alanon?* What might have happened if Chris had asked Jeremiah Williams for help on that lonesome road following the dance? It might be interesting to turn the new novel into an audio book and make copies available in the classroom library or the school library/media center.

A topic that many adolescents might choose to explore would be the hero image of sports figures who lead less than exemplary lives. Certainly, Mrs. Whittaker felt that the football players on display in the lunchroom were providing poor role models for the other students at Valley View High. A classroom might dedicate one wall to "endorsements" of athletes who conquered addictive behaviors, whether it be alcohol or other substances. Students might create cereal boxes on which to display the likenesses of such sports figures, including a biographical justification on the back of the cereal box—the side we usually read at the breakfast table. Teachers might ask for a link on the school web site on which to display their students' candidates—and ask for student and community feedback in support or disagreement of their choices.

There is also room for the traditional research assignment in connection with the issue of adolescent alcohol abuse. There are many fine nonfiction titles written at several different interest and ability levels. Nearly all have indexes and bibliographies that make further follow-up possible. Topics should be worded so that they require students to do something with the information they process. For example, students might be assigned to investigate the various types of intervention programs for alcoholics and then choose one for Chris, justifying their choice based on his particular circumstances as revealed in *Imitate the Tiger*. In addition to providing a written report, students might also be assigned to create a multimedia presentation for a particular audience, such as parents attending a PTA meeting. Their task might be to share the warning signs of alcoholism in adolescents.

---

*Alanon is a support group to help families and friends of alcoholics cope with the effects of alcoholism.

It seems that the concept of the problem novel and young adult literature go hand in hand. This pairing can be a real plus for classrooms in which teaming is a reality or in schools that use alternative scheduling that allows for cross-curricular studies. In this type of environment, the language arts, social studies, and health teachers might join forces in examining this issue from multiple perspectives. *Imitate the Tiger* is the perfect novel to make such collaborations successful learning experiences for young adults.

CHRIS SERBO IN THERAPY

Chris Serbo, age five when his mother died, would have been a perfect candidate for community services. In the best of all worlds, case managers and mentors would have "wrapped around" the home life provided by his Aunt Catherine and would have helped him develop into a secure, well-functioning young adult. Community intervention could have helped his father, John, to enter an alcohol treatment program, and we might then have seen his father participating in a recovery lifestyle, with support to stay sober provided by other recovering people. In this alternative scenario, Chris' father would have been there to provide healthy parenting. He would have been there to help Chris through the labyrinth of adolescence. In *Imitate the Tiger*, though, Chris has only Aunt Catherine, a realistic portrayal of a well-meaning and concerned caregiver who, like many real life grandparents and other stand-in guardians, is overwhelmed by her out-of-control charge.

Perhaps teachers, social workers, or other involved community members might have seen Chris' emotional and behavioral issues and realized the need for help with his problems. The American Academy of Child and Adolescent Psychiatry (1997) notes the following warning signs in younger children:

- A marked fall in school performance; poor grades in school despite trying very hard
- Worry or anxiety as shown by regular refusal to go to school, go to sleep, or take part in activities that are normal for the child's age
- Hyperactivity; fidgeting; constant movement beyond regular playing
- Persistent nightmares
- Persistent disobedience or aggression (longer than six months) and provocative opposition to authority figures
- Frequent, unexplainable temper tantrums.

In preadolescents and adolescents:

- Marked change in school performance
- Abuse of alcohol and/or drugs
- Inability to cope with problems and daily activities
- Marked changes in sleeping and/or eating habits
- Many complaints of physical ailments
- Aggressive or nonaggressive consistent violation of rights of others such as thefts, vandalism, or opposition to authority
- Intense fear of becoming obese with no relationship to actual body weight
- Depression shown by sustained, prolonged negative mood and attitude, often accompanied by appetite difficulty, sleeping, or thoughts of death
- Frequent outbursts of anger.

For the drug and alcohol abusers in each age category, I would add:

- Associating with other known drug/alcohol users
- Legal, school, health, or family problems associated with the consumption of alcohol or drugs.

In the Multidimensional Addictions and Personality Profile (MAPP) (1988) by John R. Craig and Phyllis Craig, a substance use disorder involves at least one of the following criteria:

- Signs of physical withdrawal, impairment, or deterioration due to prolonged or excessive use of a substance
- A psychological dependence on the effects of the substance in an attempt to avoid or cope with personal problems such as anxiety, loneliness, nervousness, depression, poor self-concept, or feelings of inadequacy
- Any abusive, secretive, or irresponsible behaviors by an individual involving the use of substances more frequently, in greater amounts, or under circumstances that are not medically or socially acceptable
- Any instance where the use of, or the effects of, the substance significantly alters or interferes with an individual's ability to function in any manner. (37)

Typically, descriptions of indicators of substance abuse or substance dependence would be applied to criteria set out in the *Diagnostic and*

Statistical Manual of Mental Disorders (DSM-IV) (1994) and a diagnosis would be determined. Paper/pencil questionnaires as well as interviews with the client, family members, or other involved persons would be administered by a health professional. Information gathered would be used to make a determination about the nature of the substance use problem. All of the information would then be used to determine the appropriate level of treatment. Depending on the severity of the problem, the client might need medically supervised detoxification, inpatient hospitalization, or residential placement in a rehabilitation center, as we saw with Chris in our story. Community centers also often provide a variety of individual/group intensive outpatient treatment or individual/group low intensity treatment, which might, for example, meet once per week. Family sessions might also be a part of any of the above services, as might referral to self-help organizations, such as Alcoholics Anonymous and Narcotics Anonymous. Aftercare or continuing care provides support at the end of the primary treatment program. As I talk with addiction specialists around the country, drug combining in all phases of use, abuse, and dependency seems to be commonplace today. Although Chris sticks to alcohol in *Imitate the Tiger*, many teenagers are also using marijuana, taking prescription drugs, and taking steroids to enhance athletic abilities.

Imitate the Tiger opens as Chris, the central character, enters a residential rehabilitation program. He is asked to produce a written journal—writing assignments are often used to accomplish particular purposes during chemical dependency treatment. These assignments allow the client to focus on specific issues such as the harmful consequences of their use of chemicals. Questions might be posed by the counselor in written or verbal form. Chris displayed facility with a diary/journal method. For some people who have difficulty concentrating due to attention deficit hyperactivity disorder or other biochemical issues, this method may present some frustrations. In some instances, sticking with verbal explorations with a partner or professional facilitator may be necessary to accomplish the goals.

Chris describes his use of alcohol in the book at various times. We see how Chris moves from the early phase where he indicates that he is preoccupied with alcohol. When he cannot get beer, he raids his Aunt Catherine's liquor cabinet. In this same phase, Chris sneaks around and lies about his use. Chris describes rapid intake, defensiveness, guilt, and increased tolerance, all early phase indicators. Middle phase signs are also seen in Chris' story. They include loss of control, alibis, grandiosity, disapproval of others, mood swings, drug-centered behavior, self-pity, school problems, resentments, family problems, and jealousy/possessiveness. Chris also shows late phase signs of protecting his supply (always knowing where to find a drink) and morning use (the hair of the dog that bit you).

As Chris endeavors to self-explore, he starts at the outer edges of remembrance and circles in to disclosures of self. Chris states that he remembers first getting drunk at age fourteen. The American Medical Association, in a March 1998 online page discussing adolescent health, states that teens typically try their first alcoholic drink around age thirteen. Chris, at age seventeen, has progressed to passing out in a ditch in his own vomit and then betraying his best friend when confronted by attackers who threaten to slit his throat while beating him bloody. Displaying the utmost in rationalization, Chris is then able to distort his feelings of shame and weakness into pride about his drinking and fighting.

Chris desperately needs to communicate honestly. Like Chris, other adolescents who are chemically involved consistently disclose in self-reports that they do not have anyone with whom they are sharing their deepest feelings—confusion, sorrow, or fear. Chris relates that he cannot deal well with his emotions. He describes lying and manipulating and his older drinking buddies who take their anger out in barroom brawls. Many chemically dependent people have never learned how to express anger or fear in appropriate ways. As he comes to understand himself better, Chris will need to experience appropriate ways to express himself. A group setting is a safe place to begin to practice new behaviors. With modeling, role-playing, and encouragement from a facilitator or counselor in a treatment program, clients can learn how to alter old self-destructive patterns, for example, by changing the people they associate with and avoiding the negative places, such as bars, that have been a part of their alcoholic behaviors.

Asking Chris to contract to change these interactions in his life would be a part of his treatment. Doing this in written form helps to clarify the issues. Spending time with people who continue to use alcohol will be problematic for him. This is especially difficult for teenagers. Maintaining social relationships and participating in peer groups are normal parts of the adolescent stage of searching for identity. Setting limits surrounding the places he spends his time will also be important. If Chris continues to spend time in bars, it is very likely that he will relapse into his former "using" behaviors. Riding around in cars, if previously an occasion when drinking took place, would also probably need to be avoided as a social activity. Also potentially problematic may be something as simple as associating particular music, especially music that actually salutes the negative behavior in its lyrics, with the drinking mood. The concern is to identify what triggers old behaviors.

Another suggestion helpful to Chris would be to return to the physical activities that have been an outlet for emotions for him in the past. In his final words, as he picks up the football again, we can see him moving in that direction. I would encourage him to join a community athletic club, many of which have scholarships. I would also love to see Chris in some kind of mentoring program. We have already seen that he wants to respond to positive attention and guidance, as given by Mrs. Whittaker and later by his sponsor, Mr. Lake. Chris will need to learn to have fun, but in the new realm of healthy activities. Swimming, bowling, basketball, and bike riding are examples of activities I would encourage him to explore.

Client H. reported seeing herself in the relapse struggles portrayed in Drew Barrymore's biographical account, *Little Girl Lost*, indicating that this first-person narrative by someone she could identify with allowed her for the first time to admit her own chemical dependency. Additionally, H. stated that, like Drew, she felt used by her using friends, who didn't really care about her well-being but enticed her back into the old routines of using, which landed her in treatment several times in succession.

Looking again at Chris' emotional state, we see that as he continues to remember, he states that he "chokes up." Being called "chicken" by the school coach taps into Chris' internal pool of fear and humiliation. During treatment the professionals would continue to assess Chris for possible dual diagnosis issues. Ongoing assessment of psychosocial functioning would be necessary to determine if there is a concurrent psychological disorder in addition to a primary chemical dependency disorder. For example, client L. experienced physical and sexual abuse as a preadolescent child. He also participated in the drug-using lifestyle of his parents, often rolling marijuana joints for them or watching them snort cocaine or shoot up heroin. Although placed with a guardian and now in a stable environment, he struggles with mental health issues along with his own chemical dependency. Although he is very bright, his borderline personality behaviors often influence his ability to participate fully in treatment efforts. His sexual acting out is also a factor that is both inspired and exacerbated by drinking alcohol.

If we have ruled out a primary or additional secondary mental health diagnosis, we would need to look at possible situation specific depression with Chris. His life events would seem to warrant some expression in depressive symptoms, like sleep problems, appetite problems, feeling empty or sad, fatigue or loss of energy, feelings of worthlessness, diminished ability to think or concentrate, or recurrent thoughts of death. In his journal Chris states that he is having thoughts of killing himself. The irresponsible behaviors he describes, such as using his friendship with Polly for selfish gain without regard for her feelings, disappointing teachers that he cares about like Mrs. Whittaker, and not sticking up for his friend Billy, have added to Chris' feelings of low self-worth. As he learns to express his caring for others and learns to care for himself, Chris will be able to rebuild his self-esteem. Once he begins to take positive steps, like making things right with those in his life, Chris' mood will stabilize.

If I were establishing a team to work with adolescents, I would want Mrs. Whittaker as a member. She exhibits the caring attitude that is a crucial component for helping kids. She is responsible and carries through on her beliefs of advocacy, even though this is not always comfortable and easy. She reports the drinking of the football team members. The attitude she demonstrates, of requiring responsibility and accountability for one's actions, is crucial for teenagers. As inspired guides, teachers are on the front line in teenagers' lives. Adolescents are on the training ground, and consequences are a necessary part of learning in this time of passage to responsible adulthood. Buffering natural consequences for teens will only compound their problems. As we see with chemically dependent adults, it appears that if the lessons are not learned early, the consequences are greater later.

In looking at the life realms that Chris will need to change, his decision to try prayer shows an area that many find to be crucial to recovery from addictions. Often you'll hear people talk of a hole in themselves, of a need to fill it. Alcohol may seem to fill it momentarily, but that illusion soon wears off with the pain that steady use of alcohol invariably brings. When drunk, Chris screams to the sky his anger about losing his girlfriend Marissa. Other than screaming in anguish, Chris seems to have no real spiritual connection. Gaining a lived spirituality can be part of a route to healing. This step may take many different forms, and there is no one right way. Chris' rediscovery of his spiritual side echoes that of many other suffering alcoholics who have either lost contact with a spiritual path, have never developed their spiritual side, or are disillusioned and dispirited by life events.

As he continues to grow, it will be crucial for Chris to learn about relationships. Family treatment, which might range from individual family problem-solving sessions to large multifamily group sessions, would be another good place to look at underlying relationship problems. T., another client, like Chris, was an athlete. He prided himself on his strength and ability to be stalwart. It was in a family group, while discussing his distant relationship with his father, that he allowed himself to cry. If these openings are used as springboards, they can be the agents of powerful change. The group process can allow for the opening, then the individual must carry on and apply what has been learned.

Parent sessions, which both support and teach, are also important. If the parents enable the addiction, they need to learn about the dynamics of manipulative relationships. If the family is stuck in modes of pain infliction, they may need more long-term ongoing family therapy in a mental health setting. If parents or siblings are also chemically dependent, intervening with the other using parties will be necessary. In one example, N.'s father brought him to treatment. N. confided to the counselor that his father was drinking heavily on a daily basis. N. asserted that he did not believe he should have to change when his father was not willing to change. N.'s father refused treatment; N., unfortunately, did not successfully complete treatment. One year later, N.'s father was still seeking treatment for the boy, but not for himself.

Among the issues that children of alcoholics may face are the inability to talk about feelings and/or problems and the confusion resulting from seeing what is happening in the family and knowing that it doesn't match up with what is being communicated. This kind of pretending can lead to distortion of reality. These children and adolescents may have problems with goal setting and with their role responsibilities. Like Chris, these young people may be embarrassed about their parents' behavior, or they may shift the blame for their own shortcomings onto their parents. Cycling from one crisis to the next may become an unrecognized way of life.

Having a sponsor, a trusted guide, in the AA (Alcoholics Anonymous) Fellowship is an excellent way to learn new ways to live life. Attendance at AA or other recovery meetings would help Chris to learn about service to others. Listening to the strength and hope of others would give him examples to follow. The twelve steps and twelve traditions, from the recovery movement, will also guide him.

Maybe, beginning to recover from the alcohol problems that have brought many battles into his life, Chris will find a peace that lasts and will learn how to live with honor. Maybe then Chris will really be able to imitate the tiger.

RECOMMENDED READINGS

Alcoholism: Fiction

Bauer, J. (1998). *Rules of the road.* New York: Putnam. ISBN: 0–399–23140–4. 201 pp. MS, HS.

While Jenna drives an elderly woman from Chicago to Texas, she discovers the strength to deal with her alcoholic father.

Brooks, B. (1989). *No kidding.* New York: Harper and Row. ISBN: 0–06020–722–1. 207 pp. HS.

Sam lives in a futuristic world in which he cares for his younger brother and makes a home for his alcoholic mother after she is released from a treatment facility.

Bruchac, J. (1998). *The heart of a chief.* New York: Dial Books. ISBN: 0–803–72276–1. 176 pp. MS, HS.

This novel is set on an Indian reservation and shows Chris, a Penacook Indian, asserting himself in issues that affect the reservation while dealing with his father's alcoholism.

Cadnum, M. (1993). *Calling home.* New York: Puffin Books. ISBN: 0–140–34569–8. 144 pp. MS, HS.

Peter, an alcoholic, accidentally kills his best friend and keeps this horrible secret as he descends into a mental breakdown.

Carbone, E. (1997). *Corey's story: Her family's secret.* Burlington, VT: Waterfront. ISBN: 0–914–52530–1. 116 pp. MS.

Corey, her mother, and her father's employer orchestrate an "alcoholic intervention" to force her father into recovery.

Cart, M. (1998). *My father's scar.* New York: St. Martin's Press. ISBN: 0–312–18137–X. 204 pp. HS.

Andy's recollections of his abusive childhood at the hands of his alcoholic father are explored as he comes to realize his homosexuality. The theme of family alcoholism is secondary to Andy's acceptance of his homosexuality.

Carter, A. (1989). *Up country.* New York: Putnam. ISBN: 0–399–21583–2. 256 pp. MS, HS.

Carl Staggers is sent to live with relatives in the country after his mother, who suffers from a drinking problem, is ordered into a recovery program after a hit and run accident. His plan for the future is seriously threatened.

Cheripko, J. (1996). *Imitate the tiger*. Honesdale, PA: Boyds Mills Press. ISBN: 1–56397–514–9. 221 pp. MS, HS.

Chris Serbo wants to know what it is to be a man—but his battles on the football field and with the bottle aren't enough to answer this consuming question. This powerful novel is the focus of this chapter.

Cormier, R. (1991). *We all fall down*. New York: Bantam Doubleday Dell Books. ISBN: 0–44021–556–0. 199 pp. HS.

While drunk, Buddy and his friends vandalize a house in his neighborhood. A silent witness stalks the vandals to avenge the crime. We see Buddy's powerless remorse as he becomes romantically involved with the daughter of the owner of the house.

Covington, D. (1996). *Lasso the moon*. New York: Bantam Doubleday Dell Books for Young Readers. ISBN: 0–440–22013–0. 196 pp. HS.

April's father is a doctor who is a recovering alcoholic. She falls in love with one of his patients, an illegal alien from El Salvador. The emphasis in this novel is on the characterizations of April and Fernando and their relationship.

Deaver, J. (1995). *Chicago blues*. New York: HarperCollins. ISBN: 0–060–24675–8. 192 pp. MS, HS.

Lissa, seventeen, must make a home for her sister Marnie, eleven, when her mother's alcoholism makes her incapable of caring for her family. Eventually, the family is reunited in an ending that is more optimistic than realistic.

Draper, S. (1994). *Tears of a tiger*. New York: Simon and Schuster. ISBN: 0–689–31878–2. 192 pp. MS, HS.

When a car crash kills his best friend, Andy can't deal with the guilt caused by his drinking and driving. His story is told in the form of letters, homework assignments, journal entries, and conversations. After watching him struggle with depression, we learn of his suicide. This novel won the Corretta Scott King Genesis Award, and some paperback editions include a reader's guide and teaching strategies.

Fox, P. (1988). *The moonlight man*. New York: Bantam Doubleday Dell. ISBN: 0–440–20079–2. 192 pp. MS, HS.

Catherine spends a summer in Nova Scotia getting to know the father she has not seen since her parents' divorce. She is emotionally torn between hate for his drunkenness and love for the beauty of nature that he shares with her.

Gelb, A. (1995). *Real life: My bestfriend died.* New York: Pocket Books. ISBN: 0–671–87273–7. 209 pp. MS, HS.

Dave tells his real life story of the traffic accident that took his friends' life and resulted in his turning to alcohol. With the help of caring friends and adults, he confronts his problem.

Grant, C. (1992). *Shadow man.* New York: Atheneum. ISBN: 0–689–31772–7. 160 pp. MS, HS.

Gabe McCloud, while drunk, slams his truck into a tree and dies. The remainder of the book deals with the first-person reactions of those who knew him in the small town in which he lived, somewhat like Edgar Lee Masters' *Spoon River Anthology.* Gabe's own journal entries are used to give further insight to his character.

Hermes, P. (1998). *Cheat the moon.* Boston: Little, Brown. ISBN: 0–316–35929–7. 167 pp. MS.

First-person narrative of Gabby, age twelve, who cares for her younger brother during the alcoholic binges of her widowed father.

Hughes, D. (1994). *The trophy.* Westminster, MD: Alfred A. Knopf Books for Young Readers. ISBN: 0–679–84368–X. 135 pp. MS.

Danny, age ten, struggles to please his alcoholic, unemployed father on the basketball court. A realistic portrayal for younger adolescents.

Lynch, C. (1996). *Dog eat dog.* New York: HarperCollins. ISBN: 0–060–27210–4. 144 pp. MS, HS.

The *Blue-Eyed Son* trilogy focuses on Mick and his alcoholic brother, Terry, and is set in an Irish American working-class neighborhood in Boston. The story revolves around Mick and his attempts to rise above the racism and violence in which his brother Terry takes such pleasure.

Martin, N. (1997). *The eagle's shadow.* New York: Scholastic. ISBN: 0–590–36087–6. 176 pp. MS.

Told in the first person, this novel recounts the story of Clearie, who helps stop liquor sales among the Tlingits of Alaska when she must live with relatives while her father is in the army.

Martinez, V. (1996). *Parrot in the oven*. New York: HarperCollins.
    ISBN: 0–060–26704–6. 216 pp. MS, HS.

This National Book Award winner focuses on a Mexican American family
through the eyes of Manny, the younger son, who wants to be a "vato firme,"
a man to respect, in spite of his family's problems. Many of those problems are
brought on by the father's alcoholism.

McCourt, F. (1996). *Angela's ashes: A memoir*. New York: Scribner.
    ISBN: 0–684–87435–0. 363 pp. HS, Adult.

Although this memoir would be appropriate only for adolescents reading on an
adult level, the images of the family's poverty, caused largely by Frank Mc-
Court's father's alcoholism, are truly bleak.

Passey, H. (1989). *Speak to the rain*. New York: Atheneum. ISBN: 0–
    689–31489–2. 167 pp. MS, HS.

Janna's father turns to alcohol following her mother's death. Janna's horror
swells as her sister is possessed by the spirits of an Indian tribe.

Quarles, H. (1998). *A door near here*. New York: Doubleday. ISBN: 0–
    385–32595–9. 208 pp. MS, HS.

Fifteen-year-old Katherine is in charge of the household and her three younger
siblings while her alcoholic mother retreats to her bed, incapable of dealing with
her divorce and job loss. The novel's strength is Katherine's inventiveness when
it comes to dealing with everyday problems.

Rodowsky, C. (1994). *Hannah in between*. New York: Farrar, Straus and
    Giroux. ISBN: 0–374–32837–4. 151 pp. MS, HS.

Hannah becomes aware of her mother's drinking problem through a litany of
erratic behavior. An accident forces her mother to confront her problem in a
realistic portrayal of withdrawal. (ALA award winner)

Ryan, M. (1995). *The trouble with perfect*. New York: Simon and Schus-
    ter Books for Young Readers. ISBN: 0–689–80276–5. 170 pp. MS.

Thirteen-year-old Kyle seems to just miss in everything he tries—especially
under the scrutiny of his demanding, alcoholic father. Light reading with engaging teen characters.

Tabor, N. (1999). *Bottles break*. Watertown, MA: Charlesbridge Pub-
    lishing. ISBN: 0–881–06317–7. ES.

Although this is a picture book, its simple tissue art illustrations are wonderful. Bottles become the image of alcoholism in the mind of the child. The dialogue is more adult-oriented and might be used to create an introduction and discussion point for older students.

Wershba, B. (1997). *Whistle me home.* New York: Henry Holt. ISBN: 0–805–04850–2. 160 pp. MS, HS.

When Noli discovers that the young man she has fallen in love with is gay, she turns to alcohol to escape her devastation.

Wood, J. (1994). *A share of freedom.* New York: Putnam. ISBN: 0–399–22767–9. 256 pp. MS, HS.

Told in first-person narrative, this is the story of Freedom Jo Avery, who searches for the true identity of her father after her mother's drinking problem lands Mama in rehab and Freedom and her brother in foster care.

Zindel, P. (1995). *David and Della.* New York: Bantam Doubleday Dell Books for Young Readers. ISBN: 0–553–56727–6. 176 pp. MS, HS.

David Mahooley is handicapped by his writer's block, and Della Jones by her drinking. The focus here is on Zindel's wild characterizations.

Alcoholism: Nonfiction

Barbour, S., ed. (1998). *Alcohol: Opposing viewpoints.* San Diego: Greenhaven Press. ISBN: 1–56510–675–X. 218 pp. HS.

Part of the outstanding Opposing Viewpoints Series, this volume examines both sides of the various issues surrounding alcohol use and abuse. A strong bibliography and index are included.

Barrymore, D., with Todd Gold (1990). *Little girl lost.* New York: Pocket Books. ISBN: 0–671–68923–1. 303 pp. HS.

Drew Barrymore's celebrity status as well as the story of her move from drinking alcohol at age nine to experimenting with marijuana and cocaine will interest adolescent readers. The use of alcohol as a gateway drug is very realistic.

Chiu, C. (1998). *Teen guide to staying sober.* New York: Rosen Group. ISBN: 1–568–38249–9. 64 pp. MS, HS.

Causes, effects, and preventive policies for teen alcoholism.

Claypoole, J. (1997). *Alcohol and you*. New York: Franklin Watts. ISBN: 0–531–11351–5. 143 pp. MS, HS.

This text discusses all aspects of alcohol use by teenagers, including cost to society and its position as a gateway drug. The bibliography and index are supplemented by a list of sources to contact for further information and help.

Harris, J. (1994). *This drinking nation*. New York: Simon and Schuster. ISBN: 0–027–42744–7. 196 pp. MS, HS.

This book deals with the history of drinking in the United States. The text covers contemporary issues such as media perceptions and teenage drinking. Unfortunately, a previous title, *Drugged Athletes* (1987), is out of print but may be available in libraries.

Landau, E. (1994). *Teenage drinking*. Hillsdale, NJ: Enslow. ISBN: 0–894–90575–9. 104 pp. MS, HS.

In addition to a discussion of the causes and effects of teenage drinking, Landau begins each chapter with firsthand accounts to stimulate discussion and thought.

Lee, M., and R. Lee (1998). *Drugs and codependency*. New York: Rosen Publishing Group. ISBN: 0–823–92744–X. 64 pp. MS, HS.

One of the stronger volumes in the Drug Abuse and Prevention Library, this text deals with alcohol in part, but emphasizes the co-dependent personality. This series is aimed at reluctant readers.

McGovern, G. (1997). *Terry: My daughter's life and death struggle with alcoholism*. New York: NAL/Dutton. ISBN: 0–452–27823–6. 224 pp. HS.

A family memoir by Senator George McGovern that chronicles the tragedy of his daughter's death at age forty-five. Terry was found frozen to death where she had collapsed while drunk.

Mitchell, H. (1997). *Teen alcoholism*. San Diego: Lucent Books. ISBN: 1–560–06514–1. 96 pp. MS, HS.

This text discusses alcohol as a drug, giving information on all aspects of its use, effects, treatment, and prevention. Contains not only index and bibliography but also glossary and other endnotes.

Taylor, B. (1996). *Everything you need to know about alcohol*. New York: Rosen Publishing Group. ISBN: 0–823–92316–9. 64 pp. MS.

This volume in the Need to Know Library provides an elementary discussion of alcohol, its use, and its effect on the body. A bibliography and index are included.

Trapani, M. (1997). *Inside a support group: Help for teenage children of alcoholics*. New York: Rosen Publishing Group. ISBN: 0–823–92508–0. 64 pp. MS, HS.

Essentially, this is an introduction to Alateen, a support group based on the principles of Alcoholics Anonymous. This series is aimed at reluctant readers.

Wekesser, C., ed. (1994). *Alcoholism*. San Diego: Greenhaven Press. ISBN: 1–565–10074–3. 250 pp. HS.

This volume in the Current Controversies Series provides thoughtful essays reflecting the pros and cons of various issues surrounding alcoholism and its causes and treatment. Bibliographical references and index are provided. This is an especially good source for debate.

Winters, Paul, ed. (1997). *Teen addiction*. San Diego: Greenhaven Press. ISBN: 1–565–19536–2. 176 pp. HS.

This volume in the Current Controversies Series deals with the larger subject of addiction and provides solid source materials for use by older students. The variety of sources and formats is a plus.

INTERNET RESOURCES

While it is true that web sites often disappear, the following are maintained by organizations that will not likely abandon their web presence without appropriate forwarding information.

Higher Education Center for Alcohol and Other Drug Prevention: *http//www.edc.org/hec/*

This site offers consultation services, publications, interactive discussion, forums, and current news on alcohol and other drugs.

National Clearinghouse for Alcohol and Drug Information: *http://www.health.org*

This site offers resources, research and statistics, databases, publications and catalogs, available conferences, and related links to other information on drugs and alcohol.

National Institute on Drug Abuse: *http://www.nida.nih.gov*

This site offers survey results for students and teachers, information updates, and teaching support materials.

VIDEOTAPE

AIMS Multimedia (producer). (1998). *Binge drinking blowout: The extreme dangers of alcohol abuse.* Chatsworth, CA: AIMS Multimedia.

This program utilizes first-person accounts of teens who have learned the dangers of alcohol and the impairment it causes to decision making.

REFERENCES

Craig, J. R. and P. Craig (1988). Multidimensional Addictions and Personality Profile.

Alcohol and Drug Abuse (1997). http://www.aacap.org/about/glossary/alcohol.htm.

CHAPTER 13

Going Backwards: A Family Systems View of Alzheimer's

Joyce Graham and Scott Johnson

Adolescence is a time of stress. Beyond the pressures placed on young adults by their peers, by their families, by society, both in fact and as portrayed in the media, the stress of their home lives bombards many young adults. For many, home is not a place of security and certainty, but one of confusion and chaos. Quite often this upheaval is created as a response to difficult family situations caused by mental or physical health issues.

My own nephew Mark, my sister's son, is caught in the difficult web of living in a household in which much frenzy comes from dealing with his father's failing health, the result of advanced Alzheimer's disease. Mark, now twelve years old, is the only child from this marriage; he has four half brothers and sisters ranging in age from twenty-five to forty-two. As I've watched Mark deal with his father's deterioration, which began with a massive heart attack when Mark was eight years old, I've seen him become more reclusive, less interested in school, and more sullen. Much of his frustration is directed at his mother, who faced, and met, the difficult decision of having to place her husband in a nursing home because she could no longer care for him at home. This gut-wrenching choice, as well as the rapidly declining health of her husband, has placed a burden on her and on their household. Mark has gone from being a bright-eyed, happy, honor roll fourth grader to a frequently difficult adolescent. His struggle, though unusual because of the age of his parents, is certainly not unique. Increasingly, young adults are encountering the complex issues of living in a home where one or both parents are involved in caring for a relative stricken with the mental and physical deterioration that comes with Alzheimer's. So, my interest in looking at this disease and its impact on young adults is intensely personal. I have come to this project in my work with Scott Johnson in the hope of learning more about what I can do to better support my family as they continue the struggle of caring for and letting go of someone they love.

The book we have read, *Going Backwards* by Norma Klein (1986), tells the story, in first-person narrative, of Charles Goldberg's life as a sixteen to seventeen-year-old growing up in an affluent family in Manhattan. Charles lives with his father, a pathologist; his mother, a part-time caterer; his gifted ten-year-old brother, Kaylo; and his grandmother, Gustel. Another character central to the book is Josie, who has worked as the housekeeper and cook for the Goldberg family for many years. Gustel, who has lived with the family only a short time, is suffering from failing mental and physical health due to Alzheimer's disease. Charles' mother, Megan, grows increasingly angry that she and her sons must deal with the bizarre actions of her mother-in-law. As she grows angrier, Sam, her husband, becomes more frustrated with his inability to keep everyone happy. Meanwhile, Charles is a senior at a highly competitive high school for the fine arts. As he struggles to adjust to life with Grandma, he must also face his fumbling ways with girls, his budding sexuality, and his future college and career prospects.

Klein's book provides the reader with layers of family problems and issues to face; these are certainly compounded by the responsibility of caring for a family member living and dying with Alzheimer's disease. In this chapter, we will first examine how Klein portrays Alzheimer's. Then we will look at how the Goldbergs are coping with this problem, particularly in light of the dynamics that already exist within the nuclear family. From here we will explore Charles' confrontation with experiences common to adolescence. In the final section, Scott will present an analysis of the family dynamics and suggest ways Charles and his family can be better equipped to deal with the personal difficulties he faces.

SOME SYMPTOMS OF ALZHEIMER'S DISEASE AS SEEN IN *GOING BACKWARDS*

Numerous behavior problems are typical of Alzheimer's disease; these problems emerge at different times as the deterioration continues. Among others, the following behaviors identified by the Alzheimer's Association are seen in *Going Backwards*: concealing and denying memory loss;

exhibiting stubbornness and repetitive behavior; wandering; hiding, losing, and hoarding things; following people, particularly the significant caregiver; directing insults and accusations toward others; and experiencing sleep problems. As I know from my family, these and numerous other behaviors characterize the debilitating changes one goes through as one declines through the stages of Alzheimer's. Charles, in *Going Backwards*, like my nephew, wrestles to understand what is happening to his family. Charles, however, is in mid to late adolescence, and the loved one afflicted with the disease is a grandmother, not a parent, and a newcomer to the family home. Nonetheless, Charles struggles to be patient and kind to his grandmother while working to come to and maintain his own identity.

As the book opens, Charles' grandmother, Gustel, has recently moved in with the family because she is suffering from memory loss and can no longer remain in the retirement community where she had lived with her husband prior to his death. Charles' father, Sam, is completely devoted to his mother; he feels that she struggled and sacrificed throughout her life so that his father and he and his sister could have greater success. Sam's adoration for his mother is returned; however, her failing memory causes her frequently to forget Sam's name, where she lives, who the rest of the family members are, and virtually any event that isn't from the distant past, an example of short-term memory loss characteristic of Alzheimer's patients. As the book begins, Gustel has crept quietly into the library, where Charles is studying. When he notices her, Gustel asks him what his father's name is. Charles answers the question, as he does each time she asks one, but his frustration is evident when he realizes that she asked the same question only twenty minutes ago. Charles is so frustrated by his grandmother's inability to remember that he decides to prod her memory by recounting family trips and long walks on the beach. He even goes to his closet and pulls from it his treasured shell collection gathered during those family holidays. Among the shells, he finds an interesting and beautiful one and reminds Gustel that she had found it for him on one of their beach walks. Their frustration is evident when Gustel is unable to pull the memory forward. Such self-awareness is common in the early and middle stages of Alzheimer's. I recall the startled look that used to cross Mark's dad's face when he seemed to understand how little he understood. As with my brother-in-law, Gustel quickly slips further away from the ability to recall much from her life.

My personal awareness of Alzheimer's disease makes me understand that all will not be well in the Goldberg family, despite the assurances

Charles and his father frequently give each other and Gustel, as a way to console her and themselves, that all will be well. Although the reader can certainly sympathize with Charles' struggle to console his grandmother, it is obvious that the Goldberg family's problems will only increase. Alzheimer's is a degenerative disease, as both Scott and I have seen in our own families, and Gustel's condition is sure to decline even further. Declining health is the source of stress and loss for both the person directly affected and those who love them. And, as family systems work, as one person changes, people around them must adapt to the changing dynamics within the family.

COPING WITH ALZHEIMER'S DISEASE

Families struggling to care for a loved one with Alzheimer's disease have an immensely difficult task. Not only does the afflicted individual require ever-increasing amounts of care, but at the same time, the individual with the illness is less and less able to participate in the family. As we both have seen in our own families, alliances are drawn between the immediate caregivers and the ill member of the family. Isolation becomes a serious problem as the family stays at home more to care for their loved one and because of the difficulty of taking the Alzheimer's patient out in public. Thus, relationships within the family become more important at the same time that it becomes more difficult for many individuals to respond in predictable ways to each other. As changes continue in the family dynamic, different individuals establish alliances.

In *Going Backwards*, Charles has one reliable relationship, with Josie, the housekeeper and cook who has worked for the family for years. They provide a haven for each other amid the continually bizarre happenings in the Goldberg household. For example, when Gustel accuses Josie of stealing a set of pearls, although she had never owned pearls, Charles is able lend a sympathetic ear. Gustel's behavior here is typical of the changes in mood or behavior that the Alzheimer's Association lists as one of the ten warning signs of this disease. Gustel frequently becomes frustrated and/or angry, yet often has difficulty expressing these feelings in language, another indicator of the illness.

One evening Charles is suffering from insomnia and has wandered into his father's study to talk. While Charles and his dad are talking, Kaylo comes in and tells them that his grandmother has come into his room and is in his closet. When Sam helps Gustel from the closet she tells him that she has been writing the story of her life. The markings, written in Hebrew, are unintelligible to Sam. After helping Gustel back to bed and giving her a "snack" of Valium, Sam confides in Charles that he does not think his mother can continue to live with the family. Then he asks Charles to accompany him to visit a few potential nursing homes nearby. Charles is perplexed by this request, because his dad has never before sought out his advice; however, he agrees to go along.

A few days later, Charles' father asks him to visit a nursing home in the Bronx with him the next Saturday. As he wonders about his father's request that he accompany him for "moral support," Charles realizes that his father doesn't want to move Gustel into a home because she won't know where she is. Charles understands that his grandmother suffers from "disorientation of time and place," another warning sign of Alzheimer's disease. Like my nephew Mark with his father, Charles must face the changes in his grandmother. Doing so, however, is hard when the memories he holds of her are so different from the person she has become. "In a way it's as though my real grandmother had died and this other person is standing in for her, but not doing a very convincing job, forgetting her lines, wearing the wrong costumes. What's it like for her? Does she remember the way she used to be? Maybe it's only weird for the people who are watching and remembering" (96). Anyone who has been acquainted with someone with Alzheimer's disease can certainly relate to these thoughts. The uncertainty of what the individual dealing with this disease must be experiencing frequently haunts family members struggling to adapt to the emerging unfamiliarity of their loved one. While adolescence is a time that calls for stability and steadiness, living with an Alzheimer's patient means chaos and complete uncertainty for all family members, including young adults living in a household that is serving as the primary caregivers for an ill family member who is experiencing significant changes in personality.

Part of the uncertainty Charles must cope with is the anger and frustration his mother is experiencing with having Gustel live with the family. In particular, she is concerned because Kaylo, the precocious ten-year-old, who is musically gifted, is being traumatized by Gustel's presence. Kaylo is having difficulty falling asleep since Gustel's arrival, and he frequently suffers from nightmares. One night he dreams that a witch comes into his room and sits on his bed. When he retells the "dream," his mother realizes that the witch is actually Gustel, and that she had indeed disturbed Kaylo's sleep yet again by wandering through his room another night.

Mrs. Goldberg is not alone in her frustration. Josie must continually deal with Gustel's taunts, racist remarks, and false accusations. Gustel continually accuses Josie of being a whore and of stealing her possessions. Klein's representation of this prejudice, and Josie and Charles' reactions to it, seem believable and disturbing. Josie seems to feel powerless because of her position as an employee of the family. Charles is portrayed as a young adult trying to clarify his own attitudes and beliefs about life. What he knows is that he finds Gustel's comments about Josie to be intolerable.

Incidents such as the accusations aimed at Josie and Gustel's disturbing Kaylo during the night cause Charles' mother to grow angrier and angrier with her husband for his inability to place Gustel in a nursing home. Sam assures her that he will find a solution if only she will be patient, and soon everyone will be happy. However, it is obvious that this is an unrealistic goal; everyone cannot be happy in this family, and Dr. Goldberg is both unwilling and unable to realize the impossibility of their household situation.

As Megan's frustration escalates, she reminds her husband that "one of the tenets of marriage is to choose your wife and children over your mother" (34). As she leaves the room, Charles' father advises him, "Never have a mother. Never have a wife" (34).

Although Charles seems to understand that his father is having difficulty dealing with the decision, over strong objections by Charles' mother, to bring Gustel into their home, Charles adopts his father's approach to life. As he comforts his grandmother as she once again forgets where she is, Charles reassures her in the same tone and words his father uses time and again. Sam's words, however, do not convince him, and his doubts about his family are evident throughout the work. This is especially true when Charles thinks about his friend Kim's family, which seems sane and quiet in comparison to his own. Kim lives with his mother, father, sister, and eighty-seven-year-old grandfather. Charles talks openly with Kim and shares his concern that he may inherit his grandmother's illness. This is a horrible fear for a sixteen-year-old to hold, yet one that seems quite believable for the many young adults dealing with this illness in their own families.

DEALING WITH ADOLESCENCE

At no other point in a person's life does one experience such rapid physical and emotional changes as during adolescence. Among other developmental issues, teenagers must deal with tremendous changes in their bodies, try to understand their emerging sexuality, and work to develop an individual identity. Klein certainly captures much of adolescence in *Going Backwards*. In spite of the chaos in his family, Charles is also dealing with very typical maturation experiences for a sixteen-year-old boy. Early on we discover that Charles is frustrated by the assumptions that his parents hold about his responsibilities as a babysitter for Kaylo. He is tired of having to care for his younger brother. He also realizes that he is experiencing significant physical changes. Charles' self-effacing attitude is evident throughout the book. He continually doubts his looks, his intelligence, his ability to have a girlfriend, his musical talents. Perhaps this lack of confidence is the aspect of the book that will be the most familiar to adolescents; Charles is struggling with his identity, and he feels overshadowed by his peers and his sibling, although in his case the sibling is much younger than he.

Charles relies on his relationship with Kim to provide an outlet for many of his thoughts. Kim seems quite realistic, in spite of Klein's stereotypical portrayal of him as Korean: "he has a mind like a steel trap. He's the best in our class in math and pretty good at everything else, too" (9). Kim, a devoted musician who practices several hours a day, feels comfortable visiting Charles. In fact, he is the only friend who visits Charles at home throughout the novel, yet another sign of the isolation Charles is experiencing.

The one area that Charles does not particularly feel comfortable discussing with Kim is girls. Kim seems to be uninterested in having a girlfriend yet, and in the midst of struggling with a complicated family situation, Charles is becoming more and more interested in girls. Sam has pushed Charles for years to pursue girls, encouraging him to make sexual advances, and has talked about birth control and sexually transmitted diseases with him since he was thirteen. That the conversations did not include information on AIDS is telling of the book's 1986 publication date. Charles, now sixteen, is still a virgin, and feels awkward around all girls; however, Wendy Wolfe, a classmate who is a dancer at the arts school that he attends, is becoming attractive to him. Charles first realizes his attraction to her during a class critique of a recent dance recital by Wendy; he realizes that he is fantasizing about her sitting naked before the class. Charles' isolation, as is typical with many adolescents, is quite evident when he decides that, as much as he would like to, he cannot discuss this phenomenon with Kim. Josie also pushes Charles to find a girlfriend, and she is the only one who will listen as he expresses his doubts about his ability to both establish and maintain a relationship. Josie, however, is always encouraging, and she and Charles spend much time in the kitchen talking about relationships and life.

Charles thinks frequently of Wendy and begins to talk with Josie even more about relationships. His self-doubt is clear when he tells Josie, "I'm not charming, I have lousy skin, I'm fat" (55). Josie's seeming lack of understanding and continual prodding from his father to chase girls cause Charles to become even more frustrated with his lack of experience. Finally, he decides to ask Wendy for a date. When she accepts, they decide to go to a Broadway show the following Saturday. Charles spends lots of money on tickets and dessert after the show, only to have the conversation with Wendy bring up many negative issues for the two of them. Charles' observation that Wendy does not eat much results in her insulting him because of his weight. Their conversation over dessert after the performance reveals that Wendy had been out of school for four months and hospitalized for part of that time due to anorexia. Although the date is disastrous for Charles, he and Wendy realize that they share many of the same fears and anxieties about attempting to have a relationship with someone of the opposite sex. Both express the stereotypes they hold for the other sex, and the two of them are surprised that they share so many of the same fears and that they enjoy each other's sense of humor.

Charles spends the next three days after his first date in bed with a fever and stomach virus. When Josie confronts him on Monday, the second day of his illness, and insists that he shower and come to the table for breakfast, Charles decides that his "whole life has been warped by my being always surrounded by women of superhuman strength. No wonder I'm a neurotic mess" (72). The influence of women in his life is more evident when his mother insists that he go to school for Kaylo's recital on Tuesday, even though he is still quite ill. Charles sleeps during much of the concert, but does manage to stay awake long enough to hear Kaylo's standing ovation performance. His mother's elation is evident as she celebrates the performance with her friend and with Kaylo's teacher. As Charles dozes in the back seat of the car after the recital he overhears his mother confide to her friend that Charles has always had problems. Charles is, of course, annoyed by his mother's reaction. Once again, the reader is given a good view of the Goldbergs' unrealistic expectations. Charles is an outstanding student at a school with a selective admissions policy. He has been accepted on early decision at Cornell. He has good friends and is a responsible member of the family, and yet his mother and her friend do not recognize his achievements. Obviously, this would be frustrating and insulting for any adolescent.

Perhaps the greatest gift Charles ever receives from his father comes one night after his first date with Wendy. Suffering from insomnia, Charles wanders into his father's study late, only to find his dad reading. Charles is thinking about how much his father loves classical music, and when he apologizes that he probably is not going to be good enough to make it as a professional musician, his dad reassures him by saying, "So, you'll do something else" (81). This reassurance is the only explicit sign Charles receives from his parents throughout the entire book that they have confidence in him. It is no wonder, then, that Charles turns to Josie for support and encouragement.

As Scott points out in the next part of this chapter, families do indeed divide into groups, and Charles is well aware that an important link in the group for him is Josie. This alliance becomes even more important when Wendy invites Charles home to study with her after school one day. Finally, Charles has his first opportunity to experiment with a girl, and amid talk about tomorrow's test, he and Wendy make out. Josie is the only person he can talk to about his fears and desires.

Just as Charles is making progress with Wendy, the time arrives for him to go with his dad to visit the nursing home. They are mostly silent as they tour the facility. Perhaps the most unsettling event of the tour occurs when an elderly woman approaches Sam, thinking he is a friend of her son's, and pleads with Sam to help her find her son, who, according to the nurse, had died the year before. When the woman is scurried back to her room by a member of the staff, Sam abruptly excuses himself and says he will get back in touch.

Charles and Sam return to the family only to face many questions from Charles' mother. When it is clear that Sam has many reservations about placing Gustel in the home, his wife insists that Sam's first responsibility is to his wife and children and that he must move Gustel into the home immediately. Sam's anger and sense of helplessness are evident when, a week later, he phones the home, only to learn that a room will be available within ten days for his mother. Surprised by the sudden availability of space, Sam begins to make preparations to move Gustel. On the night before she is to actually go, Sam helps Gustel pack her things and get ready for bed. He calls Charles to come in to say goodnight to his grandmother. Realizing that he will be telling his grandmother good-bye before her move, Charles takes her his favorite shell, the one she had found for him.

Charles' good-bye to his grandmother is even more poignant when the reader is told a few pages later that his grandmother has died in her sleep. Learning this upon his return from school, Charles is warned by Josie that his father is despondent over Gustel's death and cautions him to be careful with his father, who is overcome by grief and isolates himself from the rest of the family throughout the two days surrounding the wake and burial.

Klein moves the story to Charles' enrollment the following fall at Cornell. Just before Thanksgiving, Charles receives a phone call from his mother telling him that his father had died an hour before. Charles assures his mother that he will catch the next flight home, and within a few hours he is back in New York for his father's funeral. Charles' lack of response to his father's sudden death is even more startling than his father's intense reaction to Gustel's death. During the next day, he listens to his mother without emotion, walks with Kaylo in Central Park, phones his new girlfriend, whom he met that fall at Cornell, and goes with his mother, Kaylo, and Josie to a private funeral for his father. Kim and Wendy, dating each other now and both students at Harvard, are home for Thanksgiving; the three friends spend time together walking, talking, and visiting their old high school.

Charles returns home to spend the evening with his mother and Kaylo. After dinner, Charles and his mother go into his dad's study to talk. As they sit in the small room sipping brandy, Charles' mom, after a long period of silence, tells him that his father gave Gustel an overdose of Valium the night she died. The news, startling as it seems, does not surprise Charles. When Charles asks his mother why she felt he had done this, her response is, "Out of love. That's one thing I'm sure of. He adored her and he couldn't bear to see her suffer. He hated those nursing homes. He knew he could get away with it, if that's the right expression, because she had no money, she was elderly, he gave her just the right amount" (180). No matter from what perspective one looks at this incident, Charles is left to deal with the fact that his father has killed his grandmother. At the same time, the book closes as Charles is dealing with the loss of his father. Throughout the book, Klein gives numerous warnings that Charles would lose his father, whom she describes as looking ten years older than he is. Charles frequently talked or thought about how much his father smoked and drank. Yet, the ending turns the reader's attention away from Alzheimer's disease and opens another difficult trauma for the family.

Perhaps the most gripping part of the novel is the isolation experienced by all of the members of the Goldberg family. Since we only come to know them at the very time that Gustel moves in, we do not really have an adequate picture of the family before her arrival. Yet, it seems clear that the feelings of isolation and frustration experienced by all of the Goldbergs did not begin with Gustel's arrival.

We are left to hope at the end of the book that Charles will be okay, though my colleague, Scott, is not so sure. In the next part of this chapter, Scott looks at ways in which Charles and the Goldberg family can become better equipped to deal with life.

A FAMILY SYSTEMS VIEW OF THE GOLDBERGS

One of the classic tools of family therapists to help us understand what is happening in families is called a genogram. A genogram is a little like a family tree—it shows who was married to whom, who were whose parents and whose children—but it doesn't stop there. It also attempts to show what those various relationships were qualitatively like—who was close to, or distant from, whom; who was in conflict with whom; who may have had an affair with, or was divorced from, or was merely dating whom; who lived with whom, even if they were not nominally part of the same family; who lived in what location, or did what kind of work; who was seen by others in what kind of way—who was the nominally favored child, the neglected, the happy, the rebellious; who may have died from, or suffered with, what kind of emotional disturbance or disease. These are some of the issues a genogram attempts to survey and express.

Looking at a genogram, at least at a well-constructed one, one begins to see not simply chains of individuals and events but relational patterns, many of which may appear repeatedly. Individual behavior that may have seemed confusing at first glance suddenly begins to fit into a larger scheme. A pattern of sexual affairs or drug abuse carried through several generations no longer seems the singular weakness or evil of a particular family member. A pattern of self-sacrifice repeated through grandparents, parents, and children no longer strikes us as the special goodness of a single woman or man. Wonderful or horrible things people may have done lose some of their wonder or their terror when placed in the context of the behavior of other family members over time.

Genogram of the Goldberg family at the outset of *Going Backwards*

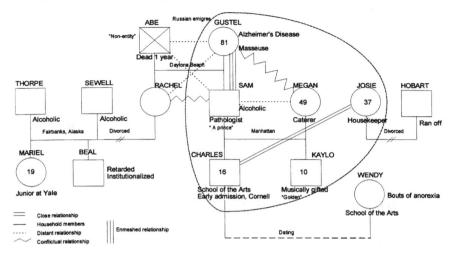

At least that is how, as a family therapist looking at the genogram of the Goldberg family in Norma Klein's novel, *Going Backwards*, I tend to look at things (see diagram). For me, and, I suspect, most other family therapists, this is not a story of a troubled adolescent but of a troubled family, one whose difficulties started long before the novel's central character, Charles Goldberg, was born, yet who now, as the story unfolds, is living with those problems' consequences.

At the outset of the novel, Charles' grandmother, Gustel, who suffers from Alzheimer's disease, has recently come to live with his family in their twelve-room apartment. Yet, in the simplest terms, this is a story less of a family struggling with a member suffering from Alzheimer's disease than of a family struggling with the residue of a marriage between Charles' grandparents in which one partner, Gustel, was seen as dynamic and vital and creative and powerful, and the other, her husband, Abe, was seen as a "non-entity." Spanning three generations, it is a family in which Charles' father Sam was "adored" by Sam's mother, while Sam's sister, Rachel, was viewed as unimportant; a family in which Sam became, in his mother Gustel's eyes, a substitute for her ineffectual husband and "unimportant" daughter, and thus was delegated, as family therapists say, to succeed in their stead.

And it is a family in which Sam, having been beatified by his mother, feels obligated to repay her by having her come live with them, even at the cost of the peace of his own wife and children. In part, to deal with the repercussions of this choice, Sam numbs himself to the conflict that Gustel's living in his house causes by remaining inebriated throughout most of the tale and by keeping Gustel drugged on Valium much of the time. In addition, to lessen criticism from his family, he routinely over-medicates his older son with narcotics as well.

It is also the story of a family in which the second generation of parents, Sam and his wife, Megan, have essentially repeated Sam's parents' mistakes by again singling out one child, Charles' brother, as "gifted" while viewing Charles as still needing some way to distinguish himself. It is, moreover, a family in which Sam attempts to cover his own abuse of alcohol by encouraging drinking by sixteen-year-old Charles and to resolve some of his own sexual frustrations by pushing Charles to become sexually active. And it is a family, finally, in which the nominally less valued child, Charles, appears to feel as attached to the family housekeeper, Josie, as he does to his own mother.

Thus, while the nominal family problem of the story is the grand-mother's Alzheimer's disease, and while her condition exacerbates Charles' family's difficulties, it in no way creates them. In fact, it is a wonderful smoke screen to divert attention from them. Let us look at this story in more detail.

TROUBLED FAMILIES

Troubled families can be, in some ways, a lot like spy rings. They have secrets they want to keep—or that at least some members want to keep—and they go to great lengths to keep them. One of the time-tested ways that spies keep important secrets safe is by leaking less important ones. If you want, for example, to make sure that no one knows that you have the enemy's nuclear weapons' codes, perhaps you'll let people find out that you have information on their new long-range cannon. The in-formation on the cannon may be relatively minor—perhaps all you know is that they have one—but that is unimportant. What matters is that your enemy knows you have it, and so will worry about that rather than about the much more damaging information they don't know you have. The essence of the tactic is diversion, and that is often how members of troubled families behave.

In Charles' family, this means that friends and neighbors know that Charles' grandmother who suffers from Alzheimer's is living with them and that she can't remember family members' names or take care of herself, but that they don't know many other, more devastating things about life with the Goldbergs. There is a scene early on in the story, for example, where Charles and his classmate, Kim, are studying calculus together at Charles' house, when they are interrupted by Gustel, who repeatedly wanders into the room where they are studying. After several more disturbances by Gustel, Charles calls his father at the dinner party, who tells him to give Gustel more Valium, even though she has already had a fair amount, along with sleeping pills.

Charles does as his father suggests, but a short time later he and Kim hear a thud from another room. They find Gustel sitting on the floor with purple stains on her nightgown and on her arms and legs. Gustel, heavily doped, has fallen while trying to drink a glass of grape juice. There is broken glass, her head is cut, and grape juice is staining the room. The juice has soaked her nightgown, so that her breasts and belly are exposed. Kim begins picking up broken glass while Charles tries to clean her and cover her up. It is exactly the kind of embarrassing scene anyone would dread, and particularly an adolescent's nightmare, but it is also the kind of situation in which most people would be embarrassed by the wrong things.

For what is telling in the scene is not so much that a woman with Alzheimer's wanders the house making life difficult for her grandson, or even that she has fallen and hurt herself and her grandson has to clean her up, but that the mother of a medical doctor living in his own house would receive such inadequate, even negligent care. A physician who told the grandson of a different Alzheimer's patient over the phone to give the patient more Valium after the patient already had a large Valium dose, along with other debilitating drugs, who then had the patient fall and cut herself, would be flirting with malpractice. Charles, at sixteen, sees little beyond his own and his friend's embarrassment, and never questions his father's judgment.

ALCOHOL AND DRUG ABUSE

Alcohol abuse and substance abuse, in this story, have a life of their own. Charles' father, Sam, drinks heavily at dinner, and at other times. Megan pleads with him one evening at the dinner table to slow down his drinking so he won't die early. Sam promises, but his drinking does not change. And he does die, we find out, at the story's end. His encouragement of Charles' drinking, of course, makes sense in this regard, for it normalizes and masks his own problem.

But then it is in everyone's interest in the Goldberg family to make drinking look as normal as possible in order to make Sam's drinking appear acceptable. Even Megan's plea to Sam at dinner is to drink less— not so that he won't become a drunken bum, kill a patient, lose his practice and his medical license, and ruin his family, but the much vaguer dread that somehow drinking will affect his health and he'll die prematurely. It is the plea of someone who really doesn't want to face the reality of being married to an incipient alcoholic. In the simplest terms, the family is in denial about Sam's alcohol abuse.

There is also plenty of denial and ambivalence involving prescription drug abuse. Abusing medication, of course, is especially easy for physicians to do—as a group they have a relatively high rate of it. But while Sam may or may not be abusing prescription drugs himself, Klein gives several examples of Sam's overmedicating his mother. Valium, an anti-anxiety drug, is particularly powerful when given to the elderly and should be prescribed for them with great restraint and very low dosages. Yet, according to Charles, Sam gives his mother "a half bottle" a night. Even allowing for teenage exaggeration, this is troubling. Gustel's earlier mentioned fall, during which she spills grape juice and cuts her head, clearly appears to be a classic symptom of Valium overdose. And of course, there is every possibility that Gustel has become dependent on Valium—the fact that she constantly takes so much of it makes this nearly a certainty, though her illness tends to mask its effects.

Sam's abuse of his prescription privileges and his Hippocratic oath to "first, do no harm" is not limited, of course, to his mother. He also, Charles reports, "gives me Dalmane," a hypnotic drug used for insomnia, "as well as Valium" to help him sleep. Both are addictive, and Charles' father's suggestion to alternate so he doesn't become addicted, while perhaps reasonable in some clinical circumstances, here sounds like nothing more than the verbal sleight of hand all pushers use to convince their addicts their dope is safe. And, while Valium is prescribed for insomnia, its primary use is to ease anxiety. It is as if Sam on some level really knows how disturbed his family is, and is basically trying to numb everyone to their emotional distress.

Charles again seems not to understand his own behavior, or how much his father's "help" has undermined him. A sixteen-year-old who alternates periodic use of Valium and Dalmane over the course of at least a year is, without question, "into drugs" and so close to dependence that one wonders if the difference really matters. If he doesn't have a dependency yet, he's doing his best to develop one. As is often the case with people whose substance abuse centers on prescription medicine rather than common street narcotics, no one in the family recognizes this behavior for what it is.

The ultimate example of the use of drugs to manage stress in the novel, of course, occurs the night before Gustel is to enter the nursing home in which Sam has finally, reluctantly, agreed to place her. When Charles wakes the next morning to learn that his grandmother is dead, all he is told is that Gustel has died in her sleep. Later in the tale, after his father's death, his mother reveals the truth.

One does not have to be a crusader against physician assisted suicide—something that I personally support—to recognize that Sam's behavior is little short of murder. A man who regularly anesthetizes himself and other members of his household with drugs and alcohol fits no one's image of a sober, caring physician helping a debilitated patient die, nor of a devoted son, committing parental euthanasia after painful and deliberate reflection.

INTIMATE RELATIONSHIPS

To suggest that the meaning of the word "love" in the Goldberg family is distorted is to engage in understatement. This is not to say that there is no affection whatsoever in this family, no genuine acts of kindness or altruism, but simply to observe that what the family members often assert to be acts of affection and selflessness generally do not, on inspection, hold up to their claims.

Sam's repeated assertion, for example, that he wants Gustel to live with them out of love for her is impossible to square with his constantly giving her overdoses of Valium. It is, in fact, difficult not to speculate from a clinical point of view that, rather than lessening the symptoms of his mother's Alzheimer's and making her life more livable, Sam's doping of Gustel very probably increases her loss of memory and weakens whatever slim connection she may have with the world. But a less drugged Gustel also would obviously mean a more difficult, more uncontrollable Gustel, a Gustel, more than likely, whose behavior would so obviously be beyond Sam and his family's ability to manage that he would have no choice but to place her immediately in a nursing home where she could be cared for without being thoroughly narcotized.

Yet to admit that, Sam would have to admit that he is unable to help the mother who calls him "a prince." Gustel's idolizing of her son is not a blessing but a trap for Sam, since everyone knows that a gentle, kind man would never put his mother in a nursing home, would he? In essence, Sam's act of "love" in taking in Gustel ultimately is meant mainly to maintain Sam's image of himself as a caring son, not to ensure the best treatment for his mother. It is, in short, less an act of love than of insecurity and simple guilt.

Sam's blatantly false argument that all nursing homes are "hell holes" is designed in some sense merely to make it impossible for his wife or children to argue in favor of placing Gustel in a professional care facility. The nursing home he and Charles actually visit seems far from hell in Klein's narrative—far less hell, certainly, than the Goldbergs' home. Yet, again, for Sam to admit that Gustel might be better off in someone else's hands would be to give up his own need to be needed—Sam's co-dependency, as therapists like to say. The attention of the world, in Sam's sad universe, is limited. It must be saved largely for Gustel, the queen, and her son, the prince.

HUSBAND AND WIFE

While Charles acknowledges how weird the relationship of his grand-mother and father is, he seems singularly unaware of the obvious dis-tance between his mother and his father. Few, if any, interactions between Megan and her husband in the book seem warm or even friendly. By and large the two seem in conflict, primarily over Sam's drinking and Gustel's presence in the house. Even Charles' description of what his father thinks is a "perfect" evening—sitting alone in his study, drinking wine and listening to Brahms—suggests volumes about the state of his parents' relationship. And when her husband prematurely dies at the novel's end, Megan seems notably undistressed. While she cries briefly when telling Charles about Sam's death on the phone, her reactions (and the rest of the family's, except perhaps for Kaylo's), seem muted, even allowing for her still being in shock. Yet Charles asserts in several places that his parents have a great marriage.

Depending on our perspectives, Sam and Megan's relationship may be viewed in any number of ways. They are not divorced, they do not appear to physically abuse each other, they rarely shout or say unkind things. They have a comfortable, wealthy life, into which little unpleas-antness not of their own making intrudes. As Joyce rightly points out in her discussion, these facts are important to Charles, for they are some of the few assurances he has of family stability.

Charles' exaggerated view of his parents' happiness seems of a piece with many of the other distorted views the Goldbergs have of their actions and relationships. In this sense, to some extent Charles acts as what therapists call a "gatekeeper," telling others how they should see his family's interactions rather than letting outsiders draw conclusions of their own. This is a normal function; all families have them. But it becomes problematic when the way that the gatekeeper believes the family should be seen and the actual reality are out of sync with each other, as they repeatedly are here.

None of this is to suggest that there is no real caring in the Goldberg family, no sense of the welfare of others, and Joyce notes several examples of genuine tenderness and care, such as Sam's crucial reassurance of Charles toward the middle of the novel that he has confidence in Charles' ability to succeed. Sam and Megan, and Sam's parents, Gustel and Abe, clearly have many flaws as parents and as couples, but there is no question that on some level they want good things for their children and themselves. The problem is simply that the actions that they take to secure their own and their children's welfare often have exactly the opposite effect from what they intend, frequently because they themselves are afraid to examine the motives for their behavior. But nothing in their past prepares them to ask such questions, and the result is a quiet, well-mannered tragedy. And where, in all this angst, shall we put Alzheimer's disease, the nominal focus of Klein's tale?

ALZHEIMER'S DISEASE

Alzheimer's disease is a type of dementia generally found among the aged. It tends to strike more women than men and is a progressive disorder for which there is no known cure and few if any effective treatments. It is also, as few people realize, an invariably fatal disorder, a fact often masked by the advanced age of most of its victims. Its hallmarks are sudden memory loss and confusion, and it is a disease with relatively distinct stages. The early phases are generally only discernable in retrospect, and then principally by relatives and friends—the repetitive or nonsensical questions so-and-so would ask, the time our father forgot to call on our birthday and then didn't remember not calling, the car accident that our aunt felt couldn't possibly have been her fault even though her own description suggested that it must have been. In its later but still early phases there are often heated arguments.

Slowly, after enough of these events, someone may suggest a trip to a doctor. Alzheimer's symptoms typically surface several years before it is ever diagnosed, and the only way a definitive diagnosis can be made is by an autopsy. Some of its symptoms can be mimicked by reactions to a variety of medications and conditions like high blood pressure, and a working diagnosis is basically a process of eliminating other possibilities. The later stages of Alzheimer's can be relatively tranquil, if individuals are receiving professional care or their family caregivers are not overly stressed. Later stage sufferers tend to lose some of their defensiveness and can become much less demanding, though this is not always the case and families should not live in the hope that this invariably will happen.

But this is an important point to bear in mind, for it speaks directly to the issues of euthanasia and assisted suicide Klein's novel explores. While in the earlier stages of the disease the obvious suffering of its victims and those around them often makes suicide or euthanasia seem a reasonable course of action, such alternatives can become far less rational as the progress of the disease ironically robs victims of their consciousness that anything is really wrong, and thus their mental decline becomes somewhat less of a burden for both patients and those who tend to them.

Individuals experiencing Alzheimer's in the early stages, however, typically try to cover up the fact, which often makes their behavior seem even more bizarre. They sometimes vehemently fight the idea that there is anything wrong with them until they have to be declared incompetent by a court of law. Adding to the problems of treatment is the fact that many families simply do not see Alzheimer's as an illness, regarding it as a normal part of the aging process, which it is not, and so mistakenly attempt to manage it largely by themselves.

The difference between normal aging and Alzheimer's disease is most apparent in Klein's contrasting portrayals of Charles's chaotic family life and the sane and stable household of his friend Kim. It is easy to misread this part of the story as simply a contrast of cultures between an essentially nuclear Jewish American family and a Korean American household's more extended relationships. But it is also a crystalline warning that we should not confuse caring for a physically frail but mentally competent elderly relative—Charles pointedly describes Kim's grandfather as seeming to have "a million movies" stored in perfect order in his head—with attempting to play nursing home to someone like Gustel suffering from an extremely complex, severe, long-term, and progressive mental disease.

Klein's description of Alzheimer's itself and its symptoms is, as Joyce observes, dead on target. Gustel's memory loss, her incontinence, and her paranoia are common middle-to-late-stage Alzheimer's symptoms. What many readers may unfortunately not grasp, however, is Klein's intentional portrayal of Sam's mistreatment of her disease.

Even in the mid-1980s, treating Alzheimer's through massive doses of narcotics would have been questionable practice. Alzheimer's patients may occasionally need restraint—some can become violent—and they unquestionably need twenty-four-hour, close supervision, but they do not need constant sedation. As I have noted earlier, Sam's overdosing of his mother likely increases her confusion and memory loss. Keeping her at home, though ostensibly a noble sacrifice, can also tend to increase the isolation of both sufferers and caregivers, unintentionally hastening the patient's inevitable deterioration and diminishing the caregivers' ability to deal with it.

THE GOLDBERGS IN THERAPY

Treating a family like the Goldbergs involves addressing multiple problems. While Alzheimer's is one of them, it is certainly not first on the list. Helping the family see that would certainly be one of therapy's larger challenges.

The most difficult problem in therapy frequently is simply getting family members to attend. Megan would be most likely to initiate treatment, and Charles and Kaylo presumably would come with her. Sam would not be easy to get to participate, as a physician who calls hospitals "prisons" is unlikely to be comfortable in therapy, and therapy might well have to proceed without him. Personally, I would make it a point to have Megan ask Josie to take part. She is seen by Megan and Charles as a member of the family, and many of her insights would be valuable.

A second issue would be gathering the kind of information Klein gives us in the novel. Few therapists ever have access to anyone's thoughts on the scale that we do as readers. But starting by gathering the family history and perspectives that make up the genogram would make sense. Even any lack of information family members might come up against would be important, as it could cause Charles or Megan in particular to go home with questions for Sam or others about who their relatives are and what their relationships were like. Certainly one would ask many more questions about Megan's family and its influences on Goldberg life, a topic that Klein does not explore in any depth.

Genograms are particularly valuable interventions because they are based directly on information from clients, and they tend to speak for themselves. Often, family members themselves will make important observations about family patterns, such as Sam and Kaylo both being seen as "gifted" while Rachel and Charles, clearly bright and accomplished, tend to be overlooked.

Helping Megan and Charles understand the serious nature of Sam's alcohol abuse and the general abuse of narcotics in the family would be paramount. The issue of caring for Gustel comes after this and could be put in a fairly blunt way: Do you really think a family with dependencies on alcohol and Valium is in any position to care for an eighty-one-year-old woman with Alzheimer's? While this question primarily needs to be addressed to Sam, it wouldn't matter that he wasn't there. In fact, it would have far more power coming from Megan or Charles than from a therapist. It's the kind of question, too, that just might get him involved in therapy.

An equally difficult issue would be the question of Sam's continuing to practice medicine until he undergoes evaluation and possible treatment himself for alcohol abuse and for the possible misuse of his prescription privileges. Any responsible therapist would have to raise this question with the family and try to prepare them for the potentially severe consequences of Sam's suspect behavior. He might also conceivably need to be reported by the therapist for abuse of both a minor and an incapacitated adult, with similar consequences. While all this might not be an immediate issue, the family would need to be prepared to face it, with or without Sam's help.

Somewhere in this tangle is the question of finding good care for Gustel. Apprising the family of the unintended but real harm Sam is doing to her in a form they might be able to bear would be important, along with noting the obvious damage they are doing to themselves. One of the greatest difficulties in caring for someone with Alzheimer's is simply that it is terribly expensive, since it requires around-the-clock supervision. For the Goldbergs, however, money is not an immediate problem. Fear and ignorance, however, are.

Helping them understand that Alzheimer's is not invariably the worst thing in the world either for the sufferer or those around him or her would be a central part of this work. Preparing them for her eventual death, including exploring their own fears of aging and dying and their beliefs on assisted suicide and euthanasia, would be especially important. When and whether they would be able to act on the fruits of this exploration is a different question, but the aim of therapy would be to help them see choices in their perspectives and their actions, something they haven't really had.

Even if I were working in a school system I would hesitate to work at any length with Charles alone. The problems, after all, are not really his, though he suffers with their consequences. Occasionally, one must help a young person like Charles whose parents are unwilling to take part in therapy understand what some of the difficulties in his family are and to help him see that, though he may have a role in them, they are usually not of his making. Helping him become less dependent on narcotics through specific drug treatment and to behave in an age appropriate way regarding alcohol would be important tasks as well.

Should therapy come after Gustel's or Sam's death, one adds grief work to helping them retroactively understand the recent difficulties of family members' lives. One might also add the problem of a family member reaching the conclusion that Sam was not Gustel's savior but her murderer, and therapy most likely would have to address the large amounts of rage, ambivalence, sorrow, confusion, and pain that in some degree all family members would feel.

There is no magic to be done here, but there is the possibility of introducing some clarity into the lives of people whose sense of choice and action has been seriously distorted and limited by their pasts. One can hold out the chance of change, and hope, at least, that some or all of them may take it.

CONCLUSION

It is easy to read or misread *Going Backwards* and come away with the idea that Alzheimer's and aging are simply sheer hell, always destroyers of family life. Make no mistake, Alzheimer's disease is a terrible affliction, and few things are more painful than watching a loved one suffer with its symptoms, as both Joyce and I have done. But it is not invariably unmitigated torment, either for the sufferer or for those who care for her or him, particularly for families like the Goldbergs who can afford good outside care. It is part of the tragedy of this particular family that they fail to see it in a more hopeful way.

Families who understand that Alzheimer's is an illness, not normal aging; families who do not bring to the table the festering mix of substance abuse, guilt and resentments, and distorted views of family relationships carried by the Goldbergs; families who do not equate love with personal suffering and competition; and families who can talk about and negotiate the differences of their members have a much better chance of weathering such a trying but invariably time-limited problem.

Klein's story ultimately is not about the damage caused by Alzheimer's to the Goldberg family but of the underlying family damage that long predates it and that Gustel's illness simply brings into the light. It is in that sense that Charles and his family are going backwards, and there is, sadly, little indication as the novel ends that their direction has substantially altered or is all that likely to change. The novel lends itself, for educators and therapists, to rich discussion and introspection. The issues are relevant for every adolescent and would generate insightful journals, poetry, research projects, artwork, and music.

RECOMMENDED READINGS

Alzheimer's: Fiction

Cargill, K (1997). *Nana's new home.* Abilene, TX: KrisPer Publications. ISBN: 0–9660–5660–4. 32 pp. ES.

This comforting story about a child's grandmother explains Alzheimer's disease to young children.

Chetkovich, D. (1993). *Danger at Rocky River: The NeuroExplorers in a memorable misadventure.* Houston: Baylor College of Medicine. MS.

Several young adolescents form a club called the NeuroExplorers in which they learn about the brain, nervous system, and memory. One of the members has a grandfather with Alzheimer's disease who wanders away from his nursing home, and the NeuroExplorers come to his rescue.

Dyjak, E. (1990). *I should have listened to Moon.* Boston: Houghton Mifflin. ISBN: 0–3955–2279–X. 144 pp. MS.

A twelve-year-old girl must come to terms with growing up and growing old when her best friend develops an interest in makeup and boys, and her somewhat confused and forgetful grandmother moves in to share her bedroom.

Graber, R. (1986). *Doc.* New York: HarperCollins. ISBN: 0–0602–2064–3. 160 pp. MS, HS.

Brad, a high school sophomore, experiences feelings of embarrassment, guilt, and grief in dealing with his grandfather Doc, who has Alzheimer's disease and exhibits realistic behaviors such as throwing tantrums, forgetting to dress, and suffering from incontinence.

Hickman, J. (1994). *Jericho*. New York: Greenwillow Books. ISBN: 0–6881–3398–3. 144 pp. MS.

An account of twelve-year-old Angela's visit to help take care of her great-grandmother who has Alzheimer's disease alternates with the story of the old woman's life. As a result of caring for her great-grandmother, Angela gradually learns to appreciate the journey that lies ahead.

Howe, N. (1988). *In with the out crowd*. Boston: Houghton Mifflin. ISBN: 0–3807–0472–2. 208 pp. HS.

Sixteen-year-old Robin begins to question her values and friendships as she finds herself ousted from the most popular group in school, and at the same time spending time with her grandfather, who has Alzheimer's disease.

Kelley, B. (1996). *Harpo's horrible secret*. Prairie Grove, AR: Ozark Publishing. ISBN: 1–5676–3059–6. 130 pp. ES, MS.

Harpo is a fourth grader who, while sharing his bedroom with his great-grandfather, who has Alzheimer's disease, begins to see many of his great-grandfather's symptoms in himself.

Klein, N. (1986). *Going backwards*. ISBN: 0–590–40328–1. 182 pp. HS.

This story of a family's struggle with Alzheimer's is discussed in this chapter.

Mahy, M. (1988). *Memory*. New York: M. K. McElderry Books. ISBN: 0–6895–0446–2. 288 pp. HS.

Nineteen-year-old Jonny Dart is haunted by feelings of guilt about his sister's death, and through a chance meeting with Sophie, an old woman suffering from Alzheimer's disease, is able to come to terms with his loss. While he deals with the horrible realities of Alzheimer's disease, he is still able to recognize Sophie's dignity and courage.

Skurzynski, G. (1989). *Dangerous ground*. New York: Bradbury Press. ISBN: 0–0278–2731–3. 128 pp. MS.

While taking one last driving tour of Wyoming before moving out of state, eleven-year-old Angela accompanies her beloved seventy-eight-year-old great-aunt Hil to Yellowstone National Park, where Hil's strange behavior suggests she may be suffering from Alzheimer's disease.

Woodbury, M. (1997). *Jess and the runaway Grandpa*. Regina, SK: Co-teau Books. ISBN: 1–5505–0113–5. 208 pp. MS.

Twelve-year-old Jess has a few problems—her cat was hit by a car, her best friend Brian has turned into an obnoxious fool and, worst of all, her next door neighbor, "Grandpa Ernie," can't remember who she is. Set against a backdrop of Alzheimer's disease, this is a story with universal themes of love and friendship.

Young, A. E. (1986). *What's wrong with Daddy?* Worthington, OH: Willowisp Press. ISBN: 0–8740–6066–4. 176 pp. MS, HS.

This story follows Jen, a teenager whose father is suffering from Alzheimer's disease, through the several phases of dealing with her father's illness, beginning with embarrassment and ending with acceptance and the help of a support group and friend.

Alzheimer's: Nonfiction

Beckelman, L. (1990). *The facts about Alzheimer's disease*. New York: Crestwood House. 0–896–86489–8. ES, MS.

Part of the Facts About series, this book discusses the symptoms, possible causes and treatments, and long-term effects of this degenerative disease in language appropriate for upper elementary and middle school children.

Check, W. A. (1989). *Alzheimer's disease*. New York: Chelsea House. ISBN: 0–7910–0056–7. 116 pp. MS.

The author explores a number of topics related to Alzheimer's disease: possible causes, symptoms, treatment, care, and financial and legal issues. This book, a title in *The Encyclopedia of Health: Medical Disorders and Their Treatment*, includes a bibliography of additional resources.

Frank, J. (1985). *Alzheimer's disease: The silent epidemic*. Minneapolis: Lerner Publications. ISBN: 0–8225–1578–4. 80 pp. ES, MS.

The author explains how Alzheimer's disease progresses, gives case histories of victims, and describes some of the problems their families face.

Gillick, M. R. (1998). *Tangled minds: Understanding Alzheimer's disease and other dementias*. New York: Dutton. ISBN: 0–5259–4145–2. 224 pp. HS.

This book, written for adults, can also be useful and meaningful for young adults who want to know about the effects of Alzheimer's disease on individuals and their families, and about the changing attitudes toward and scientific theories on aging and diseases related to it. By creating a composite patient with Alzheimer's disease, the author illuminates the suffering that accompanies this disease and advocates accepting people with Alzheimer's just as we accept those with physical disabilities.

Gold, S. D. (1996). *Alzheimer's disease*. Parsippany, NJ: Crestwood House. ISBN: 0–8968–6857–5. 48 pp. ES, MS.

The author discusses the causes, effects, and treatments of Alzheimer's disease in language appropriate for elementary and middle school children and includes a bibliography for further study.

Landau, E. (1996). *Alzheimer's disease*. New York: Franklin Watts. ISBN: 0–5311–1268–3. 112 pp. ES, MS.

This book, put out by a respected publisher of children's nonfiction books, examines the possible causes, social effects, and personal trials of Alzheimer's disease. There is a bibliography of other resources suitable for upper elementary and middle school children.

Index

AA (Alcoholics Anonymous), 252, 256, 263

The Abduction, 22

About Handicaps: An Open Family Book for Parents and Children Together, 23

Accident, 42

Accommodations, 55, 59, 62–63, 64–65, 119, 127

Acquired immunodeficiency syndrome. *See* HIV/AIDS

Activities, classroom, 122, 143–45; relating to alcohol abuse, 248–50; relating to anorexia, 203–5; relating to chronic illness, 78, 79, 85–92, 100–101, 102; relating to disabilities, 2, 14–18, 37–40, 41

ADD. *See* Attention deficit hyperactivity disorder (ADHD)

A.D.D. Warehouse (Web site), 129

Addabbom, Carole, 70

Adderal, 116

ADHD. *See* Attention deficit hyperactivity disorder (ADHD)

ADHD Owner's Manual (Web site), 129

Adolescence: body image in, 32, 98, 103, 148, 176–77, 184, 186, 188, 189, 191, 193, 207, 208, 210; characteristics of, 7, 36, 40–41, 68, 98, 141, 149, 150, 154–56, 161–62, 173–74, 270–71; choices during, 100, 101, 102; identity issues during, 4, 5, 6, 8–9, 27, 30, 35, 37, 40, 52, 57, 60, 62, 64, 102, 106, 151, 154–55, 156, 159, 163, 169, 171, 172–73, 246, 253, 271; self-concepts/self-image during, 5, 8–9, 36, 62, 68, 103, 151, 161, 163, 176, 184, 186, 189, 191; self-esteem during, 6–7, 8–9, 30, 31, 35–36, 40, 48, 60, 61, 100, 104, 117–18, 128, 169, 172, 190, 194, 207, 212, 255. *See also* Adolescents; Adolescents, chronically ill; Adolescents, physically disabled

Adolescents: alcohol abuse among, 31–32, 33, 39, 102–3, 107, 113–14, 156, 243–64, 257, 258, 259, 261–63, 277, 278–79; attention deficit disorder (ADHD) among, 111–30, 138, 155, 252; attitudes toward death of others, 77–78, 79–80, 84, 94, 95–96, 135–37, 138, 140, 145, 146, 147, 148, 156, 167, 168, 169–70, 170, 171, 173, 232–33, 234, 235–36, 257, 259, 274, 288; attitudes toward own death, 11–12, 13, 16, 19, 22, 83–84, 92–93, 114, 155–56, 167, 174, 202, 224, 258; depression among, 117, 138, 151–74, 208, 255, 258; drug abuse among, 31, 107, 114, 156, 252, 254, 261, 263–64, 277, 279–80, 284, 285, 286; eating disorders among, 98, 103, 105–6, 138, 173, 174, 175–216; and HIV/AIDS, 217–40; isolation/loneliness among, 31, 46, 51, 65, 72, 99, 101, 103, 142, 151, 155, 169, 170, 171, 173, 225, 230, 268, 271, 275, 284; mental health in, 137–38, 139, 145–50; rebellion among, 142, 154–55, 160, 170, 173, 200, 201; relations with friends, 139–41, 142, 146, 148, 154–55, 167, 169, 170, 171, 172, 184–85, 186, 189, 214, 223, 231–32, 234, 235, 236, 245, 246, 253, 255, 259, 271, 274, 287, 288; relations with ill relatives, 79–80, 92, 93–94, 94, 95, 96, 109, 148, 169, 172; relations with opposite sex, 31, 36, 37, 81, 95, 98, 99, 102–3, 105, 113, 120–21, 140, 146, 155, 156, 158–59, 166, 184, 186, 190, 202, 205, 224, 232, 233, 245, 246, 255, 258, 261, 266, 271–72, 287; relations with peer groups, 5, 6–8, 31, 35–36, 40, 68, 98, 101, 102, 104–5, 109, 113, 129, 154–55, 158, 161, 166, 171, 253, 288;

relations with siblings, 127, 147, 168, 170, 223, 224, 271, 288; sexuality in, 31, 36, 37, 48, 107, 140, 141, 142, 146, 173, 181, 198, 201, 219, 220–22, 232, 233, 234, 244, 254, 257, 261, 271, 277; and suicide, 19, 114, 136, 155–56, 167, 170, 171, 174, 191, 202, 224, 255, 258. *See also* Adolescence; Adolescents, chronically ill; Adolescents, physically disabled; Parents; Teachers
Adolescents, chronically ill: adjustments to illness, 83–84, 98–100, 103–6; relations with friends, 80, 81, 92, 94, 98, 99, 100, 101, 148; relations with parents, 80–81, 82, 84–85, 93, 98–99, 103, 106–7, 108; relations with siblings, 93, 94–95, 107; school environments for, 100. *See also* Adolescence; Adolescents, physically disabled
Adolescents, physically disabled: accommodations for, 55, 59, 62–63, 64–65; adjustments to disabilities, 7, 34–35, 41, 59–60, 62, 64; challenges for, 5–6, 51–52; community attitudes toward, 29–30, 45–46, 52, 53, 55, 58, 59, 61, 63, 64–65, 66; fiction relating to, 18–23, 41–47; films relating to, 48; nonfiction relating to, 23–24, 47–48; relations with counselors, 1, 2, 8, 9, 12, 13–14, 18; relations with friends, 1, 2–5, 11, 23, 32–33, 36, 38–39, 46, 47, 62, 70, 72; relations with non-disabled students, 12; relations with parents, 4, 22, 23, 27–28, 31, 32, 44, 55, 58, 60–61, 62, 63, 64–65, 73; relations with siblings, 43, 44, 61; relations with teachers, 28, 30, 34; school environments for, 9–13,

28, 33, 34–35, 37, 52. *See also* Adolescence; Adolescents; Adolescents, chronically ill
After the Dancing Days, 45
AIDS. *See* HIV/AIDS
AIDS: Everything You and Your Family Need to Know But Were Afraid to Ask, 240
AIDS: Ten Stories of Courage, 238
AIDS and HIV: Risky Business, 237
Alanon, 249
Alateen, 263
Alcohol: Opposing Viewpoints, 261
Alcohol abuse, 160; among adolescents, 31–32, 33, 39, 102–3, 107, 113–14, 156, 243–64, 257, 258, 259, 261–63, 277, 278–79; and anger, 246–47; fiction relating to, 257–61; Internet resources relating to, 263–64; nonfiction relating to, 261–64; among parents, 245, 249, 257–61, 263, 277, 278–79; and psychotherapy, 250–56; symptoms, 250–53; treatments, 249, 252, 253. *See also* Adolescents, drug abuse among
Alcoholics Anonymous (AA), 252, 256, 263
Alcoholism, 263
Alcohol and You, 262
Aldape, Virginia T., 47
Alder, C. S., 145
Alexander, Charlene, 149
Alexander, Sally H., 67
All the Days of Her Life, 97–107, 109
Alzheimer's Association, 266, 268
Alzheimer's disease, 265–90; fiction relating to, 287–88; nonfiction relating to, 289–90; symptoms, 266–67, 268–69, 282–84, 288, 289
Alzheimer's Disease (Check), 289
Alzheimer's Disease (Gold), 290

Alzheimer's Disease (Landau), 290
Alzheimer's Disease: The Silent Epidemic, 289–90
American Academy of Child and Adolescent Psychiatry (AACAP), 141, 149, 250
American Anorexia/Bulimia Association (Web site), 195
American Diabetes Association, 97
American Disability Association (Web site), 40
American Institute for Teen AIDS Prevention, 240
American Psychiatric Association, 197
Americans with Disabilities Act, 47, 222
American Sign Language (ASL), 53–54, 66, 70, 71, 72
Amputation, 31–36
And the Band Played On, 240
Andrews, Jean F., 70
Angela's Ashes: A Memoir, 260
Anger, 128, 151, 152–53, 170, 171; and alcohol abuse, 246–47; management of, 157, 160–67
Anne Frank: The Diary of a Young Girl, 248
Annerton Pit, 67
Anorexia nervosa, 175–83, 197–213, 272; causes, 180–81, 195, 197, 198, 199, 200–201, 214; and counselors, 185–86, 198, 199, 205–7, 212–13, 216; fiction relating to, 188–92, 213–14; Internet resources relating to, 195–96; nonfiction relating to, 192–96, 214–16; symptoms, 208; and teachers, 185, 198, 199, 207–13; treatments, 177–80, 181–83, 194, 195, 207, 216
Another Season: A Coach's Story of

Raising an Exceptional Son, 22–23

Anseltine, Lorraine, 70

Apostolides, Marianne, 192

Apple Is My Sign, 52, 54, 65–66, 73

Archambault, John, 68

Are You Alone On Purpose, 46

The Arizona Kid, 218, 234

Armstrong, Jennifer, 70, 167

Arrick, Fran, 220, 222–23, 231

As I Am, 48

Ashe, Arthur, 238

ASK about ADD (Web site), 130

Attention!, 130

Attention deficit disorder. *See* Attention deficit hyperactivity disorder (ADHD)

Attention deficit hyperactivity disorder (ADHD), 111–30, 138, 252; diagnosis, 112, 115–116, 122–24, 155; fiction relating to, 126–27; nonfiction relating to, 127–30; and teachers, 111–15, 116, 118–19, 124, 125; treatments for, 114–15, 116–19, 124–26, 127, 128; Web sites relating to, 129–30

Autograph, Please, Victoria, 126

Axell-Crowne syndrome, 189

Baby Alicia is Dying, 219, 235

Banks, Peter, 109

Bantle, Lee, 218, 219, 220, 231–32

Barbour, Scott, 261

Barden, Renardo, 149

Barrymore, Drew, 254, 261

Barry's Sister, 44

Baskin, Barbara, 23

Batson, Trent, 63–64

Bauer, Joan, 188, 257

Beach Center on Families and Disability (Web site), 40

Beatty, Monica A., 107

Because She's My Friend, 47

Beckelman, Laurie, 289

Becoming Naturally Therapeutic: A Return to the True Essence of Helping, 199, 209, 216

Beethoven, Ludwig van, 74

Beethoven Lives Upstairs, 74

Behavior modification, 118

Behrman, Carol H., 47

Bell, Alexander Graham, 73

Bell, Ruth, 173

Belonging (Kent), 68

Belonging (Scott), 73

Bennett, Cherie, 189

Bennett, James, 167

Bergman, Eugene, 63–64

Bernieres, Louis, 195

Bess, Clayton, 220, 232

Be Still My Heart, 218, 219, 233

The Best Little Girl in the World, 176–83, 191, 199

Betschart, Jean, 107

Between Madison and Palmetto, 192

Between a Rock and a Hard Place, 108

Bibliotherapy, 157–58

BIDS (Body image distortion syndrome), 214

The Big Way Out: A Novel, 148

"Big Two-Hearted River," 81, 89–90

Binge Drinking Blowout: The Extreme Dangers of Alcohol Abuse, 264

Bipolar disorders, 117, 122

Birth defects, 47; fiction relating to, 18–23; nonfiction relating to, 23–24

Bitter, Cynthia N., 192

Blake, Jeanne, 236

Blindness/visual impairments, 47, 51–53, 54–65; fiction relating to,

67–70; films relating to, 74; non-fiction relating to, 67
Blubber, 189
Blume, Judy, 18, 189
Bode, Janet, 205, 214
Body image distortion syndrome (BIDS), 214
The Body Betrayed: A Deeper Understanding of Women, Eating Disorders, and Treatment, 216
The Body Project: An Intimate History of American Girls, 215
Bordo, Susan, 214
Boskind-White, Marlene, 194
Bottles Break, 260–61
Bowler, Tim, 41
Brancato, Robin F., 41–42
Bridgers, Sue E., 167
Bring Back Yesterday, 148
Brisman, Judith, 195
Brooks, Bruce, 257
Brown, Christy, 18–19
Bruch, Hilde, 201, 202, 214
Bruchac, Joseph, 257
Brumberg, Joan Jacobs, 197, 199, 215
Bulimarexia, 194
Bulimia: A Guide for Family and Friends, 195
Bulimia nervosa, 98, 103, 105–6, 175–88, 198, 207; causes, 195, 214; fiction relating to, 188–92; Internet resources relating to, 195–96; nonfiction relating to, 192–96; treatments, 177–80, 181–83, 185, 186–88, 194, 195, 216
The Bumblebee Flies Anyway, 19
Bunting, Eve, 71, 92
Bushman, John, 14
Bushman, Kay Parks, 14
Butterflies Are Free, 74

Cadnum, Michael, 257
Calling Home, 257

Calvert, Patricia, 46, 145
Cancer, 77–92, 88, 146; fiction relating to, 77, 82, 92–96
Cancer, 96
Carbone, Elisa, 257
Cargill, Kristi, 287
Cart, Michael, 257
Carter, Alden, 257–58
Carter, Alden R., 108
Carver, 69
Casas, J. Manuel, 149
The Cay, 69
Center for Eating Disorders of University of Maryland (Web site), 196
Centers for Disease Control (CDC), 217, 219, 221, 240
Cerebral palsy, 18–19, 20, 22, 23, 44, 47
CF in His Corner, 22
Changing Bodies, Changing Lives, 173
Cheat the Moon, 259
Check, William A., 289
Checkers, 169–70
Chelsey and the Green-Haired Kid, 42
Cheney, Glenn, 47
Cheripko, Jan, 243, 244, 258
Chetkovich, Dane, 287
Chicago Blues, 258
Children and Adults with Attention Deficit Disorder (Web site), 130
Children with Diabetes (Web site), 108
Children of a Lesser God, 74–75
Children's Hospital Immunodeficiency Program (CHIP), Denver, CO (Web site), 240
Chiu, Christina, 261
Christainsen, C. B., 92
Christopher, Matt, 108
Circle of Giving, 20

Classroom activities. *See* Activities, classroom
Claude-Pierre, Peggy, 194
Claypoole, Jane, 262
Cleaver, Bill, 19
Cleaver, Vera, 19
Climbing Up from Depression, 153–54
Coerr, Eleanor, 92–93
Cognitive-behavioral therapy, 118
Cohen, Leah H., 71
Cohen, Miriam, 218, 220, 232
Colman, Hila, 42
Conduct disorders, 117, 122
Confess-O-Rama, 147
Conflict and Connection: The Psychology of Young Adult Literature, 174
Cook, Sally, 22–23
Coping in a Dysfunctional Family, 149
Corey's Story: Her Family's Secret, 257
Cormier, Robert, 19, 258
Costin, Carolyn, 194, 198, 215
Counselors/counseling, 1–2, 8–9, 12, 13–14, 17, 18, 36, 152; and diabetes, 100–101, 102–7; and eating disorders, 185–86, 198, 199, 205–7, 212–13, 216. *See also* Psychotherapy; Teachers
Count Us In: Growing Up With Down Syndrome, 23
Covington, Dennis, 46, 258
Craig, John R., 251
Craig, Phyllis, 251
The Crazy Horse Electric Game, 146
Creech, Sharon, 168
Cruise, Beth, 189
Crutcher, Chris, 146, 151, 153, 157, 168, 189, 225

Cunningham, Anne M., 239
Cystic fibrosis, 20, 22

Dancing on the Edge, 148
Danger at Rocky River: The NeuroExplorers in a Memorable Misadventure, 287
Dangerous Ground, 288–89
Dare to Be, M.E.!, 190
Dating, 31, 36, 37, 81, 95, 102–3, 105, 272
David and Della, 261
Davis, Deborah, 219, 232
Deaf community, 53–54, 71
Deaf Like Me, 73
Deafness/hearing impairments, 51–54, 64, 65–66; fiction relating to, 70–73; films relating to, 74–75; nonfiction relating to, 73
De Angeli, Maguerite, 42
Dear Dr. Bell, your friend, Helen Keller, 73
Death, 82–84, 88, 218, 260, 281, 283; of others, 77–78, 79–80, 84, 94, 95–96, 135–37, 138, 140, 145, 146, 147, 148, 156, 167, 168, 169–70, 170, 171, 173, 232–33, 234, 235–36, 257, 259, 274, 288; of self, 11–12, 13, 16, 19, 22, 83–84, 92–93
Deaver, Julie, 258
Dedication to Hunger: The Anorexic Aesthetic in Modern Culture, 215–16
Deenie, 18
Depression, 117, 138, 151–74, 208, 255, 258; and anger, 152–53, 157, 160–67; fiction relating to, 167–73; nonfiction relating to, 173–74; symptoms, 154
Dessen, Sarah, 146
Dexedrine, 116
Diabetes, 97–107; fiction relating

to, 107, 108–9, 148; nonfiction relating to, 107, 108

Diagnostic and Statistical Manual of Mental Disorders (DSM-IV), 112, 115–16, 251–52

Diana, Princess of Wales, 197–98

Diary of an Anorexic, 193

Diary of an Eating Disorder: A Mother and Daughter Share Their Healing Journey, 193

The Diary of LaToya Harper, 248

Dickens, Charles, 203

Dickinson, Emily, 171, 203

Dickinson, Peter, 67

Di Matteo, Richard, 126

Dina the Deaf Dinosaur, 70

Dineen, M. H., 127

Dinky Hocker Shoots Smack, 213

The Dinosaur Tamer and Other Stories for Children with Diabetes, 109

Disabilities, physical. *See* Adolescents, physically disabled

Distant Drums, Different Drummers: A Guide for Young People with ADHD, 128

Diversity training, 37

Diving for the Moon, 218, 219, 220, 231–32

Dixon, Ellen, 128

Do Angels Sing the Blues, 169

Doc, 287–88

Dodge, Bernie, 40

Dog Eat Dog, 259

Doherty, Berlie, 19

Donnie Makes a Difference, 108

Don't Die, My Love, 95

Don't Feed the Monster on Tuesdays! The Children's Self-Esteem Book, 128

Don't Rant and Rave on Wednesdays! The Children's Anger-Control Book, 128

A Door Near Here, 260

The Door in the Wall, 42

Dorris, Michael, 51, 52, 54, 63, 67

Down syndrome, 21, 22–23

Draper, Sharon, 39, 258

The Dreams of Maihre Mehan, 167

Drug abuse. *See* Adolescents, drug abuse among

Drugged Athletes, 262

DSM-IV (Diagnostic and Statistical Manual of Mental Disorders), 112, 115–16, 151–52

Durant, Penny Raife, 219, 233

Dwarfism, 47

Dyjak, Elisabeth, 287

Eagle Eyes, 127

Eagle Kite, 219, 233

The Eagle's Shadow, 259

Earthshine, 219, 235

Eating Disorder Center of California, 198

Eating disorders, 98, 103, 105–6, 138, 173, 174, 175–216; fiction relating to, 188–92, 213–14; Internet resources relating to, 195–96; nonfiction relating to, 192–96, 214–16

Eating Disorders: New Directions in Treatment and Recovery, 194

The Eating Disorder Sourcebook, 194

Eliot, George, 19

Emerson, Ralph Waldo, 203

Empathy, 210, 211

The Essential Guide to the New Adolescence: How to Raise an Emotionally Healthy Teenager, 173

Ethridge, Kenneth, 20

Euthanasia, 274, 280, 283, 285

Everything You Need to Know about Alcohol, 262–63

Fables, 39
The Facts about Alzheimer's Disease, 289
Faenza, Michael, 138
Falling in Love Is No Snap, 119–22, 126
Families, 84, 120–22, 148, 149, 169, 170, 173; and alcohol abuse, 256, 257–61; and Alzheimer's disease, 265–87; and anorexia nervosa, 176, 177, 178–80, 181, 190, 191, 195, 204–5; and chronic illness, 93–94, 95, 167; and HIV/AIDS, 222–30, 232–33, 235–36; and physical disabilities, 30, 31, 32, 38–39, 42, 43, 60–61; psychotherapy for, 275–77, 284–86. *See also* Parents
Fasting Girls: The Emergence of Anorexia Nervosa as a Modern Disease, 197, 199, 215
Fat Chance, 176, 183–88, 191
Father Figure, 171
Fears and Phobias, 149
Feminism, 199, 204, 214
Ferris, Jean, 93
Fiddler to the World: The Inspiring Life of Itzhak Perlman, 47
Fighting Back: What Some People Are Doing about AIDS, 237
Five Summers, 93–94
The Flawed Glass, 45–46
Flipovic, Zlata, 168
The Flying Fingers Club, 70
Foley, Jane, 119
Foley, June, 126
Food Fight: A Guide to Eating Disorders for Pre-Teens and Their Parents, 205, 214
Ford, Michael T., 236–37, 238
A Formal Feeling, 171
Fox, Paula, 219, 233, 258–59
Frank, Julia, 289–90

Frank, Lucy, 190
Franklin, Kristine L., 146
Freak the Mighty, 1–18, 22
Friendship. *See* Adolescents, relations with friends; Adolescents, chronically ill, relations with friends; Adolescents, physically disabled, relations with friends
The Friends, 138–45, 146
Froelich, Margaret W., 42
Frost, Robert, 203

Gardner, Howard, 17, 91
A Gathering of Flowers, 172
Gehret, Jeanne, 127
Gelb, Alan, 259
Gender issues, 78, 85–86, 120, 152, 163, 169, 198, 199, 214–215
Genograms, 275–76, 284–85
Gentlehands, 72
Gertz, Alison, 238
The Ghost of Tomahawk Creek, 70
Giff, Patricia R., 108
The Gift of a Girl Who Couldn't Hear, 73
The Gift of the Pirate Queen, 108
Gillick, Muriel R., 290
Glaser, Elizabeth, 238
Gleitzman, Morris, 218
Go Ask Alice, 239
God, the Universe, and Hot Fudge Sundaes, 20–21
Going Backwards, 266–87, 288
Gold, Susan D., 290
Golden Daffodils, 20
The Golden Cage: The Enigma of Anorexia Nervosa, 201, 214
Gone from Home, 147
Gonzales, Doreen, 238
Goodbye, Paper Doll, 192
Good-bye Tomorrow, 218, 235
Good Enough, 192
Gopaul-McNicol, Sharon-Ann, 149

Gordon, Michael, 127
Gorman, Carol, 42
Gould, Marilyn, 20
Graber, Richard, 287–88
Granny Was a Buffer Girl, 19
Grant, Cynthia D., 93, 146, 259
The Great Gilly Hopkins, 69
The Great Santini, 157
Greenberg, Jan, 93
Greenberg, Joanne, 71
Grilled Cheese at Four O'clock in the Morning, 109
Gross, Melissa, 238
Guccione, Leslie D., 71
Guernsey, JoAnn, 93–94
Guest, Judith, 168
Gulf, 148
Guy, Rosa, 138, 146

Haines, Sandra, 108
Hall, Arsenio, 239
Hall, Liza F., 190
Hamilton, Dorothy, 42–43
Hamilton, Virginia, 190
Hanauer, Cathi, 190
Hannah, 69–70
Hannah In Between, 260
Haring, Keith, 238
Harnishfeger, Lloyd, 20
Harpo's Horrible Secret, 288
"The Harringtons' Daughter," 172
Harris, Jonathan, 262
Harris, Karen, 23
Hasta Luego, San Diego, 70
Hautzig, Deborah, 213
Hayden, Torey L., 147
Head Over Wheels, 43
The Heartbeat of Halftime, 96
The Heart of a Chief, 257
The Heart Is a Lonely Hunter, 72
Helping Teenagers into Adulthood: A Guide for the Next Generation, 173

Hemingway, Ernest, 81, 89
Hermes, Patricia, 94, 218, 219, 233, 259
Hero of Lesser Causes, 43
Hesse, Karen, 147
Hesser, Terry S., 147
Heywood, Leslie, 215–16
Hickman, Janet, 288
The Hidden Treasure of Glaston, 21
Hide Crawford Quick, 42
Higher Education Center for Alcohol and Other Drug Prevention (Web site), 263
Hinton, S. E., 169
HIV/AIDS, 217–40; discrimination related to, 228, 233, 234, 235, 236, 237, 239; fiction relating to, 217–20, 231–36; incidence in adolescents, 217, 221; Internet resources relating to, 240; modes of infection, 218–21, 237, 244, 271; nonfiction relating to, 236–40; prevention, 222, 234–35, 237; as subject in young adult literature, 217–20; symptoms of AIDS, 218, 239; treatments, 217–18, 222, 226–27, 228–31, 237, 239
HIV and AIDS Information for Children: A Guide to Issues and Resources, 238
Hodge, Lois, 71–72
Hodgkin's lymphoma, 95
Holbrook, Sara, 39
Holland, Isabelle, 169
Holman, F., 20
Holmes, George H., 173
Hornbacher, Marya, 193
How I Changed My Life, 214
Howard, Ellen, 20
Howe, Norma, 20, 288
How It Feels to Live with a Physical Disability, 47
Hudson, Rock, 240

Hughes, Dean, 259
Hughes, Monica, 77, 85, 94
Hugo, Victor, 21
Human immunodeficiency virus.
    See HIV/AIDS
Humming Whispers, 147
Humphreys, Martha, 234
The Hunchback of Notre Name, 21
*Hunger Pains: The Modern
    Woman's Tragic Quest for Thin-
    ness*, 195, 199
Hunger Point: A Novel, 191
Hunt, Irene, 21
Hunter in the Dark, 77, 80–82, 83,
    84–85, 89–90, 91–92, 94
Hunting, 78–82, 85–88, 89
Hurwin, Davida, 94
Hydrocephalus, 21

I'm Deaf and It's OK, 70
I'm Somebody Too, 127
I Am an Artichoke, 190
I Can Hear the Mourning Dove,
    167
Identity. *See under* Adolescence,
    identity issues during
I Hadn't Meant to Tell You This,
    173
I'll Be Seeing You, 68
Imitate the Tiger, 243, 244–56, 258
*In Control: A Guide For Teens with
    Diabetes*, 107
Independence, 48, 52, 60, 61, 141,
    154–55, 156
Individuals with Disabilities Educa-
    tion Act of 1997 (IDEA), 52
I Never Got to Say Goodbye, 218,
    236
Ingersoll, Barbara, 128
Ingold, Jeanette, 67–68
In with the Out Crowd, 288
Inside a Support Group: Help for

Teenage Children of Alcoholics,
    263
Integration of disabled adolescents
    vs. isolation, 52, 53–54, 55, 57–
    58, 64, 65–66, 71
Internet. *See* Web sites
In This Sign, 71
Invincible Summer, 93
Invitational education, 9–10
Ironman, 151, 153, 157, 158–67,
    168
I Should Have Listened to Moon,
    287
Isolation: among adolescents, 31,
    51, 72, 99, 101, 103, 142, 151,
    155, 169, 171, 173, 225, 230,
    268, 271, 275, 284; integration of
    disabled adolescents vs., 52, 53–
    54, 55, 57–58, 64, 65–66, 71
It Happened to Nancy, 239
*I Would If I Could: A Teenager's
    Guide to ADHD/Hyperactivity*,
    127
Izzy, Willy-Nilly, 31–36, 47

*Jake's the Name, Sixth Grade's the
    Game*, 72
Jamiolkowski, Raymond, 149
Janover, Caroline, 126
Jepson, Jill, 72
Jericho, 288
Jessi's Secret Language, 72
Jess and the Runaway Grandpa,
    289
Jewett, E., 21
"The Jilting of Granny Wetherall,"
    203
Johnson, Angela, 94, 147
Johnson, Earvin E. "Magic," 237,
    238, 239
Johnston, Julie, 43
Joni's Story, 48

Journal writing, 88–89, 143–44,
    248, 252
Jussim, Daniel, 237
*Just Like Anyone Else: Living with
    Disabilities*, 48
Juvenile rheumatoid arthritis (JRA),
    27–30, 47

Kaposi's sarcoma, 218
Kaye, Marilyn, 219, 234
Keegan, Andrew, 109
*Keep Coming Back: The Spiritual
    Journey of Recovery in Over-
    eaters Anonymous*, 215
The Keeper, 148
Kehret, Peg, 94–95
Keller, Helen, 73, 74
Kelley, Barbara, 288
Kent, Deborah, 68
Kerr, M. E., 72, 213, 217, 219, 234
Kessa, 191
*Kids Explore the Gifts of Children
    with Special Needs*, 129
"Kids Who Are Different," 39
Kingman, Lee, 43
Kingsley, Jason, 23
Kinoy, Barbara P., 194
Kissing Doorknobs, 147
Klein, Michael, 237
Klein, Norma, 266, 271, 288
Knots on a Counting Rope, 68
Knowles, Anne, 21
Knowles, John, 156
Koertge, Ron, 147, 218, 234
Kolodny, Nancy J., 194
Konigsburg, E. L., 43
Koop, C. Everett, 240
Kossacoff, Lillian S., 47
Kranz, Rachel, 195
Krasnow, Michael, 193
Krementz, Jill, 47
Kriegsman, Kay H., 47–48
Krisher, Trudy, 169

Kubler-Ross, Elisabeth, 83
Kuklin, Susan, 237

L., Elizabeth, 215
Laird, Elizabeth, 21
Landau, Elaine, 96, 238, 262
Language, 4–5, 15, 18, 78, 88, 90
Lasso the Moon, 258
Last One Chosen, 42–43
Last Summer with Maizon, 192
Laundau, Elaine, 290
Laura Leonora's First Amendment,
    218, 220, 232
Learning disabilities, 2, 19, 20, 21,
    127; and ADHD, 117, 122, 123,
    126
*Learning to Slow Down and Pay
    Attention: A Book for Kids about
    ADHD*, 128
"The Leaving," 172
The Leaving and Other Stories, 172
Lee, Mary, 262
Lee, Richard, 262
LeMieux, Anne C., 169, 190–91
L'Engle, Madeleine, 95
Leonard, Alison, 21
Letters from the Inside, 170
Leukemia, 80–82, 84, 88; fiction re-
    lating to, 77, 82, 92–93, 95
Levenkron, Steven, 176, 181, 182,
    191, 199
Levine, Ann, 174
Levitz, Mitchell, 23
Levy, Marilyn, 219, 235
Lexington School for the Deaf, 71
Libby on Wednesday, 22
Life in the Fat Lane, 189
Life Happens, 149
Life's a Funny Proposition, 95–96
Life-Size, 191
Lipsyte, Robert, 213
Lisa, Bright and Dark, 171
Listen for the Fig Tree, 68

Literary concepts, 91–92, 203–4
Little, Jean, 95
A Little Love, 190
Little Girl Lost, 254, 261
Livneh, Hanoch., 34
Lizard, 46
Logan, Carolyn, 43–44
London, Jack, 90
Loneliness. *See under* Adolescents,
    isolation/loneliness among
Loski, Diana, 108–9
Loving Ben, 21
Lowry, Lois, 172
Lynch, Chris, 259

Magazine reviews, 86–87
Mahy, Margaret, 288
Maizon at Blue Hill, 192
Major Barbara, 204
*Making the Grade: An Adolescent's
    Struggle with ADHD*, 126
Maloney, Michael, 195
*Mama's Going to Buy You a Mock-
    ingbird*, 95
The Man Without a Face, 169
Margaret's Moves, 22
Marsden, John, 169–70
Martin, Ann M., 72
Martin, Bill, Jr., 68
Martin, Nora, 259
Martinez, Victor, 260
Mary Mehan Awake, 70
Mask, 74
Masters, Edgar Lee, 259
Mathis, Sharon B., 68
Matlin, Marlee, 75
The Mayday Rampage, 220, 232
Mazer, Norma F., 147
Mazur, Marcia L., 109
McCourt, Frank, 260
McCoy, Kathy, 149
McCullers, Carson, 72

McDaniel, Lurlene, 68, 95, 97–98,
    100, 109, 219, 235
McGovern, George, 262
McKenzie, Ellen K., 68–69
Medoff, Jillian, 191
Memory, 288
Mental health, 137–38, 139; fiction
    relating to, 145–48; Internet re-
    sources relating to, 149–50; non-
    fiction relating to, 149
Mental Health Net-Child Resources
    (Web site), 150
Mercury, Freddie, 238
"The Metaphor," 172
Me Too, 19
Metzger, Lois, 44
Midget, 41
Mikaelsen, Ben, 44
Miklowitz, Gloria, 218, 235
Miller, Caroline A., 193
Miller, Judy, 109
The Mill on the Floss, 19
The Miracle Worker, 74
Missing May, 172
Mitchell, Hayley, 262
Mom Can't See Me, 67
The Monument, 44
The Moonlight Man, 258–59
*More Notes from a Different Drum-
    mer*, 24
Mori, Kyoko, 170
Moser, Adolph, 128
Mourquis disease, 2
Mueller, Evelyn, 70
Multidimensional Addictions and
    Personality Profile (MAPP), 251
Muscular dystrophy, 21
My Body Is Not Who I Am, 48
My Brother Has AIDS, 219, 232
*My Brother's a World Class Pain:
    A Sibling's Guide to ADHD*, 127
My Father's Scar, 257
My Left Foot, 18–19

My Life As a Male Anorexic, 193
My Name Is Caroline, 193
My Sister Rose Has Diabetes, 107
My Sister's Bones: A Novel, 190

Nadeau, Kathleen G., 128
Names Project Foundation (Web
    site), 240
Nana's New Home, 287
Narcotics Anonymous, 252
National Clearinghouse for Alcohol
    and Drug Information (Web site),
    263
National Council of Teachers of
    English (NCTE), 78
National Health Information Center
    (Web site), 40
National Information Center for
    Children and Youth with Disabili-
    ties (Web site), 40
National Institute on Drug Abuse
    (Web site), 264
National Institute on Drug Abuse,
    243
National Mental Health Association,
    138
Native Americans, 20, 51–65
Naylor, Phyllis R., 148
Nell's Quilt, 197, 198–205, 213,
    214
Nelson, Theresa, 219, 235
Nerd No More, 146
Neufeld, John, 171
Newman, Lesla, 176, 183, 191
Newth, Mette, 22
Next Thing to Strangers, 148
*Nicole's Story: A Book about a Girl
    with Juvenile Rheumatoid Arthri-
    tis*, 47
Nielsen, Shelly, 126
Night Kites, 217, 219, 234
No Dragons to Slay, 93
No Kidding, 257

Nolan, Han, 148
Notes for Another Life, 167
Notes from a Different Drummer,
    24
No Walls of Stone, 72
Nureyev, Rudolf, 238

Obsessive-compulsive behavior, 147
The Old Curiosity Shop, 203
O'Neal, Zibby, 171
One Bird, 170
One Fat Summer, 213
*100 Questions and Answers about
    AIDS: A Guide for Young Peo-
    ple*, 236–37
*1–2–3 Magic: Training Your Pre-
    schoolers and Preteens to Do
    What You Want*, 124–25
Only Love, 45
Opportunistic infections, 218
Oppositional defiant disorder, 117,
    122
Ordinary People, 168
The Outsiders, 169
Overeating, compulsive, 176, 207,
    213, 214, 215, 216

Paralysis, 42, 44–45, 46, 47, 48
Paraplegia, 42
Parents, 2, 140, 141–42, 233, 247,
    256, 262; alcohol abuse among,
    245, 249, 257–61, 263, 277, 278–
    79; drug abuse among, 254, 277,
    279–80, 284, 285; relations with
    adolescents with ADHD, 113–15,
    118, 120–21, 124–25; relations
    with adolescents with eating dis-
    orders, 177, 178–80, 181, 184,
    186, 190, 192, 193, 200, 204–7,
    213; relations with adolescents
    with HIV/AIDS, 223, 224, 225;
    relations with chronically ill ado-
    lescents, 80–81, 82, 84–85, 92,

93, 98–99, 103, 106–7, 108; rela-
tions with depressed adolescents,
153, 154–56, 159, 161, 162–66,
168, 169, 170, 171; relations with
physically disabled adolescents,
4, 22, 23, 27–28, 31, 32, 44, 55,
60–61, 62, 63, 64–65, 73. *See
also* Families
Parker, Harvey C., 126
Parker, Roberta N., 126–27
Parrot in the Oven, 260
Passey, Helen, 260
Paterson, Katherine, 69
Paulsen, Gary, 44, 77, 95
Peck, Richard, 171
Peer groups. *See under* Adolescents,
relations with peer groups
People with AIDS (PWA), 224,
229, 236, 240
*People in Motion: Changing Ideas
about Physical Disability*, 48
Perkins, Anthony, 238
*Perk! The Story of a Teenager with
Bulimia*, 190
Perlman, Itzhak, 47
Pfeiffer, Susan B., 171–72
Phelen, Thomas W., 124–25
Philbrick, Rodman, 1, 22
Phillips, K. A., 193
Phoenix rising, 147
*Phoenix Rising, or How to Survive
Your Life*, 93, 146
Picking Up the Pieces, 46
Picture Perfect, 189
Piper, Deb, 72
Pipher, Mary, 195, 199, 216
Places in the Heart, 74
Pneumocystis carinii pneumonia,
218
*Poets for Life: Seventy-Six Poets
Respond to AIDS*, 237
Polikoff, Barbara G., 95
Polio, 43, 47

Ponterotto, Joseph, 149
Porte, Barbara Ann, 220, 236
Porter, Katherine, 203
*Portraying Persons with Disabilities:
An Annotated Bibliography of
Fiction for Children and Teen-
agers*, 24
The Power of the Rellard, 43–44
Prisoner of the Mound Builders, 20
Probably Still Nick Swanson, 172–
73
Psychotherapy, 149; and ADHD,
111, 114, 117–18, 125; and alco-
hol abuse, 250–56; and anorexia
nervosa, 176, 177–78, 180–83,
191; and bulimia, 186–88; and
chronic illness, 102–7; for fami-
lies, 227, 275–77, 284–86; and
HIV/AIDS, 229–30, 235; and
mental illness, 143, 153, 157–58,
160–67. *See also* Counselors/
Counseling
Public Law 94–142, 52
Pursuit (Web site), 130
*Putting on the Brakes: A Child's
Guide to Understanding and
Gaining Control over Attention
Deficit Hyperactivity Disorder*,
128
PWA (People with AIDS), 224,
229, 236, 240

Quadriplegia, 44–45
Quarles, Heather, 260
Quinn, Patricia O., 128

Rabe, Berniece, 22
Radin, Ruth Y., 69
Radley, Gail, 22
A Real Christmas This Year, 46
Real Heroes, 219, 234
Real Life: My Bestfriend Died, 259

Rebellion, 142, 154–55, 160, 170, 173, 200, 201

Red Scarf Girl: A Memoir of the Cultural Revolution, 248

Reese, Luellen K., 239

Rehabilitation Act of 1973, 47

Respect, 210–11

Responding reports, 14–18

Reviving Ophelia, 199, 216

Richmond, Sandra, 44–45

A Ring of Endless Light, 95

Riskind, Mary, 52, 54, 63, 73

Risk management, 101

Risky Times: How to Be AIDS-Smart and Stay Healthy, 236

Ritalin, 116, 117, 119

Robertson, Debra, 24

Rodowsky, Colby, 148, 260

Rostkowski, Margaret I., 45

A Row of Tigers, 19

Row This Boat Ashore, 45

Rue, Nancy N., 45

Rules of the Road, 257

Rumors and Whispers, 219, 235

Running Loose, 146

Runyon, Beverly, 193

Ryan, Mary, 260

Ryan White: My Own Story, 239

Rylant, Cynthia, 172

Sadako and the Thousand Paper Cranes, 92–93

Sallis, Susan, 45

Schizophrenia, 147, 167, 171

Schools, environment in, 9–13

Scoliosis, 18, 19

Scott, Virginia M., 73

A Season of Change, 71–72

Second Star to the Right, 213

The Secret of the Dorm Attic, 70

The Secret Language of Eating Disorders, 194

Sees Behind Trees, 51–52, 54–65, 66, 67

Self-concepts/self-image. *See under* Adolescence, self-concepts/self-image during

Self-esteem/self-worth. *See under* Adolescence, self-esteem during

Sensory impairments. *See* Blindness/visual impairments; Deafness/hearing impairments

A Separate Peace, 156

Seventeen, 184

Sexism, 199

Sexuality. *See under* Adolescents, sexuality in

Shadow Man, 146, 259

A Share of Freedom, 261

A Shavian Guide to the Intelligent Woman, 204, 216

Shaw, George Bernard, 203, 204

The Shell Lady's Daughter, 145

Sherman, Roberta T., 195

Shilts, Randy, 238, 240

Shizuko's Daughter, 170

Shoot for the Hoop, 108

Shreve, Susan R., 73

Shute, Jennifer, 191

Siegel, Michelle, 195

Siegler, Ava, 154

Siegler, Ava L., 173

Silsbee, Peter, 148

Sinykin, Sheri C., 148

Sirof, Harriet, 47, 148

Sisters Long Ago, 94–95

Skurzynski, Gloria, 288–89

Slam Dunk: A Young Boy's Struggle with ADHD, 126–27

Small, Jacquelyn, 199, 209, 216

A Small Pleasure, 92

Smith, Chelsea, 193

Snyder, Anne, 192

Snyder, Zilpha, 22

Someone Like You, 146

Something Fishy Website on Eating Disorders (Web site), 196
Something Terrible Happened, 220, 236
Sommers, V. S., 58–59
Sparks, Beatrice, 239
Speak to the Rain, 260
Spina bifida, 22
Spinal cord injury, 46
Spite Fences, 169
Spoon River Anthology, 259
Spradley, James P., 73
Spradley, Thomas S., 73
Squashed, 188
Stallings, Gene, 22–23
Stargone John, 68–69
Staying Fat for Sarah Byrnes, 189
Stein, Sara, 23
Steinberg, Laurence, 174
Stern, Judith M., 128
St. George, Judith, 73
Stone, Lucy, 204
The Story of My Life, 73
Strachan, Ian, 45–46
Straight Talk about Eating Disorders, 195
Stranded, 44
Strasser, Todd, 214
Stress management, 106
Stringer, Sharon A., 174
Students Against Drunk Driving (SADD), 39
Substance abuse. *See* Adolescents, drug abuse among; Alcohol abuse
A Sudden Silence, 71
Suicide, 136, 170, 171, 191, 255; among adolescents, 19, 114, 155–56, 174, 202, 224, 258
Sullivan, Annie, 74
The Sunflower Forest, 147
Survival Guide for College Students with ADD or LD, 128
Surviving an Eating Disorder: New

Perspectives and Strategies for Family and Friends, 195
Suzuki, Lisa, 149
Sweet Friday Island, 109
Symbolism, 91–92, 201–2, 204

Tabor, Nancy, 260–61
Tada, Joni E., 48
Tait, Nancy, 70
Taking Charge, 47–48
Taking Hold: My Journey into Blindness, 67
Tangled Minds: Understanding Alzheimer's Disease and Other Dementias, 290
Taylor, Barbara, 262–63
Taylor, Theodore, 69, 109
Teachers, 1, 8, 36, 74–75, 172; and ADHD, 111–15, 116, 118–19, 124, 125; and alcohol abuse, 255; and anorexia/bulimia, 185, 198, 199, 207–13; and depression, 151–53, 160; and physical disabilities, 28, 30, 34. *See also* Activities, classroom
Teaching literature, classroom activities for. *See* Activities, classroom
Tears of a Tiger, 258
Teen Addiction, 263
Teenage Drinking, 262
Teenagers. *See* Adolescence; Adolescents
Teen Alcoholism, 262
Teen Guide to Staying Sober, 261
Teens with Physical Disabilities: Real-life Stories Meeting the Challenges, 47
Tell Me How the Wind Sounds, 71
Terris, Susan, 197, 198, 200, 204, 214
Terry: My Daughter's Life and Death Struggle with Alcoholism, 262

Tessnear, Marshall, 175, 176, 180–83
Therapy. *See* Psychotherapy
This Drinking Nation, 262
Thom, Susan, 107
Thomas, Joyce C., 172
Thompson, Ron A., 195
A Time For Dancing: A Novel, 94
Time Out: The Truth about HIV and AIDS, 239
Tina's Chance, 21
"To Build a Fire," 90
Toning the Sweep, 94
Toothpick, 20
Tracker, 77, 79–80, 82, 84–85, 95
Tracking, 90–91
Train Go Sorry: Inside a Deaf World, 71
Trapani, Margi, 263
Trevor, Nick, 239
The Trophy, 259
The Trouble with Perfect, 260
The Turnabout Shop, 148
Two Weeks with the Queen, 218

Unbearable Weight: Feminism, Western Culture, and the Body, 214
Under the Shadow, 21
Until Whatever, 234
Up Country, 257–58
Up a Road Slowly, 21
Using Young Adult Literature in the Classroom, 14

The View from Saturday, 43
Visual impairment. *See* Blindness/visual impairment
The Voices of AIDS: Twelve Unforgettable People Talk about How AIDS Has Changed Their Lives, 238
Voigt, Cynthia, 31, 47

Walk Two Moons, 168
Walter, Virginia A., 238
Warmth, 210, 212
Wasted: A Memoir of Anorexia and Bulimia, 193
Watson, Barbara B., 204, 216
We All Fall Down, 258
WebQuests, 40, 143, 145
Web sites, 39, 108, 129–30, 143, 144–45, 209; relating to alcohol abuse, 263–64; relating to anorexia, 195–96; relating to bulimia, 195–96; relating to disabilities, 40; relating to HIV/AIDS, 240; relating to mental health, 149–50
We Have AIDS, 238
Weinshel, Margot, 195
Wekesser, Carol, 263
Wenderli, Stephen, 96
Werlin, Nancy, 46
Wershba, Barbara, 261
Westall, Robert, 148
Westridge Young Writers Workshop, 129
What's Wrong with Daddy?, 289
What You Can Do to Avoid AIDS, 237
What You Don't Know Can Kill You, 220, 222–30, 231
Wheels for Walking, 44–45
Whelan, Gloria, 69–70
When Food is Foe: How You Can Confront and Conquer Your Eating Disorder, 194
When Heroes Die, 219, 233
When Morning Comes, 145
When She Was Good, 147
Whistle Me Home, 261
White, Ryan, 222, 237, 239
White, William C., 194
Wibbelsman, Charles, 149
Williams, Karen L., 46

308   Index

Will You Be My POSSLQ?, 92
Wilson, Budge, 172
The Window, 67–68
Winning, 41–42
Winters, Paul, 263
Withstanding Ovation, 36, 48
Wolfe, Digby, 39
Wolff, V. E., 172–73
Wood, June, 261
Woodbury, Mary, 289
Woodson, Jacqueline, 173, 192
Working with West Indian Families, 149
World Wide Web. *See* Web sites

A Year to Grow, 20
The Year without Michael, 171–72

Young, Alida E., 218, 236, 289
A Young Man's Journey with AIDS: The Story of Nick Trevor, 239
Your Dieting Daughter: Is She Dying for Attention?, 198, 215
You Shouldn't Have to Say Goodbye, 94
You and Your Adolescent: A Parent's Guide for Ages 10–20, 174

Zack Attacks, 108–9
Zerbe, Kathryn J., 201, 216
Zindel, Paul, 261
Zipper, the Kid with ADHD, 126
Zlata's Diary: A Child's Life in Sarajevo, 168, 248

About the Editor and Contributors

CHARLENE ALEXANDER is Associate Professor of Counseling at Ball State University in Muncie, Indiana. She completed her undergraduate and master's degrees at Creighton University and earned her Ph.D. in counseling psychology from the University of Nebraska at Lincoln. Her primary research interest is multicultural counseling.

KELSEY BACKELS received her Ph.D. in counseling psychology from Ball State University and her M.Ed. in counselor psychology from James Madison University. She is currently Associate Professor and Counseling Psychologist in the Department of Counseling and Human Development at Millersville University. She holds a psychologist's license in the Commonwealth of Pennsylvania.

CYNTHIA ANN BOWMAN is Assistant Professor of English Education at Florida State University. She was the recipient of the first James Britton Award for Inquiry in Language Arts and received her Ph.D. from Kent State University. A regular presenter at the National Council of Teachers of English (NCTE), the International Reading Association (IRA), and state affiliates, she is the Chair of the Conference of English Education (CEE) Commission for the Preparation of Teachers with Disabilities.

DANNA BOZICK is an internationally certified alcohol and drug abuse counselor. She is a licensed social worker working with adolescents and their families at the Neil Kennedy Recovery Clinic in Youngstown, Ohio.

She has taught junior high school as well as university courses in art therapy and criminal justice.

KATHLEEN CARICO is Assistant Professor of English Education at Virginia Polytechnic and State University, where she teaches courses in English teaching methods. Her research focuses on the use of multicultural literature in the classroom as well as the use of various strategies to enhance literature study: readers' responses, computer-based communication formats, and reading partners.

JAN CARLI is the guidance counselor at Alliance High School in Alliance, Ohio. She has been working with adolescents with mental health issues for over twenty years.

JAN CHERIPKO is the author of *Imitate the Tiger*, a young adult novel about a high school football player who has a drinking problem. *Imitate the Tiger* was the recipient of the Joan Fassler Memorial Book Award, presented each year by the Association of the Care of Children's Health. For the past ten years he has served as assistant to the publisher of Boyds Mills Press, a children's book publishing company owned by Highlights for Children. His duties include working with authors and illustrators focusing on the educational and library markets. Additionally, for the past thirteen years he has been an English teacher at the Family Foundation School in Hancock, New York, a private school specializing in helping at-risk teenagers. He lives with his wife, Valmy, and daughter, Julia Christina, and two dogs, Sparky and Buffy, in Bethany, Pennsylvania.

CLAIRE J. DANDENEAU is Associate Professor of Psychology and Counseling at Indiana University of Pennsylvania. She has published numerous articles on the environmental, identity, and social issues that face all adolescents.

KAREN L. FORD is Associate Professor of Secondary Reading at Ball State University in Muncie, Indiana. She earned her doctorate in literacy and curriculum and instruction from the University of Cincinnati. Her primary area of interest is using adolescent literature to enhance the general methods courses for preservice teachers. Currently, she is involved in a research project using YA novels to address literacy and essential skills issues in a professional development school.

MARGARET FORD is the district library/media specialist for Campbell City Schools in Campbell, Ohio, where she also taught English language arts for twenty-three years. She is an adjunct faculty member at Youngstown State University, past president of the Ohio Council of Teachers of English Language Arts, and co-editor of the Children's and Young Adult Literature column for the *Ohio Journal of English Language Arts*.

PHYLLIS A. GORDON is Associate Professor of Rehabilitation Counseling at Ball State University in Muncie, Indiana, where she teaches graduate courses in counseling psychology and rehabilitation therapy. She is co-editor of *The Teacher Educator*, and her research interests include issues of gender and identity in relationship to disability.

JOYCE GRAHAM is Associate Professor of English and Coordinator of English Education at Radford University. She received her doctorate at Virginia Tech and is a past president of the Virginia Association of Teachers of English. She is a frequent presenter at NCTE and an active member of CEE, the Assembly of Literature for Adolescents of the National Council of Teachers of English (ALAN), and Women in Literature and Life Assembly (WILLA).

DAVID WILLIAM HARTMAN is Chairman of the Department of Psychiatry at Lewis-Gale Hospital in Salem, Virginia. Blind since he was eight, he received his M.D. from Temple University and is the subject of the NBC made-for-television movie *Journey into Darkness*. His autobiography is *White Coat, White Cane*, and he has served on the Virginia State Board of Mental Health, Mental Retardation, and Substance Abuse Services.

SCOTT JOHNSON is Director of Clinical Training for the Marriage and Family Therapy Doctoral Program at Virginia Tech. In addition to being a licensed family therapist, he holds degrees in literature, music, and creative writing. He is past president of the Virginia Association for Marriage and Family Therapy and a member of the editorial board of the *Journal of Marital and Family Therapy*.

SUE F. JOHNSON is Assistant Professor at Indiana University of Pennsylvania, where she teaches English composition and methods courses. An active member of WILLA, she is also a regular presenter at NCTE and her state affiliate.

PATRICIA P. KELLY is Professor of English Education and Director of the Center for Teacher Education at Virginia Tech. She is a former president of ALAN and a former co-editor of the *ALAN Review*. Her publications about young adult literature frequently center on gender is-sues, for example, "Gender Issues and the Young Adult Novel" in *Read-ing Their World* and "Reading from a Female Perspective" in *Adolescent Literature as a Complement to the Classics I.* Her critical analyses of works by young adult authors include those of Margaret Mahy, Joan Lowery Nixon, Sue Ellen Bridgers, Kathryn Lasky, Rosa Guy, and Ron Koertge.

NANCY LAFFERTY received her master of arts in counseling in 1998 from Ball State University. Previously she taught speech, theater, and English in Indiana public schools. Currently she is employed as a middle school counselor in Indianapolis, Indiana.

NANCY MELLIN MCCRACKEN directs the English Education pro-gram at Kent State University and the Northeast Ohio Writing Project. Current Chair of the Conference on English Education, she is the co-editor of *Gender Issues in the Teaching of English.*

KIM MCCOLLUM-CLARK is Assistant Professor of English Educa-tion at Millersville University in Millersville, Pennsylvania. A new mother and an inveterate lover of books of all kinds, she has been for-tunate in her teachers in the public schools of North Carolina, Guilford College, and the Pennsylvania State University. Her research interests include educational policy, literature for young adults, and teacher edu-cation. She is a member of the CEE Commission on the Preparation of Teachers with Disabilities.

JOHN NOELL MOORE is Assistant Professor of English Education at the College of William and Mary in Williamsburg, Virginia, where he teaches courses in young adult literature and secondary school English pedagogy. The author of *Interpreting Young Adult Literature: Literary Theory in the Secondary Classroom*, he has published numerous articles in state and national journals and is an active member of ALAN, NCTE, and the Virginia Association of Teachers of English.

JIM POWELL is Assistant Professor of Secondary Education at Ball State University in Muncie, Indiana. He received his Ph.D. in curriculum and instruction from Arizona State University. He currently teaches mid-dle school and high school methods courses, directs a Professional De-velopment School Network in Carmel, Indiana, and, one semester each year, teaches English at the Burris Laboratory School.

NANCY PROSENJAK is Assistant Professor of English at Metropoli-tan State College of Denver. She teaches graduate and undergraduate courses in young adult and children's literature. A regular presenter at NCTE, IRA, and the state affiliates, she is also an active member of WILLA.

ALBERT SCOTT is a licensed counseling psychologist in both Pennsylvania and Ohio, a fellow of the American Board of Forensic Examiners, and a psychotherapist. Throughout his varied career, he has been a director of counseling, clinical director, hospital CEO, mental health clinic director, chief psychologist, and private practice clinician. He has taught and studied at Slippery Rock University, Duquesne University, University of Scranton, Kent State University, and West Virginia University. He has received an award for applied research in learning disabilities and consistently publishes and receives funded grants.

PAULA STANLEY is Associate Professor of Counselor Education at Radford University in Radford, Virginia, where she also maintains a part-time private practice. She is a licensed professional counselor and a licensed marriage and family therapist in Virginia and a nationally certified counselor. A frequent presenter at state and national conferences, she has also published numerous articles in refereed journals.

LAURA SULLIVAN AND DIANE HARTMAN are the social worker and nurse practitioner, respectively, working out of the Pediatric Infectious Disease Unit of Children's Hospital in Denver. This unit has established the Children's Hospital Immunodeficiency Program, a regional care system to which physicians refer HIV/AIDS patients from birth to age twenty-four as well as pregnant women who are HIV-positive.

MARSHALL D. TESSNEAR is Associate Director of the Thomas E. Cook Counseling Center at Virginia Tech. He received undergraduate and master's degrees from Wake Forest University and received his doctorate in clinical psychology from the University of Cincinnati. A licensed clinical psychologist, his specialty areas include multimodal treatment approaches to eating disorders and the impact of disabilities on mental health functioning.

A. LEE WILLIAMS is Associate Professor in the Elementary Education Department of Slippery Rock University in Pennsylvania. She teaches undergraduate and graduate courses in literacy and assessment. Her publications focus on reading and constructivist teaching. She is currently engaged in a project that brings rural preservice teachers to urban schools for field-based seminars and classroom practice for students at risk for school failure.